Contemporary Community Nursing

Edited by

Barbara Walton Spradley, R.N., M.N.

Assistant Professor
Public Health Nursing
School of Public Health
University of Minnesota
Minneapolis

Little, Brown and Company
Boston

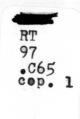

To my parents
Nathan and Lois Walton

Preface

When someone inquires, "What is community nursing?" or "What does the community nurse do?" it is often difficult to give a clear answer. There may be several reasons for this. For one thing it is a field undergoing rapid growth and development in response to the challenge of more effectively meeting health care needs. Community nursing includes public health nursing but is much broader than the traditional concept of public health nursing. In order to grasp the nature of community nursing, one must be cognizant of trends in nursing as a profession, changes in health care needs and new developments in health delivery systems.

In addition, due to the growth in scope of the nursing profession, community nursing is often defined too narrowly. Nursing educators have a monumental task in keeping up with the expansion of knowledge as well as in conveying this knowledge in an understandable form to nursing students. Community nursing instructors must often depend on their own past experiences to assist them in defining this field; so too the practicing community nurse may define community nursing in terms of her own experience. Like the proverbial blind men with the elephant, each of these practitioners may point to a limited facet of community nursing and imply it is the whole field.

Why is it important to understand the meaning of community nursing? Community nursing concepts are essential fibers in the fabric of all good nursing practice. They should be interwoven with each nursing student's experience throughout the entire preparatory period. Concepts such as prevention, the family unit, culture and community dynamics need particular emphasis because of their importance to improved nursing practice. Graduating nursing students need not only sound preparation in these areas but also a clear understanding of the career choices that lie before them. One option that frequently is not clearly explained is community nursing.

The purpose of this book is to clarify the nature of community nursing. It is written primarily for nursing students and their instructors but has considerable relevance for practicing community nurses as well. It is designed to present the important aspects of community nursing in an interesting and comprehensive manner. The articles have been carefully selected for readability and pertinence and arranged to provide a framework for more clearly understanding this field.

In Part I, "Community Nursing," the reader is introduced to an overview of the nature of this field, the principles underlying it and the changes that are currently taking place. Part II, "The Community Nurse Role and Settings," offers examples of some of the many roles of community nurses and the settings for these roles. A discussion of the expanded role and its relationship to community nursing and to other health professionals is presented in Part III, "The Expanded Nurse Role and Team Relationships." Part IV, "The Cultural Dimension of Community Nursing," emphasizes the importance of undertaking cultural differences and illustrates how the community nurse can work with a number of different cultural groups. Part V, "The Nursing Process," describes problem solving as one of the most basic tools used in nursing and gives specific examples of its application to community nursing practice. Part VI, "Communication," stresses the need to communicate effectively and discusses how to recognize and deal with barriers to therapeutic communication. Part VII, "The Family in Community Nursing," emphasizes the individual as a member of a family and gives examples of community nursing practice with a variety of age and family groups. In the last part, "Community Assessment and Health Planning," the focus broadens to emphasize the nurse's need to understand the community and to become involved in the larger community health scene.

I wish to express my appreciation to my students and colleagues in Public Health Nursing in the School of Public Health, University of Minnesota. Their ideas, interest and support were valuable contributions to the development of the manuscript. Dorothy Trask, who did much of the typing, deserves special thanks. Most of all I am indebted and forever grateful to my husband, Jim, whose prompting, ideas and encouragement throughout the entire project helped to bring this book into being.

Minneapolis   B. W. S.

Contents

Preface   vii

Contributing Authors   xiii

I Community Nursing   1

1. Community Nursing in a Changing Climate   3
   Paulette Robischon

2. An Open Health Care System Model   12
   Madeleine M. Leininger

3. High-Level Wellness for Man and Society   21
   Halbert L. Dunn

4. Educational Qualifications of Public Health Nurses   29
   Council on Health Manpower

II The Community Nurse Role and Settings   35

5. Prevention and Chronic Illness   37
   Paulette Robischon

6. Community Mental Health Nursing and Consultation   46
   Mildred Mouw, Clarice H. Haylett

7. Patient Advocacy or Fighting the System   55
   Sandra Henry Kosik

8. Nursing in a Health Maintenance Organization   63
   Barbara Bates

9. The School Nurse and Drug Abusers   70
   Kathryn K. Caskey, Enid V. Blaylock, Beryl M. Wauson

10. The Occupational Health Nurse and the Patient with Trauma   79
    Hazel L. Gallaher, Ginger M. Wyatt

11. Working in a Nonhealth-Oriented Setting   88
    Janice Hitchcock

III The Expanded Nurse Role and Team Relationships   97

12. Extending the Scope of Nursing Practice   99

13. An Approach to Role Expansion — The Elaborate Network   110
    Margaret L. Shetland

14. The Doctor-Nurse Game   116
    Leonard I. Stein
15. The Primary Care Nurse — The Generalist
    in a Structured Health Care Team   125
    Eleanor Brunetto, Peter Birk
16. The Nurse as Family Practitioner   143
    Jo Ellen Murata
17. Community Nurse Practitioners — A Partnership   150
    Jocelyn Greenidge, Ann Zimmern, Mary Kohnke

IV The Cultural Dimension of Community Nursing   157

18. The Cultural Context of Behavior: Spanish-
    Americans and Nursing Care   159
    Madeleine Leininger
19. Removing Barriers to Health Care   175
    Helene R. Robertson
20. Cultural Understanding: A Key to Acceptance   182
    Rita Hoeschen Aichlmayr
21. Health Care of the Chinese in America   189
    Teresa Campbell, Betty Chang
22. Maternity Nursing and Navaho Culture   198
    Flora L. Bailey
23. The Stigma of Obesity   205
    Beatrice J. Kalisch

V The Nursing Process   213

24. The Relevant "Who" of Problem Solving   215
    Muriel Standeven
25. The Process of Contracting in Community Nursing   221
    Margaret R. Sloan, Barbara Thune Schommer
26. Crisis Intervention — The Pebble in the Pool   230
    Janice Marland Hitchcock
27. Problem-Oriented Medical Records — Not Just
    Another Way to Chart   236
    Pamela L. Schell, Alla T. Campbell
28. Adapting the POMR to Community Child Health Care   245
    Marilyn L. Bonkowsky
29. A Search for Assessment Criteria   253
    Marlene G. Mayers

30. Quality of Care: The Nursing Audit, Part A   260
    Maria C. Phaneuf

31. Quality of Care: The Nursing Audit, Part B   267
    Avedis Donabedian

VI Communication   273

32. What Is Empathy?   275
    Beatrice J. Kalisch

33. Home Visit — Ritual or Therapy?   285
    Marlene Mayers

34. Sociocultural Factors: Barriers to
    Therapeutic Intervention   292
    Donna Aguilera

35. The Interview   299

36. Talking to Patients about Death   306
    Jeanne Quint Benoliel

37. Solving Health Problems through Small Group Action   314
    Barbara Osborne Henkel

VII The Family in Community Nursing   323

38. The Nursing Process in Family Health   325
    Jayne Anttila Tapia

39. The Impact of Illness on Family Roles   333
    Robert R. Bell

40. Nursing Care of the Infant in the Community   348
    Marguerite W. Bozian

41. Adolescents and VD   356
    Mary Agnes Brown

42. The Family That Fails to Thrive   364
    Ruth F. Stewart

43. Working with Abusive Parents   384
    Anne B. Savino, R. Wyman Sanders

44. Maximizing Health Care to Families   389
    Leonard T. Maholick, Josephine Graham

45. The Family with an Elderly Member   395
    Lucille Gress

46. Family Nursing during Death and Dying   405
    Marilee Woehning, Ida M. Martinson

VIII Community Assessment and Health Planning   413

47. Assessing Community Characteristics   415
     Donald C. Klein

48. What Is Health Planning?   425
     Tasker K. Robinette

49. How to Become Involved in Community Planning   432
     Helen Jo McNeil

50. A Cultural Approach to the Nurse's Role
     in Health-Care Planning   439
     Molly C. Dougherty

51. The Core Committee: A Model for Decision-Making
     within Public Health Units   446
     Olga Roman Smiley

52. Planning for Social Change: Dilemmas for
     Health Planning   450
     John G. Bruhn

     Index   459

Contributing Authors

Donna C. Aguilera, R.N., Ph.D.
Associate Professor, Psychiatric/
Community Mental Health Nursing,
California State University,
Los Angeles

Rita Hoeschen Aichlmayr, R.N., M.S.
Director of Adult Intensive Services,
Mental Health and Family Service
Center, Vancouver

Flora L. Bailey, Ph.D.
Former Supervisor of Physical
Education, K–VI Schools, School
District of South Orange and
Maplewood, New Jersey

Barbara Bates, M.D.
Professor, Department of Medicine,
School of Medicine and Dentistry,
University of Rochester,
Rochester, New York

Robert R. Bell, M.A.
Temple University, Philadelphia

Jeanne Quint Benoliel, R.N., D.N.Sc.
Professor and Chairman,
Comparative Nursing Care Systems
Department, School of Nursing,
University of Washington, Seattle

Peter Birk, M.D.
Medical Program Administrator,
Group Health Association, Inc.,
Washington, D.C.

Enid V. Blaylock, R.N., Ph.D.
Associate Professor, Educational
Psychology Department, California
State University, Long Beach

Marilyn L. Bonkowsky, R.N., B.S.N.
Nurse Consultant, New England
Medex Training Program,
Dartmouth College,
Hanover, New Hampshire

Marguerite W. Bozian, R.N., M.S.
Assistant Professor, Community
Health Nursing, College of Nursing
and Health, University of
Cincinnati, Cincinnati

Mary Agnes Brown, R.N., M.A.
Supervising Public Health Nurse,
Maternal and Infant Care—Family
Planning Project, New York City
Department of Health, New York

John G. Bruhn, Ph.D.
Associate Dean for Community
Affairs, University of Texas
Medical Branch at Galveston,
Medical School, Galveston

Eleanor Brunetto, R.N., M.A., M.P.H.
Director, Department of Social
Ethics, Zion Bible Institute,
East Providence, Rhode Island

Alla T. Campbell, R.N., M.S.N.
Cardiology Clinical Specialist,
University Hospital,
Augusta, Georgia

Teresa Campbell, R.N., M.S.
Professor of Community Health
Nursing, Department of Nursing,
California State University,
San Francisco

Kathryn K. Caskey, R.N., B.S.
Former Assistant Professor,
Department of Nursing, California
State College, Long Beach

Betty Chang, R.N., M.A.
Assistant Professor, Department
of Nursing, California State
University, San Francisco

Avedis Donabedian, M.D., M.P.H.
Professor, Department of Medical
Care Organization, School of Public
Health, University of Michigan,
Ann Arbor

Molly C. Dougherty, R.N., Ph.D.
Associate Professor, Maternal-
Infant Health Nursing, College of
Nursing, University of Florida,
Gainesville

Halbert L. Dunn, M.D., Ph.D.
Epidemiologist and Former Chief,
National Office of Vital Statistics,
United States Public Health Service,
Washington, D.C.

Hazel L. Gallaher, R.N., C.O.H.N.
Headquarters Nurse, Oilwell
Division, United States Steel
Corporation, Dallas

Jocelyn Greenidge, R.N., C.R.N.A., B.S.
Graduate Student and Lecturer,
Division of Dentistry and
Community Health, New York
University, New York

Lucille D. Gress, R.N., M.A.
Assistant Professor, College of
Health Sciences and Hospital,
University of Kansas Medical
Center, Kansas City, Kansas

Clarice H. Haylett, M.D.
*Chief Psychiatrist, Child
Development Services, Mental
Health Services Division, San Mateo
County Department of Health and
Welfare, San Mateo, California*

Barbara Osborne Henkel, R.N., Ed.D.
*Professor, Department of Health
and Safety Studies, California State
University, Los Angeles*

Janice Marland Hitchcock, R.N., M.S.
*Assistant Professor, Department of
Nursing, Sonora State College,
Sonora, California*

Beatrice J. Kalisch, R.N., Ed.D.
*Professor of Nursing, University of
Michigan, School of Nursing,
Ann Arbor*

Donald C. Klein, Ph.D.
*NTL Institute for Applied
Behavioral Science,
Washington, D.C.*

Mary F. Kohnke, R.N., Ed.D.
*Assistant Professor, Division of
Nurse Education, New York
University, New York*

Sandra Henry Kosik, R.N., M.P.H.
*Chief Nurse, Project PRESCAD,
Wayne County Health Department,
Detroit*

Josephine Graham Langenberg, R.N., M.S.
*Director of Nurses, The Bradley
Center, Inc., Columbus, Georgia*

Madeline M. Leininger, R.N., Ph.D.
*Dean, School of Nursing,
University of Washington, Seattle*

Leonard T. Maholick, M.D.
Medical Director, The Bradley
Center, Inc., Columbus, Georgia

Ida M. Martinson, R.N., Ph.D.
Assistant Professor and Chairman
of Research, School of Nursing,
University of Minnesota,
Minneapolis

Marlene Mayers, R.N., P.H.N., M.S.
Director, Nursing Care Systems,
Medicus Systems Corporation,
Chicago

Helen Jo McNeil, R.N., M.N.
District Executive Officer,
Seattle—King County Health
Department, Renton, Washington

Mildred Mouw, R.N., M.A.
Former Mental Health Consultant,
Mental Health Services Division,
San Mateo County Department of
Health and Welfare,
San Mateo, California

Jo Ellen M. Murata, R.N., M.P.H.
Family Nurse Practitioner, North-
east Valley Health Corporation,
San Fernando, California

Maria C. Phaneuf, R.N., M.A.
Professor Emeritus, College of
Nursing, Wayne State University,
Detroit

Helene R. Robertson, R.N., M.A.
Assistant Director, Nursing Service,
Roosevelt Hospital, New York

Tasker K. Robinette, M.H.A.
Director, Health Consulting
Services, Pacific Northwest Region,
Arthur Young and Company,
Portland

Paulette Robischon, R.N., Ph.D.
Associate Professor and
Coordinator, Community Health
Nursing, Department of Nursing,
Herbert H. Lehman College, City
University of New York, New York

R. Wyman Sanders, M.D.
Assistant Professor and Psychiatrist,
The Neuropsychiatric Institute,
Department of Medical Hygiene,
UCLA Center for the Health
Sciences, Los Angeles

Anne B. Savino, R.N., M.A.
Assistant Clinical Professor,
UAF Nurse Training Coordinator,
The Neuropsychiatric Institute,
UCLA Center for the Health
Sciences, Los Angeles

Pamela L. Schell, R.N., B.S.
Graduate Student, School of
Nursing, University of North
Carolina, Chapel Hill

Barbara Thune Schommer, R.N., M.S.
Public Health Nurse Clinician,
Ramsey County Nursing Service,
St. Paul, Minnesota

Margaret L. Shetland, R.N., Ph.D.
Professor of Nursing, College of
Nursing, Wayne State University,
Detroit

Margaret R. Sloan, R.N., M.Ed., M.S.
Assistant Professor, Public Health
Nursing, School of Public Health,
University of Minnesota,
Minneapolis

Olga Roman Smiley, R.N.
*Associate Professor, School of
Nursing, University of Calgary,
Calgary, Alberta, Canada*

Muriel Standeven, R.N., M.A.
*Assistant Professor, Department of
Family and Community Nursing,
School of Nursing, University of
Washington, Seattle*

Leonard I. Stein, M.D.
*Director of Research, Division of
Mental Hygiene, Mendota State
Hospital, Madison*

Ruth F. Stewart, R.N., M.S.
*Associate Professor, School of
Nursing at San Antonio,
University of Texas, San Antonio*

Jayne Anttila Tapia, R.N., M.S.
*Director, Arlington Visiting
Nursing Association, Inc., and
Lexington Visiting Nursing
Association, Inc., Arlington,
Massachusetts*

Beryl M. Wauson, R.N., B.A.
*School Nurse, Unified School
District, Long Beach, California*

Marilee Woehning, R.N., M.S.
*Instructor, Public Health Nursing,
School of Public Health,
University of Minnesota,
Minneapolis*

Ginger M. Wyatt, R.N.
*Industrial Nurse, E. I. DuPont
De Nemours and Co., Inc.,
Beaumont, Texas*

Ann Zimmern, R.N., M.A.
Assistant Editor, American Journal
of Nursing, *New York*

Contemporary Community Nursing

Community Nursing

Community nursing is a specialized field of nursing practice. Until recently people tended to distinguish between public health nursing, on the one hand, and hospital nursing, on the other. This distinction emphasized the geographic location of a particular kind of nursing practice: in the hospital or in the community. But this criterion is misleading and obscures the true nature of community nursing. Three fundamental features of community nursing can help to clarify the definition of this field.

First, community nursing, as the term implies, means nursing care provided to the community. Because communities include many different kinds of people, community nursing seeks to include them all in its service. Other nursing specialties serve various populations, determined, in general, either by diagnostic group (e.g., psychiatric, maternity) or by age group (e.g., pediatric, geriatric). Community nursing encompasses all these groups but is not limited to any one. Furthermore, community nursing considers individuals, families and all special groups in the context of the larger community.

Second, community nursing combines the basic principles of nursing practice with those of public health. Instead of serving individual needs only, community nursing attempts to diagnose and to treat community health needs, which might include promotion of venereal disease education, well-baby clinics or improved transportation facilities for the elderly. Another principle of public health utilized by community nursing is health planning. Health plans must be implemented by providing comprehensive services to the community. For example, once the need for venereal disease education has been diagnosed, plans can be formulated and then carried out. Community nursing also seeks to evaluate existing health services and improve their effectiveness. For example, well-baby clinics might be operating but an evaluation may show that their existence is unknown to many mothers who might otherwise use them.

Third, community nursing seeks to give distributive care rather than episodic care. Episodic care is periodic and focuses on the patient's illness. Distributive care, on the other hand, is continuing care that maintains health. For example, community nursing might follow a patient beyond the acute phases of illness, assist him through recovery and teach him and his family about maintaining good health. Distributive care is also comprehensive in that it seeks to treat the whole person and to provide the entire range of nursing services. The articles in Part I examine the nature of community nursing, the principles underlying this field and current changes that are taking place.

Community Nursing in a Changing Climate

Paulette Robischon

Some professional fields of health care are relatively stable and easy to define. Community nursing, on the other hand, continues to change at a rapid rate and carries out its work under a variety of changing conditions. Perhaps the best way to clarify the nature of community nursing is to identify these dimensions of change. This article examines many currents of change and challenges community nursing to combat deficiencies in the present health care system through innovation.

Community health workers have long been concerned with the whole man in his total environment (before ecology became a household word) and were not concerned with just a part of his body or a category of disease. But we have been largely unsuccessful in translating this holistic concept into practice or in exciting the public about it. Now, consumers have created the excitement. They are demanding such care and this demand is the challenge to the community nurse, beginning right now.

Nursing is part of the hodgepodge health care system in this country — one which provides services that are inadequate, fragmented, inefficient, inequitably distributed, and uncoordinated. Partly because of the character of our nation, we have no unified national policy on health. Our health care system has developed in a pluralistic society, combining private and public efforts with a strong tradition of voluntary action, states' rights, and local autonomy. These aspects of our social structure have made positive contributions but they also have generated problems — one of them the crazy quilt of our present health system.

But change is coming, as consumers now protest against skyrocketing costs, as the low quality of care is criticized, and as the public insists on a better distribution of services, geographical and social. The machinery of government is being used increasingly as a tool for restructuring society's institutions, and the responsibilities of the private and public sectors are shifting. Health team members are realigning their responsibilities and new workers are being added.

The recipient of health care is changing, too. He is smarter, with more sophisticated goals, more critical of things as they are, and insisting on an adequate response to his health needs. He demands to be involved in his own care. Through a growing sense of his own power, he has determined to build a better life and has shown willingness to group with others to achieve new goals.

At the same time, the population is growing and is becoming more mobile. Family life styles are changing. Poverty persists, and deteriorating environmental conditions bring new health threats. Long-term illness and conditions stemming from the individual's behavior have become prominent health problems. Dr. Roger O. Egeberg of [HEW] recently ranked the nation's most serious health problems, in order of severity, as health care delivery; population control and cleanup of the environment (of equal importance); need for support of basic research; and alcoholism and other addictive diseases.

Finally, there is a changing concept of health. It is no longer the mere absence of disease and disability — not just not being "sick." It is a more positive view of health as a condition that offers an individual the greatest capacity to live happily and productively — a goal that becomes possible as past health problems are conquered.

All of these changes have been reflected in the altered emphasis in public health, beginning in the 1960's, on involving the community in planning and carrying through a program of health care. This community — of consumers, health workers, and representatives of public and private sectors — is in partnership to develop solutions for the problems inherent in delivery of health care.

CHANGE IN NAME

The very nomenclature is changing, as *public* health nursing is becoming *community* health nursing. The term "public health nursing" can be confusing, for it often incorrectly denotes nursing performed by an official or government agency (the public agency), whereas nurses in voluntary or nongovernmental health agencies are generally called visiting nurses. The new term not only helps eliminate the confusion but, more important, it stresses the focus of this field of nursing — toward the community.

However, the new name may itself be misleading; community health nursing is not limited to care of persons outside the hospital. Nor does it merely encompass prevention, case-finding, continuity of care, total family care, and patient and family self-direction — concepts implicit in *all* sound professional nursing practice today.

Rather, according to Freeman:

Community health nursing is seen as a population-based obligation, realized through a multidisciplinary, ecologically oriented effort and utilizing concepts and skills that derive both from generic nursing and from public health practices. It focuses on nursing the *community* in contradistinction to nursing *in* the community. Family nursing care is seen as an essential aspect of health care of the population, and the community health nurse's responsibility is seen as encompassing but not being limited to this aspect of the program.[1]

The American Nurses' Association defines community health nursing practice as:

A synthesis of nursing practice and public health practice applied to promoting and preserving the health of populations. The nature of this practice is general and comprehensive, rather than limited to a particular age or diagnostic group; it is continuing, rather than episodic. The dominant responsibility of community health nursing is to the population as a whole. Therefore, nursing directed to individuals or groups becomes a valid component of community health nursing practice only as it is intrinsically related to and contributes to the care of the population as a whole.[2]

The most obvious of the various obstacles to putting into action these concepts of community nursing is lack of manpower. A survey of agencies and nurses engaged in public health made in 1968 by the U.S. Public Health Service showed that 48,742 nurses were employed in 9,995 agencies in this country.[3] Local official health agencies employed the largest single number of community nurses (39 percent), and close behind were boards of education, with 38 percent. Voluntary non-official agencies (mainly VNAs) employed 13 percent of the total community nursing personnel, and national and state agencies and universities employed the other 10 percent.

OPPORTUNITIES FOR COMMUNITY

Opportunities for employment in community nursing have expanded steadily in recent years, spurred by federal legislation that has helped to establish and expand school health services, programs for the sick in the home, and neighborhood multiservice centers, all of which employ nurses. Community nurse power has increased almost 4 percent a year during the last decade, in contrast to an increase in the general population of only 1.4 percent. For every 100,000 persons in 1938, there were 15 nurses in community health work; by 1968 there were 21 such nurses. The greatest gain in this period was in the number of nurses employed by boards of education.

Despite the steady gain of nurses prepared for and working in the community, manpower resources still do not meet service demands. This discrepancy will continue, particularly in view of impending national health insurance legislation which will add to the demands. As in other instances of nursing "shortage," some of this problem results from misuse of manpower.

Take school nursing, for instance. One study of school nursing showed that 35 percent of the nurse's time was spent on activities requiring clerical or housekeeping skills.[4] Other schools require the nurse to be always in the school building, thus curtailing her work with families and others in the community. Some school nurses are caught up in routine and static practices. They may spend inordinate amounts of time weighing and measuring children and recording the data, without any purposeful use made of the data.

Sometimes nurses are trapped by the rules and procedures of their agencies. One supervisor of a well-child clinic required a staff nurse to adhere strictly to the agency procedure book, which specified that at each visit she complete a section of the child's record that reviewed developmental milestones and provided anticipatory guidance cues. Admittedly, this was an important phase of well-child counseling. But this busy nurse, working with many families who had multiple problems, was trying to set priorities to do what was most urgently needed and wanted. A set procedure only handicapped her. She was imaginative, concerned, and energetic, and — not permitted to use her knowledge, skills, and personality to the best advantage — she resigned in frustration and moved to a comprehensive child care center where role flexibility and use of judgment and creativity were encouraged. Within a year she won an award as being the prime mover behind the development of a vital new service for children and their parents at the center.

Some nurses in official agencies follow the custom of delivering all birth certificates to new parents at home — a sure way to meet these newcomers and one that served its purpose in the past, and still may in some areas. But this practice persists without consideration of the other problems and events in the community that need the attention of nurses.

Nurses in occupational health settings sometimes function only as administrators of first-aid or as truant officers, because management sees them in this role. And there are nurses in VNAs who are caught up in providing routine morbidity care to one person in a family to the exclusion of other members; they dash from home to home caring only for the sick person in each. This latter situation has many causes: pressures of Medicare and Medicaid, need for the agency to do only that job for which it will be reimbursed, lack of judicious use of nonprofessional and auxiliary personnel, organizational problems, and, perhaps, a lack of belief in the validity of the total family approach to care. Such instances of wasted manpower in community nursing have similar counterparts in institutional nursing.

AGENCY SIZE — A FACTOR

Agency structure is another factor that influences community nursing practice. Because of the small size of many political jurisdictions, there are numerous small official health units and voluntary nursing agencies. Nationwide, 36 percent of all local agencies are one-nurse agencies, and over 10 percent employ only part-time nurses. Consequently, there is often difficulty attracting qualified personnel and providing administrative direction and nursing supervision.

At a time when prepared nursing supervisors and administrators are in short supply, we find some of them working in agencies of five nurses or less. Other agencies lack nursing supervision altogether. To overcome this shortage, it has been suggested that the qualifications be lowered for supervisory and administrative positions in home health agencies so that agencies can become certified for Medicare purposes. A more practical solution, and one that would serve the patient and community better, would be to merge or pool resources.

In other areas, local autonomy or home rule dominates and slows up regionalization, amalgamation of agencies, and pooling of resources. For example, in one town of less than 1,000 population that is adjacent to a large city but under its own political jurisdiction, the town nurse resigned. The town has only one small elementary school, and its population is shrinking as old housing is replaced with industrial concerns. It *could* have contracted for school health and department of health nursing activities from an established accredited VNA in the bordering city, which already covered the town's need for bedside nursing. Instead, the town hired a nurse — unqualified — to fill the position to satisfy the town fathers who wanted their *own* nurse.

LOOKING TO THE FUTURE

Over the last 30 years, despite the persistence of local autonomy, the number of nonofficial community health nursing agencies has decreased 50 percent. The decrease reflects reorganization and amalgamation of small agencies into more centralized administrative units, but the change has been slow. In the 1970's large nursing agencies will probably continue to expand their services and many will change their operating centers and become parts of a comprehensive health service. Small agencies will continue to fall by the wayside.

Hospital-based community nursing services also become more numerous as hospitals take on new functions as community health agencies. These extended services into the community, we hope, will not carry on the hospital's past emphasis on sickness only. These services have the potential for breaking down barriers between hospital and community and encouraging the movement of nurses from one setting to another.

The nurse in the future may care for groups of families in sickness as well as in health, in various settings, with the main concern on *health*. For example, the Health Insurance Plan of Greater New York is conducting a study in which several community health nurses function as primary care agents for a selected group of patients. These nurses follow patients in and out of the hospital, through extended care facilities (including nursing homes), or back to the patient's home. Health promotion and maintenance are their primary concern.

In the '70's health service areas will increasingly be identified not by political boundaries but by such factors as geography, population numbers, and population characteristics. Community health nursing agencies, too, will be so organized, rather than by arbitrary and meaningless boundaries. They will pool their resources in the interest of better business management and effectiveness in meeting community needs.

EXPANDING HEALTH TEAM

The original public health team consisted of physician, nurse, sanitarian, and clerk, to which were then added the nutritionist, social worker, physical therapist, health educator, and statistician. Now, many more disciplines are represented, and ancillary personnel have become part of the health unit. There are specialties within disciplines and subspecialties within these. Medicine has 30 recognized specialties; and, among the other 125 professional, technical, and vocational specialties in the allied health field, there are some 250 subspecialties.

The newest category of workers is the physician's assistant who is being prepared in more than 30 programs with 20 different titles. In addition, 15 more physician assistant programs are in the planning stage, adding six new titles to the 20 existing ones.[5] We should soon reassess the wisdom of creating this multitude of new types of workers in response to the health crisis in our country. We may find we have a monster that makes coordination of care impossible.

The complexity of the health team requires a common effort beyond merely working harmoniously with others on the same problem. The working operation of a number of people from various backgrounds and with differing preparation and concepts of the job to be done frequently leads to multiple services that are expensive and fragmented, rather than comprehensive. A grouping of workers does not necessarily make a team. Even if it did, the question of who should be the leader would remain unanswered. Peplau suggests that the health discipline structure must change from a pyramid (with the physician always on top) to a pie-shaped structure, with each discipline having a piece carved out, each interrelated with the other to form a whole, which is health care.[6]

Confusion among health workers will arise as they redefine roles and carve out new ones. Overlaps of knowledge and skills will occur, as well as instances where any of several disciplines might intervene in the patient's behalf. It is not so important to establish exact role boundaries as it is to keep roles flexible, to collaborate with other disciplines, set up ground rules, and stop worrying about who is sloughing off tasks or encroaching on whose territory.

We must use to advantage the skills and talents of all available personnel. Is a qualified community nurse necessary for every home visit? We know this is impossible and, more important, it may not be necessary. Use of indigenous workers who can narrow the cultural distance between worker and family has shown that they may be best suited for certain situations. The patient requiring long-term care at home may be well served by the worker who has had minimum training, thus reserving the professionally prepared nurse for guidance and supervision of this worker.

On the other hand, not every patient or family needs, wants, or will accept a concerted team attack on his health-related problems. One team member or discipline may be able to meet an immediate need and depart, saving other members' time and the family's patience. However, there are instances where community nursing must reach out to and accept not only the groups it has traditionally served but other cultures and subcultures as well. These include alienated and estranged young people, the isolated aged, citizens of skid row, loners of all ages, hippies, migrants, and addicts. Community nursing must find ways to provide all these people with nursing care acceptable to them and compatible with their mores, values, and life style.

REACHING THE NONACCEPTING

How do we reach those who are distrustful of established health care facilities — for example, victims of drug abuse, or those who live in communes? New social institutions are emerging to meet these groups' needs, like the "free clinic" movement, which operates outside of the organized medical and public health establishment. These clinics offer informal, nonjudgmental, and youth-oriented care, and are directed and operated by the people who use them. Other avenues include making services available at the times of day when people can use them and, in the case of migrants, having health care personnel follow these workers in their travels.

Offering primary care through ambulatory facilities that are accessible to the recipient is becoming a popular way to "reach out." However, these services are often limited to medical diagnosis and treatment, whereas many other health services are needed. Neighborhood centers must be responsible and responsive to the needs of people, not the professionals. Several new family health care centers based in large urban hospitals unfortunately follow the traditional clinic pattern — a doctor's workshop. There is the huge waiting room, the clerk overseeing the crowd, the medical specialty offices, and nurses fixing dressing trays and running about readying examination rooms. They provide no areas where toddlers can be supervised while parents confer with health personnel, or where group teaching and nurse-patient conferences can take place. In fact, they often fail to provide for any kind of family approach, where teams of physicians, nurses, social workers, and others care for groups of families on a continuing basis.

We are learning — with difficulty — that health professionals are no longer the guardian of the recipient's interest in health services. Community nursing pioneered consumer representation on its boards and councils, but often those who participated did not represent or speak for the people served. The Economic Opportunity Act of 1964 made explicit provision for recipients of federally funded health care to be involved in program decisions. We were then forced to reassess our relations with those who used our services. No longer could we shut ourselves off from honest feedback from those we served or from those we did not reach with our services.

HEALTH PROMOTION

It is said that we must change our present "last line of defense," acute-care approach, which is essentially passive, to one that stresses early detection of disease and keeping people out of hospitals. It is true that we must do so, but this is a negative approach. Our greatest thrust, I believe, should be toward health promotion. We must accentuate wellness rather than illness; become health-oriented rather than pathology-oriented. At present we give lip service to this concept while we continue to stress the provision of palliative measures:

caring for the ill, repairing the ravages of disease, and preventing the spread of disease. We must not underrate the value of these activities, but neither should we give them disproportionate emphasis.

Everyone, at any one time, is somewhere on the health-illness continuum. Health promotion activities can help the person move toward the health end by assisting him to become a fully functioning individual. This may be accomplished by promoting adequate nutrition adjusted to his developmental phase, fostering healthy personality development, educating him in positive health practices, and working to make his environment a healthy one.

We cannot speak of health promotion without considering health teaching. Our teaching has been based on the assumption of man as a rational being, his actions guided by knowledge and the implications of this knowledge. Providing health information was sufficient, we thought, to induce him to act intelligently in health matters. But we were wrong. For man is not a shell waiting to have new ideas poured into him. His health behavior is determined by various and complex psychosocial and biological factors. We must move from givers of information to change agents of behavior. For example, we must learn how to help young people refrain from establishing unhealthy habits of overeating, physical lethargy, and smoking — habits that set the stage for crippling or fatal diseases in middle life.

We must spur voluntary individual and group action for health promotion. How do we do this? We know now that we cannot act for people — only they can bring change in their behavior. But we can stimulate them to think of change as desirable and possible. If widespread change is needed, we must learn how to develop group consciousness of a problem. Here is an example.

DIETARY PATTERNS UNCHANGED

Last year, while conducting a study in a New York City ghetto area, I made some observations that I compared with similar ones I had made 20 years earlier as an undergraduate student in the same area. The nursing practice of intensive individual instruction of mothers about children's diets, used then as now in a well-child clinic, has been apparently ineffective in altering dietary patterns of this population. The families still placed high value on milk and used too much of it in the diet. Milk was used excessively also as a pacifier in the nursing bottle. There was still not enough lean meat and vegetables and too much carbohydrate (also used as a pacifier, such as potato chips) in the diet.

Some things *had* changed in the 20 years — mothers were better dressed; they had more education, and better jobs. But some things had *not* changed. In addition to housing, much of which was still deplorable in that area, I was struck by the persistence of these fixed dietary patterns. They are deeply ingrained and pass from generation to generation.

We must change our methods and aim our health teaching at populations, rather than individuals. The community nurse of the future, if she is to be skilled as a change agent in promoting health, will need more knowledge about sociocultural patterns, what purposes they serve, how they persist, and how they change. She will also need better understanding of theories of group dynamics, learning, and motivation.

Although we face many problems, there are encouraging developments. Some community health nurses are extending themselves, refusing to be bound by rules and outdated procedures, aggressively establishing their new and expanding roles, making themselves accessible to people, pioneering new methods, and collaborating in a truly interdisciplinary approach to health care.

In an age of excessive specialization, compartmentalization, and categorization, I see the community health nurse as a strong positive force for holding man together, for this nurse is a "generalized specialist," one who has an overall concern for the whole man, his family, and his community.

REFERENCES

1. Freeman, Ruth B. *Community Health Nursing Practice.* Philadelphia, W. B. Saunders Co., 1970, p. 111.
2. Members asked to review new practice definition. *Community Health Nurs.* (ANA Community Health Division on Nursing Practice) Spring 1969, p. 1.
3. American Nurses' Association. *Facts about Nursing.* New York, The Association, 1969, pp. 31—35.
4. Doster, Daphine D. Utilization of available nurse power in public health. *Am. J. Public Health* 60:25—37, Jan. 1970.
5. Physicians assistant programs (list) *RN* 33:43—46, Oct. 1970.
6. Peplau, Hildegard. Nurses as a collectivity must take a stand. *Am. J. Nurs.* 70:2123—2124, Oct. 1970.

2
An Open Health Care System Model

Madeleine M. Leininger

Community nursing cannot be considered apart from the context in which it takes place. As the health care system changes and adapts to meet patients' needs more effectively, so too will the role of the community nurse change. Madeleine Leininger proposes a health care system model that is consistent with trends in community health. It is patient-centered and designed to utilize effectively health resources and personnel.

This is the decade in which our American health care practices are being challenged for change: a time for critical evaluation of our present health care system and for the development of imaginative new ones that will provide the best possible health services to meet the diverse health needs of the diverse cultural groups that make up our society. If we are to accomplish this goal, however, we must substitute for our present closed, uniprofessionally controlled system one that is open, flexible, diverse, and oriented to the client and the community. Even more important, we need a system that will acknowledge, utilize, and distribute to best advantage the skills and services of all health professionals concerned with patient care.

Our current crisis in health care, I contend, is largely attributable to two factors: (1) inadequate identification, utilization, and distribution of the health manpower personnel now available and lack of recognition of their full potential; and (2) the fact that our present care system is operated and controlled by the medical profession.

The second factor, obviously, goes a long way toward explaining the first one. Despite the many statements that have been made to the contrary, I seriously question whether there is an actual shortage of health manpower personnel. Rather, it is our present system, with its uniprofessional dominance, that stands in the way of optimal, or even reasonable, utilization of the health care personnel already available. Nor do I believe that the encouragement and proliferation of "new" types of health workers will do much to alleviate the situation. These workers may extend the physician's services, but they will not necessarily provide clients with the more varied and appropriate range of services that are both needed and lacking.

The trend in our society to produce large numbers of health workers to solve health problems is quite congruent with our cultural norms, in that we tend to produce more of everything that seems socially desirable and possible. The more numbers we have, we seem to believe, the more likely we are to meet our needs. Careful planning for the best use of what we already have, however, before producing more is *not* one of our established norms.

We also tend to get rid of an object (and sometimes humans) after a few years of use for a seemingly "bigger, brighter, and more effective object" — one that usually has a new label and at least one attractive new feature. This norm is certainly in operation in relation to our present production of "new" types and numbers of health manpower workers. Unfortunately, many of these so-called new personnel and programs are rapidly emerging without full recognition of the professional health personnel already available and the educational programs that have prepared these workers for many years. Many of these "new" health workers are already performing activities comparable to those that have been traditionally performed by such professional personnel as the nurse and physician.

In addition, we need a system(s) to which the client can have prompt and ready access through a variety of routes; a system or subsystems that are small enough to be humanely manageable, without undue bureaucratic restraints, and capable of offering a personalized kind of service; and, finally, systems that will be truly community-oriented and will not only allow but encourage citizen input into their development, maintenance, and evaluation. Our present system has none of these characteristics -- hence, my advocacy of a new and open system.

What do I mean by a "closed system"? According to general systems theory, a closed system is one in which there is limited or no interchange in components such as materials and energy within the total environmental context. Here, we can draw an analogy with the limited interchange between health manpower resources and energy with the environmental needs or situation. Closed systems tend to function in an insulated way and to level out differences in their structure in the interest of maintaining equilibrium. Open systems, on the other hand, encourage and accommodate a continuous interchange and flow of inputs from the total environment with differential effects and processes.

A CLOSED SYSTEM

Thus, our present health care system, which permits only limited, if any, exchange of varied health manpower resources and potentials with community demands, is a closed one. And this is because it is predominantly controlled — economically, politically, and professionally — by the medical profession. The resultant sets of expectations that have developed between physicians and "their" patients further maintain the system as a closed one. There is no free exchange; instead, inputs of skills and services from other health personnel are largely controlled, regulated, and overshadowed (socially and professionally) by physicians. This closed physician-patient system is evident in federal support of health service and educational programs and is reflected by the communication media, in professional role expectations, and in many other ways.

Therefore, members of other professional disciplines — nurses and social workers, for instance — lack legitimate authority to practice in an open and fairly independent way. Instead, they usually have "to work around" the system in order to provide the kinds of health services which the public expects of them — and has a right to expect of them.

Consumers, too, come under the control of one professional person — namely, the medical man — since it is the only way in which they can enter or leave the system. As Norris has pointed out, ". . . everyone — patient and professional alike — *must wait* until the physician has seen the patient. The physician is the gatekeeper of the health care system and he continues to marshal continual support to maintain that role. Not only does he control the entry *into* the health care system; he provides the only pathway *through* the system."[1] Yet, if clients are to receive appropriate help through appropriate types of professional workers, those workers *must* have direct access to the client, and vice versa.

Furthermore, even in situations where other than the physician does provide the health services, third-party payers usually require the physician to sign papers to the effect that the client *did* receive health services under his authority. For many years nurses have provided direct health services to clients, and yet it has been extremely difficult for them to receive any form of direct payment (except for private duty nursing) through second- and third-party insurance payments. Payment for nursing services through Medicare and Medicaid is equally difficult to obtain, and most health insurance policies cover primarily physician services and not nursing services.

Recently, though, there is some indication that the consumer of health services now wants to pay only the professional person who actually provided his health care. One client, for instance, refused to pay the physician whom he did not see and who did not provide him direct services. Instead, he insisted upon paying the nurse who gave him direct health care services. If consumer demands such as this one accumulate, then perhaps the consumer will give impetus to changing the system in order to render payment to those who give him service.

Another sense in which our health system is closed is that information about the client is expected to filter in and out from the physician exclusively. Seldom do most other health professionals feel free to retain or act upon this information entirely alone. Instead, there is the implicit expectation that the physician should know about "his" patient and have exclusive rights to all patient information. This circumstance tends to create a strong dependency role for the other health care personnel. In the strictest legal sense, we have no system for a free exchange of patient information with shared responsibility by health professionals except as controlled by the physician. Although we know that this rule is often impractical and frequently broken, it is done in an under-the-counter way and represents a dysfunctional practice outside the established norm.

Friedson, in his *Professional Dominance: The Social Structure of Medical Care,* has aptly summarized the situation in saying that

... professions in general and medicine in particular cannot live up to their professed ideals as long as they possess thorough-going autonomy to control the terms and content of their work and as long as they are dominant in a division of labor. In essence, I [have] suggested ways to which professional dominance and autonomy could be tempered by administrative accountability, by accountability to the individual patient himself, and by the deliberate encouragement of workers who can compete with the medical practitioner.[2]

The closed system, therefore, seriously limits the full rendering of health services to clients by professional groups (other than the physician) and according to each professional's particular expertise. As a result, authority and accountability for professional services to clients tend to be seriously hampered, weakened, and confused. Although the physician delegates all kinds of "responsibility" or "tasks" to others, he seldom delegates the full authority to make independent judgments in relation to the carrying out of those responsibilities.

AN OPEN SYSTEM

An open health care system, on the other hand, would offer the client a choice of services from several health disciplines and not limit him to physician services only. It would most surely offer him earlier, prompter, and easier access to services according to his health problem; for instance, he might not need to see a physician at all if his problem could effectively and appropriately be handled by a nurse or social worker.

Such a system should also result in a substantial reduction in the cost of health services — especially those routine, minor, noncomplex kinds of health services that can be provided by other than a physician. Additionally, the system would permit professional contributions from many different health groups, all of them expected to assume responsibility and accountability for their services to clients, whether provided independently or in collaboration with other disciplines. In other words, an open system could and should maximize the contributions of all available health personnel according to their professional skills and knowledge.

Furthermore, personnel functioning in an open health system learn to live with differences in needs and do not try to maintain the balanced equilibrium — the status quo — that characterizes a closed system; instead, an open system is always responsive to change. It would encourage, for instance, an open exchange of ideas among all health disciplines. And it would look for feedback, too — both positive and negative — from individuals and the community to the care providers (this could work both ways) in order to improve and further develop a system sensitive to any inputs from within and outside it. Modifications could then be made according to client, community, and professional needs.

Finally, an open system fosters the development of multiple kinds of client-professional relationships and permits comparisons of different kinds of health

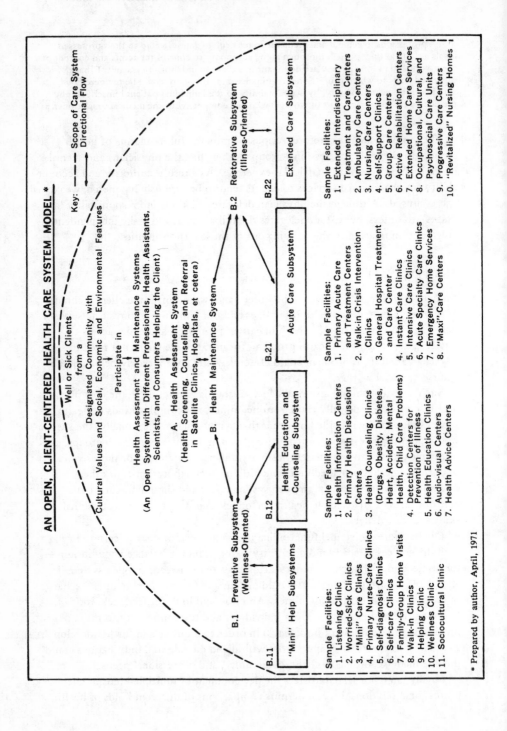

AN OPEN, CLIENT-CENTERED HEALTH CARE SYSTEM MODEL *

Key:
- - - - Scope of Care System
⟷ Directional Flow

Well or Sick Clients
from a
Designated Community with
Cultural Values and Social, Economic and Environmental Features

Participate in

Health Assessment and Maintenance Systems
(An Open System with Different Professionals, Health Assistants, Scientists, and Consumers Helping the Client)

A. Health Assessment System
(Health Screening, Counseling, and Referral in Satellite Clinics, Hospitals, et cetera)

B. Health Maintenance System

B.1 Preventive Subsystem (Wellness-Oriented)

B.11 "Mini" Help Subsystems

Sample Facilities:
1. Listening Clinic
2. Worried-Sick Clinics
3. "Mini" Care Clinics
4. Primary Nurse-Care Clinics
5. Self-diagnosis Clinics
6. Self-care Clinics
7. Family-Group Home Visits
8. Walk-in Clinics
9. Helping Clinic
10. Wellness Clinic
11. Sociocultural Clinic

B.12 Health Education and Counseling Subsystem

Sample Facilities:
1. Health Information Centers
2. Primary Health Discussion Centers
3. Health Counseling Clinics (Drugs, Obesity, Diabetes, Heart, Accident, Mental Health, Child Care Problems)
4. Detection Centers for Prevention of Illness
5. Health Education Clinics
6. Audio-visual Centers
7. Health Advice Centers

B.2 Restorative Subsystem (Illness-Oriented)

B.21 Acute Care Subsystem

Sample Facilities:
1. Primary Acute Care and Treatment Centers
2. Walk-in Crisis Intervention Clinics
3. General Hospital Treatment and Care Center
4. Instant Care Clinics
5. Intensive Care Clinics
6. Acute Specialty Care Clinics
7. Emergency Home Services
8. "Maxi"-Care Centers

B.22 Extended Care Subsystem

Sample Facilities:
1. Extended Interdisciplinary Treatment and Care Centers
2. Ambulatory Care Centers
3. Nursing Care Centers
4. Self-Support Clinics
5. Group Care Centers
6. Active Rehabilitation Centers
7. Extended Home Care Services
8. Occupational, Cultural, and Psychosocial Care Units
9. Progressive Care Centers
10. "Revitalized" Nursing Homes

* Prepared by author, April, 1971

16

services. Certainly, different professional services meet different client health needs, and this could lead to a refinement in matching clients' needs with specific professional services.

For example, client needs for psychophysiological comfort, interpersonal support, and empathy are often best met by professional nurses, whereas needs for various kinds of community services might best be met by social workers. An open system would therefore make for more options, less cost, readier access to health services, earlier and better care, active consumer input, and more interdisciplinary participation, plus a delineation of professional areas of responsibility and accountability.

To date only a paucity of health care models have been proposed as alternatives to our present system. Granted, there has been much talk about the need to change health care systems, but few advocates have offered any new designs. Yet it would seem essential to explore several models in order to see which ones offer the best potential for generalized and specialized uses.

Encouragingly, Garfield has provided a noteworthy health care model that provides a fairly comprehensive scheme of health care services.[3] His model has several favorable features, such as separating the well from the sick, a multihealth screening plan, subsystems to meet certain needs of clients, and the potential use of paraprofessionals in the health care system.

Its major limitation is the lack of emphasis upon the use of cultural, social, and community data and the role of the client in the model. Also, it depicts physicians in a central and controlling position, with other professionals in typical subordinate positions, and tends to see the hospital setting as the central focus for health care services. In contrast, the model proposed in this article focuses primarily on the client and his community and emphasizes the roles of various health disciplines and community groups within the system.

MODEL FOR CARE

The open, client-centered model that I am proposing is presented in diagram form on page [16]. As I see it, it has several important features.

First, it focuses upon client(s) coming from a designated community with its particular social structure, cultural norms, economic conditions, political interests, and other features that relate to the client's health status, treatment care, and health maintenance. Staff working in this open system will support an active interchange of ideas with the client and his community so that the client's life style and health values, as well as those of his community, will be given full consideration. In addition, professional staff, community workers, social scientists, environmentalists, and many other persons will be expected to contribute their viewpoints and knowledge toward effective understanding of and work with the client. Since wellness states are largely defined by the culture and community in which one lives, these factors need to be given more consideration than is presently the case and are therefore emphasized in this model.

Second, this model will provide for a broadly conceived health assessment plan in which the client may have a choice as to the professional person he and his family (or social group) wish to have help him with his health problem; he is not limited to entering or leaving the system through a physician. Moreover, he may seek the services of different health professionals at different points in his health maintenance program. If he is uncertain about the appropriate person for his health care problem, health consultants are available to assist him.

Both generalists and specialists in various disciplines may be called upon to assess the client's needs and provide care as indicated, but the professional person with whom the patient first initiates the contact will maintain responsibility to and for him and will coordinate and follow through on his health plans or needs.

While many varieties of multiphase assessment subsystems will undoubtedly be present in large urban multiservice institutions, satellite health assessment systems on a smaller scale will probably be established in rural communities. Health screening, counseling, and referral will be carried out by different kinds of health professionals and will vary according to their respective skills and interests. Independent and collaborative health assessment practices will co-exist.

Third, the proposed model places major emphasis on health maintenance and on its two important subsystems: prevention (the wellness-oriented subsystem), and restoration (the illness-oriented subsystem). The wellness subsystem, as the diagram indicates, will emphasize "mini" kinds of helping services, as well as health education and counseling. The illness subsystem will be concerned with acute and extended care. These two subsystems, however, are not mutually nor totally exclusive. Clients may need to move between them from time to time — hence, the directional arrows shown on the diagram.

Attention to wellness behavior and to the cultural ways in which people maintain a healthy state seems particularly important. In some cultures of the world, for instance, people strive for a wellness orientation and resist illness behavior, whereas in other cultures a pattern of sickness behavior tends to be the mode of living. What factors contribute to these contrasting life styles? As more knowledge accumulates about wellness behavior, we can predict that there will be less need for practitioners for the ill and more need for "wellness" practitioners — a shift from our present directions.

Fourth, the model supports a refinement in the division of labor to areas of professional accountability and responsibility without at the same time supporting a high fractionization of health care services. Health personnel with both specialized and generalized skills will be responsible for their own decisions and actions. Professional staff could be prepared to function in either the wellness or illness subsystems, rather than be an expert or generalist in both.

Clients with a "mini" health problem would not need to enter the restorative system but would seek the services of a wellness-oriented health worker. For example, clients who are lonely and want social contacts could come to the "wellness" or sociocultural clinics and would not need to play a sick role in order to get help or attention. The prevention subsystem would focus upon early assistance with minor and noncomplex health stresses in order to prevent crisis and complex health problems at a later time.

Some client problems could be handled primarily by one professional person, while another kind of problem might require collaborative work. Thus there would be many opportunities for several disciplines to work together on particular clients' problems, or on general problems that require a team effort for their solution. The model, then, encourages the maximum utilization of present and emerging health practitioners and uses the skills of all health-related scientists in an effective partnership way.

Fifth, the model supports the concept of providing diverse kinds of health care resources and facilities to meet the diverse health needs of people in our society. Several examples of facilities are offered in the model to stimulate thinking about the various ways in which people might be helped. Some of these facilities already exist, others are being considered, and still others will need to be developed.

Sixth, the model encourages social and natural scientists, humanists, and consumers, as well as health profession practitioners, to become active participants, developers, and evaluators of an open system of care. Distributive authority and control, as well as coordinated and independent areas of responsibility for health practitioners, characterize the proposed mode of operation. Consumers, health scientists, and professional disciplines (other than medicine) are all seen as having a part in controlling and maintaining the open system.

Since consumers will be "buying into" or investing in the system, they merit an equally active part in shaping and developing it. A coordinating professional health specialist with no vested interest or biases in any profession (and not necessarily a physician) will coordinate the health services, with focus upon the consumer obtaining the best health services available in view of the health manpower resources, skills, and money.

The model supports the idea of expanding, contracting, or modifying health services according to the health needs of people in a designated community. A large- or small-scale delivery model could be developed from the present one, as both the process and structure are apparent. Furthermore, this model permits study and comparison of the effectiveness and costs of each health care subsystem, as well as comparison of this model as a total health delivery system with other models. Thus, the model was constructed with a view toward providing health maintenance and comprehensive health care services from both the wellness and illness frame of reference and as important parts of a total health care delivery system.

Within such a proposed open system, changes are inevitable, and so professional staff must change to meet the demands and resources of the people. Role modification and role expansion are both expected and encouraged to meet new societal forces and consumer needs. Accordingly, there will be opportunities to develop new kinds of health facilities (as indicated in the sub-systems of the proposed model), and to terminate dysfunctional health facilities that are no longer needed.

The educational implications of this model are multiple, exciting, and important in the preparation of health professionals, especially according to an inter-disciplinary education model.[4] There is no doubt that with this open system, professional nurses, as the largest health manpower group, will move more significantly into the health prevention subsystem and assume greater responsibility for health practices in the restorative subsystem. The nurse will assume increasing responsibility for primary health care and will also continue to refine her role responsibilities and skills in the care of people with chronic illnesses.

All health disciplines will need to examine their changing roles and to prepare future health practitioners accordingly, through changes in their respective educational and professional patterns. Overlapping and collaborative health role areas will need to be identified — among other reasons, to reduce competitive behavior and role conflicts.

SUMMARY

In summary, an open, client-centered health care system has been presented as a model to stimulate new directions in conceptualizing future health services. The criteria of increasing accessibility and availability of health services, with focus upon reducing health costs and fully using all available health personnel (especially the professional nurse), have been emphasized. It is my belief that we need health care models which will conceive health services of the future in broad terms, rather than from a unidisciplinary perspective.

While this model might appear quite futuristic to some, an open health system *can* become a reality if consumers, professionals and others are interested in and committed to the idea; there are already some beginnings and efforts in this direction. The public must become more cognizant of ways to alleviate the health crisis, and health professionals must honestly face the problem inherent in our present closed health system and search for ways to change it. Ideas planted today can bear fruit tomorrow, if nourished in a committed, active, and supportive manner.

REFERENCES

1. Norris, C. M. Direct access to the patient. *Am. J. Nurs.* 70:1006, May 1970.
2. Freidson, Eliot. *Professional Dominance; Social Structure of Medical Care.* New York, Atherton Press, 1970, p. 234.
3. Garfield, S. R. The delivery of medical care. *Sci. Am.* 222:15–23, Apr. 1970.
4. Leininger, Madeleine. This I believe . . . about interdisciplinary health education for the future. *Nurs. Outlook* 19:787–791, Dec. 1971.

High-Level Wellness for Man and Society

Halbert L. Dunn

*A fundamental aspect of community nursing is the promotion of good health.
This includes the prevention of illness. Beside the obvious benefits of reducing
health care costs and discomfort to the consumer, promotion of positive health,
or wellness, is a means of ensuring productive, self-actualized persons. What
are the factors that contribute to good health and how does one assess these
factors in patients and families? Among public health professionals the
community nurse has a primary responsibility to undertake this assessment and
implement a plan for promoting health. Halbert Dunn offers a pragmatic
approach to positive health that can further enhance the effectiveness of
community nursing.*

The awakened interest of public health circles in full-time local health departments and in the family and community programs of health maintenance is an
indication that health workers are becoming more "health oriented." This shift
in emphasis is in accord with the frequently quoted fundamental objective
expressed in the Constitution of the World Health Organization, "Health is a
state of complete physical, mental, and social well-being and not merely the
absence of disease and infirmity."

To most of us, this concept of positive health is "seen through a glass darkly,"
because our eyes have been so long turned in a different direction, concentrating
fixedly on disease and death. When we take time to turn our gaze in the opposite
direction, focusing it intently on the condition termed good health, we see that
wellness is not just a single amorphous condition, but rather that it is a complex
state made up of overlapping levels of wellness. As we come to know how to
recognize these levels objectively, more or less as we now diagnose one disease
from another, we will realize that the state of being well is not a relatively flat,
uninteresting area of "unsickness" but is rather a fascinating and ever-changing
panorama of life itself, inviting exploration of its every dimension.

It is my thesis, therefore, that both medicine and public health must undertake a multiple and thoroughgoing exploration of the factors responsible for
good health. Without prejudice to the importance or the continuation and
support of existing medical and health programs involving preventive, curative,
or rehabilitative research and activities, it seems clear that many of today's and
tomorrow's problems call for the stimulation and development of a new major
axis of interest directed toward positive health — one strong enough to activate
physicians, health workers, and others in devoting a substantial segment of

From *American Journal of Public Health*, Vol. 49, No. 6, pp. 786–792, 1959. Reprinted
by permission of the publisher and the author.

their time, resources, and creative energies toward understanding and culturing good health in a positive sense.

WHY A NEW HEALTH AXIS IS NEEDED

The need for this new axis of interest is rooted in the changing demographic, social, economic, and political character of civilization. These changes are well known, although their significance is usually not fully appreciated. They might be summarized thus:

1. *It is a shrinking world.* Communication time has shrunk to the vanishing point. Knowledge of events can span the world in seconds and can be known to the masses in a matter of hours. Travel time from the farthermost reaches of the earth has diminished from years and months to a matter of days and hours.
2. *It is a crowded world.* Turned loose in an all-out assault upon disease and death, the medical and health sciences have brought about generally falling death rates without a corresponding reduction in birth rates. The consequent "epidemic" of population growth has reached towering proportions in many parts of the world and brings with it new health problems arising from population pressures and the scarcities of materials and living space.
3. *It is an older world,* in terms of its people, productivity, and resources. A consequence of the revolution brought about by the health sciences is that relatively more people live to an older age. The per capita demand for the output of the economic and productive machinery is steadily advancing. Consequently, it is probably a fallacy for us to assume, as so many of us have done, that an expansion in scientific knowledge can indefinitely counterbalance the rapidly dwindling natural resources of the globe.
4. *It is a world of mounting tensions.* The tempo of modern life and its demands on the human being and his society are steadily increasing with no corresponding readjustment and strengthening of the inner man and the fabric of his social organizations.

Due to these four factors among others, the problems which face the medical and public health professions have changed character drastically in the last few decades. Chronic illness and mental disease are far more prevalent. A great range of neurotic and functional illnesses, which seldom destroy life but which interfere with living a productive and full life, are on the increase.

The preventive path of the future, both for medicine and public health, inevitably lies largely in reorienting a substantial amount of interest and energy toward raising the general levels of wellness among all peoples. This calls for spelling out in objective terms what high-level wellness actually means for the individual, the family, and the social structure.

THE HEALTH GRID

In order to concretize the goal of high-level wellness, it is essential to shift from considering sickness and wellness as a dichotomy toward thinking of disease and health as a graduated scale. For the purposes of this paper, this scale is conceptualized as one axis of a "health grid" (Figure 1). The health grid is made up of (1) the health axis, (2) the environmental axis, and (3) the resulting health and wellness quadrants, that is, (a) poor health in an unfavorable environment, (b) protected poor health in a favorable environment, (c) emergent high-level wellness in an unfavorable environment, and (d) high-level wellness in a favorable environment. The environmental axis includes not only the physical and biological factors of the environment but also socioeconomic components affecting the health of the individual. The health axis ranges from death at the left

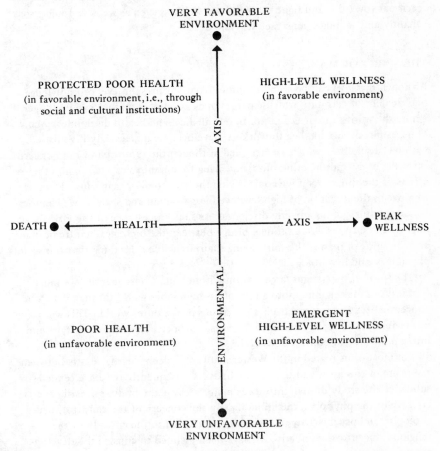

Figure 1. The Health Grid, Its Axes and Quadrants (Source: U.S. Department of Health, Education, and Welfare, Public Health Service, National Office of Vital Statistics)

extremity to "peak wellness" at the right. The area in between the extremes proceeds through serious and minor illnesses into the area of positive health or freedom from illness. Thereafter, it moves into an area of good health at present largely uncharted and undifferentiated, toward a goal as yet but dimly perceived which is indicated as peak wellness. This goal represents the extreme opposite of death, that is, performance at full potential in accordance with the individual's age and makeup. To make effective headway toward this goal, we need to crystallize our concept of what the goal is, not only for the individual but also for the family, the community, and society generally.

Since the nature of this goal is ever changing and ever expanding, we will probably never reach it in absolute terms; but we can come to know and appreciate its essential characteristics in relative terms. As the goal, at first seen far above us, becomes clearer and stirs response from deep within us, we will reach out toward it and fight for high-level wellness even as we have fought so valiantly and so long against sickness and death.

THE SPIRIT OF MAN

Although this goal can be seen but dimly from our present level of knowledge, one element of certainty which emerges in clear relief is that we can no longer ignore the spirit of man as a factor in our medical and health disciplines. Many of us, as physicians and health workers, have become increasingly dissatisfied with our disciplines, which are designed as though the sum total of our concern is for the body and the mind of man, leaving to metaphysics and religion the affairs of the spirit. As if we could divide the sum total of man thus! If we are to move in the direction of high-level wellness for man and society, we cannot ignore the spirit of man in any discipline. In fact, the essence of the task ahead might well be to fashion a rational bridge between the biological nature of man and the spirit of man — the spirit being that intangible something that transcends physiology and psychology.

The spirit of man stems largely from within him. Consequently, we must find ways of making him more aware of his own inner world through which he conceptualizes and interprets his perceptions of the outer world. This will bring us inevitably, sooner or later, into the arenas of social and religious affairs and into a multitude of controversial issues.

For most of us reared in the Western culture, a deep cleavage exists between the realm of the spirit and that of the body. Consequently, we have tended to subdivide the study of man into three major areas — the body, primarily the concern of the physician; the mind, largely the concern of the educator, psychologist, and psychiatrist; and the spirit, entrusted to the custody of the religious preceptors. Similarly, we have been inclined to consign the development and maintenance of man's physical, social, and economic environment largely to economic and political leaders.

This fragmentation of man into areas over which various groups struggle to maintain their jurisdiction appears to be nonsensical, since it tends to defeat the purposes of each group, which strives for the enrichment and fulfillment of that particular segment of man's nature over which it undertakes to maintain jurisdiction. Harmony between jurisdictions can come to pass only when each special interest group realizes that it does not and cannot have a monopoly over a particular area of the nature of man. Harmony will result when the fact is faced that man is a physical, mental, and spiritual unity — a unity which is constantly undergoing a process of growth and adjustment within a continually changing physical, biological, social, and cultural environment.

It is natural that the religious leader, for example, express his particular concern for the spirit of man, but this should not lead him to ignore the body and mind of man or the environment in which man lives, since all these elements affect the well-being of the spirit. Nor should it lead him to the exercise of a monopoly over the spirit of man. The physician, on his part, must take into account spiritual as well as physical considerations if he is to do an effective job of helping his patient toward good health of body and mind. For no person can be well physically if he is sick spiritually.

It is natural for each group competent in a special field of knowledge to approach the study and care of the well-being of man from its own particular point of vantage, but this must not preclude considerations of the unity of man as a whole living within a constantly changing total environment. High-level wellness can never be achieved in fragments, ignoring the unity of the whole.

To the study of man as a unity living within a total environment, the fields of medicine and health have much to offer. To adventure along this pathway of study and responsibility calls for the creation of methods by means of which various levels of wellness can be recognized objectively. Since this proposal has been developed more fully elsewhere,[1] it suffices here to say that, from the standpoints of medicine and health, the principal disciplines contributing to such a science will probably be biochemistry, physiology, and psychology.

The types of questions needing answer are: How do we distinguish and classify degrees or levels of wellness? What are the effects of age, sex, and race on these levels? In what ways can we recognize a particular level in and of itself so as to be reasonably sure we are dealing with a homogeneous group?

If an objective yardstick of wellness can be calibrated in biochemical, physiological, and psychological terms, it would soon become a powerful new tool for the physician, enabling him to recognize low-level wellness and to develop therapies to raise lower levels to higher ones.

If and when it becomes possible to differentiate between levels of wellness, all the indexes now available to us in the measurement of disease and death will become available to us in the area of positive health.

Wellness levels would then become susceptible to measurement in terms of prevalence rates much in the same way we now measure morbidity. Furthermore, we should be able ultimately to calculate the frequency constants of such measurements, correlating them with related social and economic phenomena.

STEPS WHICH CAN BE TAKEN TO QUANTIFY POSITIVE HEALTH

Even though such diagnoses of levels of wellness are not now available, much can be done to quantify positive health, for example:

1. Effect refinements in incidence and prevalence rates to demarcate more clearly the area of positive health from that of illness and disability.
2. Develop susceptibility indexes through the use of biochemical and functional tests to differentiate groups of persons most susceptible to specific diseases and conditions.
3. Establish precursors-of-disease indexes, closely related to the foregoing and designed to show variations from the normal.
4. Select groups of people who are disease-free and who are making full use of their talents, capacities, and potentialities; then measure them by biochemical, functional, and psychological tests to establish the characteristics of those enjoying a high level of wellness. Such groups would need to be selected so as to be representative of the various ages, sexes, and racial combinations.

Possibilities of measuring levels of wellness in the family have been set forth elsewhere.[2] They involve special studies aimed at obtaining answers to four major areas of assessment: (1) What are the day-to-day functional and emotional interrelationships of the family members? (2) What activities occupy the family and its members? (3) What values are important to the family and its members? (4) To what degree does the illness or wellness of a family member reflect the health status of the family as a unit?

It is worth pointing out that, if and when it becomes possible to diagnose levels of wellness in the individual, a very great advantage will accrue to social science technics. For instance, the researcher trying to evaluate the effect of different types of community life on the family or on the individual could select a sample of individuals and measure the effect on their levels of wellness of varying community conditions.

Once the concept of high-level wellness as a health goal has been crystallized and enriched by many minds contributing to it from their own points of reference, the battle for wellness in man and society will be joined. There must be many points of engagement if the battle is to be won.

KNOW THYSELF

It is the author's view that the central bastion to be conquered involves teaching people how to "know themselves." Psychology tells us through laboratory demonstrations that our perceptions of the outer world are indissolubly linked with the concepts and emotions fixed in our minds and body tissues. Without a knowledge of one's inner self, understanding of the outer world cannot have breadth and depth. A mind tortured with prejudice, hate, and fear projects itself in distorted human relationships.

Although psychiatrists have done much to relieve the twisted minds of the mentally ill, little has been undertaken to help ordinary people, classified as "well," to know themselves and thus become better balanced and able to meet their daily problems more adequately. How much of the demand for sleeping pills, alcohol, and tranquilizers is due to this deep-felt need?

It will not be easy to help some adults achieve a better understanding of self. In fact, it is quite likely that the majority of people are fleeing from a deeper knowledge of themselves. With the very young, the task will be less difficult.

Since the personality of the child is largely formed in the preschool years, we must find ways to teach parents the importance of this inner world and how best to guide and nurture the child in his plastic early years, so that he may later be capable of high-level wellness and reach a mature and secure adulthood.

This process calls for the exercise of maturity and wisdom in addition to all the guidance that science can bring to bear. Growing children need broad and diverse opportunities for self-realization. Contact of the child with a wise and mature mind during this period offers one of the best means by which insight may be gained into family and social values and objectives. Maturity and wisdom must be made available to the growing infant and child in order to encourage, temper, and season his explorings and adventurings of self.

RESOURCES OF WISDOM AND MATURITY

Untapped resources of wisdom and maturity are available to the nation among its retired people. Persons no longer active in their careers, but who have lived rich, full lives, acquiring wisdom and maturity in the process, might become part-time companions and counselors to our children, particularly in the case of the gifted child who feels lost without intellectual supplementation of his normal family and school life. Let us call on retired persons of special competence and in good health to return to active life within the community. Let us ask them to help with the children who need extra intellectual stimulus and wise understanding. Let us ask the best qualified of them to serve as advisers to the "sick" family and as special custodians of the culture of the group, so to speak. The community needs them and they need the community.

CREATIVE EXPRESSION

In the fight for high-level wellness, action to enhance the importance of creative expression in our culture is a must. Creative expression is a most important

element in the bridge between the biological nature of man and the spirit of
man. The creative spirit resides within every living person. It can be kindled in
any man, woman, or child. "What is the creative spirit?" you ask. At one time,
I defined it as "an expression of self, adventuring into the unknown in search
for universal truth."[3] However defined, we need to value it highly and nurture
it well, since man's position of dominance in the world stems more directly from
this quality than from all others.

Man finds discovery both absorbing and satisfying. With creative expression
comes intense inner satisfaction. At the same time, it permits man to contribute
of himself to the social group and thus form bonds with his fellow man of love,
trust, and security. Creative expression and love of one's fellows satisfy deep
psychological and emotional needs in our inner world and simultaneously are
radiated outward to bring us to the fullness of life of which man is capable.

When we learn how to diagnose high-level wellness through objective measures,
we shall probably find that a substantial amount of creative expression, altruism,
and love in daily life is essential for the approach to a high state of well-being.
Through the development and application of these values in daily life, we will
achieve self-confidence and faith in ourselves. This in turn will bring growth of
self, development toward fuller maturity, and a balanced wellness of body,
mind, and spirit.

The goal of high-level wellness for man and society can be achieved, though
not easily. The needs are for a clear-cut concept and dedication to it; for money
and research; for understanding, courage, and a reassessment of basic values; for
a positive orientation toward life and society. We must dare to dream, "dreams
are the seedlings of realities."

REFERENCES

1. Dunn, Halbert L. Points of Attack for Raising the Levels of Wellness. *J. Nat. M. A.* 49,
   4:225–235 (July), 1957.
2. _____. How Well Is Your Family? Scheduled for publication in an early issue of *Today's
   Health*.
3. _____. *Your World and Mine. Essays on Human Relations.* New York, N.Y.: Exposition,
   Press, 1956.

Educational Qualifications of Public Health Nurses

Council on Health Manpower

Given the changes in community health needs and the expansion of the nurse's role, how can the professional nurse prepare for practice in the community? The following report describes the educational qualifications requisite to community nursing practice. It also provides an excellent summary of the characteristics and functions of community nursing.

GENERAL SCOPE OF PUBLIC HEALTH NURSING

Public health nursing is one of the basic, organized community health services. It integrates and utilizes the philosophy, content, knowledge and skills of public health and of professional nursing. Characteristically, public health nursing provides family-centered service, and includes comprehensive nursing service to individuals, families, and communities. The pattern of service of public health nursing is vitally interwoven with those of other professional and allied workers with similar goals, and involves participation in community organization to promote and implement health action.

Current concepts of public health, with emphasis on diagnosis of community health needs, health planning, and comprehensive health services include a focus on the quality, distribution, and delivery of public health services. These concepts include a growing recognition that health should be measured in terms of wellness and that health care is a basic human right. They reflect heightened expectations of the public for health, and increased citizen participation in determining the needs for service and the patterns of delivery of health services in the community.

Expansion and other alterations in the delivery of health services are precipitating changes in various kinds of personnel providing public health nursing services. Persons not previously involved are being included on the health team. These additional personnel are from nursing, from other professions, and from nonprofessional groups.

Changes in concepts of public health and changes in patterns of delivery of health services add new dimensions to the roles and functions of practitioners. Some of the increased responsibilities of the public health nurse are to reexamine services provided, to redefine task and skill requirements, and to assign activities accordingly. The public health nurse has a major responsibility to determine training needs of all nursing personnel employed in public health.

The public health nurse has increased responsibility for making diagnostic and therapeutic determinations of patient, family, and community health needs,

From *American Journal of Public Health,* Vol. 61, No. 12, pp. 2505–2509, 1971. Reprinted by permission of the publisher.

and for participating in the provision of primary health care.[1] This expanding role requires the public health nurse to function more independently and to assume a leadership role in decision-making situations.

Nurses in public health now function in a variety of environments. On January 1, 1970 over 50,000 registered nurses were employed in public health by more than 10,000 agencies, excluding industries and other occupational settings. Of these, over 23,000 nurses were employed by State and local health departments, almost 20,000 by boards of education, and 8,000 by visiting nurse associations and hospital based home care programs. The 1970 Census of Nurses in Public Health showed slightly more than 17 percent of all these nurses in public health are in administrative, consultative, or supervisory position; the remaining 83 percent are employed as staff nurses, specialized practitioners, or coordinators of care. These groups represent a wide range of educational backgrounds and experiences, from the new graduate of a diploma, associate degree, or baccalaureate program in nursing to the experienced nurse with a master's or doctoral degree.[2]

The provision of public health nursing services requires many types of nursing personnel: aides, licensed practical nurses, and nurse technicians, among others. However, this statement is concerned with the characteristics, functions, and educational qualifications of professional nurses practicing in public health.

CHARACTERISTICS AND FUNCTIONS

The types and qualifications of nursing personnel may vary with the program responsibilities and the scope of services provided by the employing agency. There are two distinct levels of professional nurses practicing in public health: the nurse prepared at the baccalaureate level who is a generalist in nursing, and the public health nurse specialist who is prepared at the master's level.

The Public Health Nurse Generalist

Baccalaureate nursing programs provide introductory content in public health which is needed for professional nursing practice in any setting. Graduates of these baccalaureate programs are public health nurse generalists when they are practicing in the field of public health. The philosophy and recommendations of the National League for Nursing are explicit in this regard. In delineating the characteristics of baccalaureate education in nursing, the Department of Baccalaureate and Higher Degree Programs states:[3]

[1]Aradine, Carolyn R., and Hausen, Marc F., "Nursing in a Primary Health Care Setting." *Nursing Outlook,* April, 1970, p. 45.
[2]U.S. Department of Health, Education and Welfare, Public Health Service, Division of Nursing. Nurses in Public Health, January, 1970. (Unpublished.)
[3]National League for Nursing, Department of Baccalaureate and Higher Degree Programs. *Characteristics of Baccalaureate Education in Nursing.* New York: The League, 1968.

"Given an opportunity to develop their potential, these graduates can:

1. Give effective nursing care to people of all ages, in varying circumstances, and in a variety of settings;
2. Interpret and demonstrate such care to patients and their families, to associated personnel, and to members of other professions;
3. Identify the nursing care needs of patients and make critical judgments in planning, directing, and evaluating the care that is given by themselves and others working with them;
4. Assist individuals and families to identify their health needs, and collaborate with patients, families, and others in meeting these needs;
5. Identify underlying principles from the social and natural sciences, and utilize them in assessing various factors in the nursing situation and in adapting to or initiating changes in relation to these factors;
6. Recognize various forces affecting the community's social, health, and welfare programs, and participate in planning and carrying out community health programs;
7. Advance without further formal education to positions requiring beginning administrative skills;
8. Recognize the need for continuing personal and professional development."

The Public Health Nurse Specialist

Public health nurses, prepared in public health nursing at the master's level, have basic responsibility for planning, implementing, and evaluating community nursing services. As experts in public health, these nurses may be employed as administrators, supervisors, consultants, educators, expert practitioners, or researchers in family and community health. They frequently have responsibilities in two or more of these areas concurrently.

The statement of the Public Health Nursing Section of the American Public Health Association, Committee to Define the Public Health Nurse Specialist is accepted as further delineation of nursing functions. This statement asserts that the public health nurses specialist may serve as:[4]

"1. a provider of direct patient care and family care in situations requiring an unusual degree of skill;
2. a role model for nursing staff by providing family-focused and family-based community health nursing services;
3. an analyst of nursing practice with respect to problems of family and community nursing services;
4. a collaborator with clinical nurse specialists and other professionals;
5. an innovator with ability to initiate change in nursing practice through experimental and other approaches. This requires leadership skills and knowledge of the preparation, roles and functions of all nursing personnel and other health workers;
6. a health worker who, with consumers and other community and professional groups, assesses and identifies neighborhood health and related needs, thus providing the basis for determining the nature of community health nursing services required;
7. a collaborator on interdisciplinary teams in establishing objectives for the services to patient, family, and community, who
   a) influences changes in the systems for providing services, and
   b) assists in the development of systems for continuity of health care based on the risks, threats, and stresses to health throughout the life span;

[4]American Public Health Association, Public Health Nursing Section Committee, Statement on the Public Health Nurse Specialist. August, 1970 (unpublished).

8. a research-oriented worker who participates in the development of data collection systems in order to describe the health status of the population, and to analyze the relationships between the health status and program components (such as nursing), thus providing a basis for recommendations and action."

EDUCATIONAL QUALIFICATIONS

The professional services in public health nursing are provided by the graduate of the baccalaureate program in nursing who in this setting is the public health nurse generalist, and the public health nurse specialist who is prepared at the master's level.

The Public Health Nurse Generalist

The graduate of a National League for Nursing accredited program with a baccalaureate in nursing meets the educational qualifications for professional practice in public health. This undergraduate preparation includes lower and upper division courses in the behavioral, physical, and biological sciences and in the humanities; an upper division major in nursing built on preceding and concurrent courses in the sciences and humanities; and courses in nursing theory and practice which are directed toward the care of individuals and families and which include content in medical, surgical, maternal, child, psychiatric, and public health nursing.

The Public Health Nurse Specialist

The essential qualifications of the public health nurse specialist is the completion of a master's degree with a major in public health nursing. This major may be offered in a school of public health accredited by the American Public Health Association or in a graduate program in nursing accredited by the National League for Nursing. Areas of content accepted by the Public Health Nursing Section of APHA for preparation of a nurse specialist in public health as appropriate for the master's degree in public health nursing include:[5]

1. Opportunity to deepen public health background through participation in and direction of multidiscipline groups, to differentiate roles of various disciplines, and to develop skill in multidiscipline problem solving;
2. In depth study of concept of community organization and dynamics of community action;
3. Development of skill in applying principles from behavioral, physical, and biological sciences to problem situations;
4. Opportunity to study methods of assessment of community health and to develop and apply indices to measure presenting health problems;
5. Opportunity to understand man-environment stress relationship;
6. Reexamination of the philosophy which has guided public health nursing practice with particular reference to —
   a. trends in nursing practice in general and their application to the practice of public health nursing.

[5]Op. cit., American Public Health Association.

    b. concepts from behavioral sciences in relation to the development and testing of
       theories of public health nursing practice,
    c. the role and function of the public health nurse specialist;
7. Study directed to increase knowledge of the research process to improve the ability to
    critically analyze research findings of others, and to initiate and participate in studies;
8. Through collaborative arrangements between educational institutions, health agencies,
    and health centers provide opportunities to —
    a. involve each student in examining and analyzing her ability to apply principles and
       theories from the behavioral, physical, and biological sciences in advanced practice
       with families and communities,
    b. develop inquisitive skills that will foster continuing concern and action to improve
       health services and nursing practice,
    c. increase ability to evaluate, study and adjust nursing programs to the changing needs
       of society,
    d. develop those leadership skills involved in positions of advanced responsibilities.
9. Develop expertise in interviewing, counseling and communication skills to improve
    patient, family, and community responses to health and health related needs.

CAREER DEVELOPMENT

The rapid pace of both social change and scientific and technological advances
makes continued learning an essential requirement for effective nursing practice.
A career in public health nursing requires a balanced combination of continuing
education, inservice education, and varying experiences that will permit personal
and professional growth.

    Continuing education may take the form of full time advanced study, short
courses, or other planned educational programs directed toward increasing the
knowledge and the scientific base for practice. Inservice education is defined by
the National League for Nursing as "a planned educational experience provided
in the job setting and closely identified with service in order to help the person
perform more effectively as a person and as a worker."[6]

    The experience required for different levels of responsibility depends on
many factors of which education is but one. Other factors that will influence an
individual's preparedness for advanced responsibility include the quality of supervision and guidance available, the climate for growth, the type and amount of
inservice education programs provided, and the individual's demonstration of
ability to assume responsibility and to take initiative in testing appropriate
models of practice.

BIBLIOGRAPHY

American Public Health Association, Public Health Nursing Section Committee. Statement
    on The Public Health Nurse Specialist. August, 1970. (Unpublished.)
American Nurses Association. *Statement on Graduate Education in Nursing.* New York:
    The Association, 1969.

[6]National League for Nursing, Report of Steering Committee, Interdivisional Council on
Inservice Education. (Unpublished.)

Murphy, Marion. "Why a Master's — Prepared Practitioner in Public Health Nursing?"
    Nursing Outlook, Vol. 15, Part I. March, 1967, pp. 33—37; Part II, April 1967, pp.
    56—60.
National Commission for the Study of Nursing and Nursing Education. "Summary Report
    and Recommendations," *American Journal of Nursing,* Vol. 70, No. 2, February, 1970,
    pp. 279—294.
National League for Nursing, Department of Baccalaureate and Higher Degree Programs.
    Characteristics of Baccalaureate Education in Nursing. New York: The League, 1968.
National League for Nursing. *Characteristics of Graduate Education in Nursing.* New York:
    The League, 1968.
National League for Nursing. Report of Steering Committee, Interdivisional Council on
    Inservice Education. (Unpublished.)
U.S. Department of Health, Education, and Welfare, Public Health Service, Division of
    Nursing. Nurses in Public Health, January, 1970. (Unpublished.)

COUNCIL ON HEALTH MANPOWER (1971)

Charles E. Lewis, M.D., Chairman
Maggie R. Matthews, M.P.H., Staff Associate
William J. Curran, J.D.
Jack B. Hatlen, M.S.
William McC. Hiscock, M.A.
John L. S. Holloman, Jr., M.D.
Marion I. Murphy, Ph.D.
Clarence E. Pearson, M.S.P.H.
John H. Romani, Ph.D.
Quentin M. Smith, D.D.S.
Esther C. Spencer, M.S.W.

The Council on Health Manpower expresses grateful appreciation to the Subcommittee
on Educational Qualifications of Public Health Nurses which assisted with the preparation
of this report. This subcommittee consists of:

Barbara Wilcox, R.N., Chairman
Doris E. Roberts, Ph.D., Referee
C. L. Brumback, M.D.
Daphine D. Doster, R.N.
Mrs. Leah Hoenig
Joyce Lashof, M.D.
Mrs. Elizabeth D. Loosley
W. Fred Mayes, M.D.
Jean Stair, Ed.D.
Mrs. Frances E. Williamson
Mrs. Ruth Anne Yauger, R.N.

The Community Nurse Role
and Settings

*What is the role of community nurses? What do they do? There is
no single answer to this question because community nurses are
carving out new roles and redefining old ones. As pointed out in
Part I, community nurses combine professional nursing practice
with the basics of public health practice. Their goal is to provide
family-centered, comprehensive nursing service to individuals,
families and communities. Although there are a variety of activities,
in each the community nurse uses the fundamental principles of
prevention, case-finding, positive health teaching, encouraging
patient and family self-direction, continuity of care, consideration
of the total family and collaboration
with the health team.*

*The settings in which community nurses practice are as varied as
the nurses themselves. Some work in hospitals to provide a link
between patients, their families and the community. Some function
as public health nurses in official health agencies; others serve in
schools or with visiting nurse associations. Business and industry
provide additional settings for the community nurse. Health
maintenance organizations, community mental health centers, outpatient clinics and consulting roles in the community are all open to
the nurse. Some nurses are even moving into areas and organizations
that are nonhealth-oriented but which have great significance for
primary prevention.*

*The articles in this section provide examples of the varied roles
and settings of community nursing. Several themes run through most
of the articles. First, community nursing provides distributive care
rather than episodic. Contact with people is continuous and the
service ranges from primary prevention
through care of the sick.*

*Second, in the varied settings of community nursing, an important
element has become clearer — the increased independence of nurses.
This does not mean they do not have responsibility and independence in the hospital or other more traditional settings. It does
mean that many situations arise in the course of community nursing
in which the nurse does not have immediate recourse to the counsel
and support of other health professionals. This responsibility and*

independence requires self-confidence, special skills in decision making and the ability to negotiate with a wide range of people.

Finally, the nurse whose role is to serve the entire community must deal with people from many cultural backgrounds. She must develop a sensitivity to her own acquired perceptions of the world and those learned by people in different subcultures. This important aspect of community nursing will be discussed in Part IV, which is an examination of the cultural dimension of health care.

5

Prevention and Chronic Illness

Paulette Robischon

In contrast to many other health professionals, a major component of the community nurse's role is the prevention of illness. The three levels of prevention form the guidelines for community nursing action regardless of setting. The community nurse's preventive role is graphically portrayed in this chapter as it relates to chronic illness.

To cope with problems inherent in limited inpatient facilities and to permit the patient to be cared for in familiar surroundings, increasing numbers of long-term patients are cared for outside the hospital. These numbers will undoubtedly continue to multiply, with a concomitant expansion of public health nursing involvement.

Why has public health nursing committed itself to devoting a large portion of its energies to chronic illness? How has this involvement developed? In what ways is public health nursing concerned with prevention in chronic illness? How is the public health nurse instrumental in the provision of comprehensive care to the chronically ill? The answers to these questions provide the framework for this paper.

DEFINITIONS OF "PUBLIC HEALTH" NURSING

"Public health" nursing as used in this discussion primarily denotes the nursing *setting*. What were formerly the knowledge, skills, and approaches of the "public health" nurse (as differentiated from the "hospital" nurse) have become part of professional nursing in general, regardless of the setting. Public health nursing no longer connotes an *exclusive* approach to patient care. The concepts of prevention, positive health, case finding, continuity of care, total family approach, patient and family self-direction, and a cognizance of community-family-patient interrelationships are implicit in all sound professional nursing practice. Nursing views and works with man as a total being in interaction with his family and society, whether the environment is a hospital or other care institution, business or industry, school, clinic, day center, or home.

As lines of demarcation between preventive, curative, and rehabilitative nursing fade, public health nursing ceases to be a neatly contained entity. Nursing has a unity of approach and cannot be divided into these various parts and still retain its usefulness. It is in the context of this underlying philosophy that the terms "public health" or "community" nurse are used. These interchangeable terms refer to nurses in both voluntary agencies and official agencies since both are involved in chronic illness.

From "The Public Health Nurse and Chronic Illness," *Nursing Clinics of North America*, Vol. 1, No. 3, pp. 433–441, 1966. Reprinted by permission of the publisher and author.

THE PROBLEM OF CHRONIC DISEASE

Public health leaders agree that chronic disease is the major health problem of our day.[3, 4, 8]   The emergence of these diseases has followed closely the control of a host of infectious diseases. Chronic illness, increasing environmental hazards, and the need for improved health services come into view as interrelated, top priority community health problems.

With the formation of the Commission for Chronic Illness there was a turning point in care of the chronically ill. This national body functioned from 1949 to 1956 to promote an exchange of ideas and to stimulate action by individuals and organizations at every level across the country. During this period the concept of the organized home care program was further developed and expanded. The passage of the Community Health Services and Facilities Act of 1961 which pushed forward improvements in out-of-hospital services for the chronically ill and aged was another milestone. In 1964 the President's Commission on Heart Disease, Cancer and Stroke reported its findings and recommendations to narrow the gap between new knowledge of these disease processes and full utilization of the knowledge.[9] Various amendments to the Social Security Act as well as broadened definitions of "disability" have led to possibilities for care in an unprecedented variety of conditions. These innovations, which focused attention on chronic illness, have helped to implement the ideas which grew out of concern and deliberation about this wide-scope problem.

In the late 1920's nursing, as a vital health discipline, became involved in the shift of emphasis from acute and infectious diseases to chronic illness. By the 1940's the trend toward nursing care of the chronically ill gained great impetus which continues today in the home and other extrahospital settings. Public health nursing service statistics vividly attest to this: in some voluntary agencies four out of five home visits are to patients who have chronic diseases. Official community nursing services are also grappling with this problem; health department nurses are giving an increased amount of time to meet the needs of ill and disabled persons.

PREVENTIVE ASPECTS

To facilitate discussion, the public health nurse's work with chronic illness will be schematized into three interrelated phases of care or "levels" of prevention.

Primary

The primary level, or the prevention of the original occurrence of the chronic disease, poses the greatest problem. Progress in preventing, ameliorating, or positioning the *effects* of chronic disease has overshadowed progress in primary prevention. Despite this, nurses can utilize existing knowledge and skills to meet the challenge of primary prevention. The public health nurse, for instance, can be instrumental in the prevention of heart disease when she assists a woman to establish early prenatal care, so that the possible finding of a positive serologic test may lead to prompt treatment and the prevention of syphilitic heart disease. The referral of a school age child with a streptococcal infection for prompt medical care may avert an attack of rheumatic fever and possible heart damage. Early case finding and treatment of tuberculosis may prevent later pericarditis.

The nurse in industry is in a particularly advantageous position to prevent disabling conditions. She is alert to the need for, and encourages the use of, protective equipment to prevent blindness, chronic pulmonary disease, and dermatosis. The occupational health nurse is in a unique position to observe the effects of stress, which are regarded to be implicated in the multiple etiology of some chronic diseases. She can mitigate or rechannel these stresses. The visiting nurse who provides family health guidance includes accident prevention as a major area for health teaching, since vigorous efforts to teach accident prevention can avert much of the severe and permanent disability that follows many nonfatal injuries.

As nursing knowledge expands and scientific advances are achieved, it should be possible for the nurse to be effective in primary prevention of conditions such as cancer, alcoholism, hypertension, and certain birth defects.

Secondary

Case finding is the key to secondary prevention. At this level prevention means early diagnosis and prompt treatment. If the nature of the illness precludes a cure, the alternative is to retard the disease and prevent disability. To set the stage for early finding of visual and auditory impairments, the nurse in the child health conference promotes the institution of vision and hearing screening programs for preschool children.

A large number of cases of chronic disease in the earliest stages can be found when the potentialities of early detection are realized. A case in point is cancer, which is at least twice as curable as the present cure rates indicate. The salvage rate for uterine cancer could exceed 90 percent rather than the current 50 percent if available detection methods were fully utilized. Nursing must devise means of motivating individuals who do not utilize community resources for detection tests and regular health examinations.

Family and individual histories provide the alert nurse with clues which may indicate illness warranting direction into channels to health care. If persons with chronic disease are to take measures that will minimize morbidity, nursing intervention through teaching is needed.

Tertiary

Rehabilitative care is the focus in tertiary prevention. Rehabilitation is the return of the individual disabled by disease or accident to his greatest usefulness — physically, socially, emotionally, and vocationally. This involves learning to live productively with diseases and disabilities that cannot be cured. In rehabilitation the nurse modifies patient and family attitudes of hopelessness about the disease, interprets the rationale of the rehabilitation regimen, and teaches the patient and his family self-help. She also works toward the prevention of regression in the patient by teaching him and his family how to maintain the benefits gained in the intensive phases of the rehabilitation program.

Nursing activity ranges from occasional home visits for follow-up of the patient's progress with the patient and family giving the care, to more frequent nursing visits to provide intensive general care and rehabilitative measures. Patients, who span a wide age range, include the child with cerebral palsy or cystic fibrosis as well as the older adult recovering from a cardiovascular accident. Nursing activities might include vocational readjustment for the worker who has had hip surgery for arthritic disease; guiding the school child to adjust his eating patterns so that they are compatible with his diabetic condition; and providing support to the family of a patient recently discharged home from the psychiatric hospital. Many individuals bed-bound at home could benefit through institution of a rehabilitation regimen. These persons who are unknown to any community nursing service or other health or social agency are often discovered and given direction by the perceptive nurse.

Prevention of chronic illness is achieved within the framework of the public health nurse's total family health program. All levels of prevention are an integral part of the public health nurse's work with patients and families. The importance of primary prevention must not be overlooked as nursing responds to increased demands for the curative and rehabilitative phases of care. Instead, nursing needs to place even greater emphasis on the use of new scientific findings in the promotion of health.

COMPREHENSIVE CARE

Comprehensive care has been described as "... care in depth — intensive, deliberative consideration of the physical-social-emotional aspects of health in the light of needs represented by the individual as a member of a family and as a member of a community."[2] Comprehensive care is constructive, preventive, continuous, and implies adequacy of high quality service. How does the public health nurse contribute to the provision of this care?

Various geographic, cultural, social, economic, and demographic factors affect attitudes toward the chronically ill and the type of community services available. One community may be highly organized, having multiple agencies and services with a central information and service agency for chronic illness, while another offers only the county nursing agency, welfare organization, and a distant hospital as community resources. Limited facilities do not necessarily obviate, nor unlimited facilities automatically ensure, comprehensive care. In fact, the proliferation of agencies and services can lead to uncoordinated fragmented service to the patient.

The public health nurse is a key person — often *the* key person — in the pro-vision of comprehensive health care. In addition to her specialized job with the patient and family, she supports other team members, promotes their objectives, and interprets their services. Often she serves as the coordinator of the health care team. The nurse occupies a favorable position to furnish the continuity so essential to comprehensive care.

Continuity of Care

A recent study[1] points up the wasted effort and patient regression that occur when there are interruptions in service to patients with long-term illness. In another study lack of continuity of care is cited as the primary handicap faced by elderly, chronically ill patients.[6] If continuity is to be a practical reality, the public health nurse must make continuing efforts to promote the improvement of referral systems and be willing to share her knowledge of the patient's needs and progress with others caring for him. The responsibility for improving referrals is reciprocal. Just as the public health nurse expects to participate with the medical care facility in planning the patient's care upon discharge and expects prompt referrals containing adequate and precise information, so she must bring others into her planning activities with the patient, share what she knows with those involved in the patient's care, and expedite the referrals she makes. The existence of a referral system does not ensure comprehensive care. Momentum is lost, causing a gap in continuous care even with a prompt referral, when information about the patient is so scant that the new worker must gather data and make an assessment of the patient's needs before she can institute a care plan.

The public health nurse can work toward more effective referrals in many ways. Her contribution may extend from the qualitative improvement of indi-vidual patient referrals to serving on a community council where the objective is to institute a standardized referral system. The public health nurse needs to improve the quality of her communication skills and the rapidity with which she performs them, pending the day when push-button electronic communication will exist between patient, community workers, and health care facilities.

MOBILIZING RESOURCES

What are the resources that may be tapped to provide care for the homebound chronically ill patient? The primary resource is the patient. The community nurse helps him to establish appropriate goals for maintenance or improvement of his health, teaches him self-care, and supports him as he learns this care. From the onset of illness the nurse involves the family in the plan for care. The aim is to develop and strengthen patient and family capacity to cope with the situation and to achieve and sustain optimum well-being.

The Team

It may be necessary for the community nurse to plan and carry out a program of home care with a limited health team: patient, family, physician, and nurse. On the other hand the patient may be part of a highly organized home care program under the auspices of which he receives (in addition to medical and nursing service) social case work, physical and occupational therapy, nutrition counseling, podiatry service, assistance from the prosthetist-orthotist, as well as supplies, equipment, and medications. In the absence of some of these workers the nurse may need to extend her care into those areas where health disciplines have overlapping knowledge and skills. The public health nurse's team role needs to be sufficiently flexible to change with the composition of the team and the individual care situation.

Physical Needs

Many chronically ill patients require a high level of physical nursing care at home. Of particular importance is the prevention of deterioration in the bedfast patient. The nurse must consider the prevention of deformity, maintenance of muscle strength and joint mobility, and prevention of metabolic imbalances, decubital ulcers, urinary tract dysfunction, and respiratory complications.[5] The public health nurse and her nursing team, which may include a technical nurse or practical nurse and a home aide, can provide this type of skilled care on a visiting basis and can teach the patient and his family how to provide care in the interim. The nursing team improvises gadgets for patient self-help and assists him in borrowing devices and equipment from loan closets of local service clubs or health agencies.

Nutritional needs may be met by teaching the patient to prepare his own meals, by the use of a homemaker, or through participation in a community home-delivered meals program which provides regular diets or the modified diet sometimes needed by the patient with a chronic illness.

Homebound patients may need help with dental, visual, and hearing impairments which interfere with their physical and emotional well-being. They may have edentulous mouths, badly neglected teeth, or ill-fitting dentures, eyeglasses, or hearing aids. Improvised devices, such as a larger toothbrush handle, encourage self-help in mouth care. Efforts can be made to secure financial assistance with the cost of dentures, spectacles, and hearing aids through home care programs, rehabilitation programs, and local service clubs. Service at home can be sought for those patients unable to travel to a care facility for evaluation and fitting of their appliances.

Emotional Needs

Chronic illness presents emotional problems for patient and family. Depression is not infrequently observed. The patient may feel that he is a burden to others, is tolerated rather than needed, and has failed in his role in the family and society.

These feelings will interfere with his adaptation to illness and result in disturbed family relationships. A study of chronically disabled persons demonstrated the high degree of emotional support required by these patients and their intense need for communication with others.[7] Families may resent the patient for the burden his illness imposes.

The public health nurse can provide support and can tap other helping resources when expert case work appraisal and care are indicated. These resources would include counseling services provided by a family service agency, the mental hygiene clinic, the social worker on the home care team, and the religious adviser. The patient may be in need of diversional activities, companionship, and stimulation to prevent intellectual and emotional deterioration. These needs may be met through friends, "friendly visitor" volunteers, and church members. The family, occasionally relieved from the responsibility of patient care, may find time for much needed personal recreational and social outlets.

The Environment

The disabled patient may need modifications in housing adapted to his special needs. Relocation into a specially designed facility for independent living may be required or certain modifications to present housing may be made. Room and furniture rearrangement, borrowing or purchasing a special bed or chair, installation of hand grips, building of ramps, and removal of door sills are possible adaptations to minimize physical exertion and maximize safety. The public health nurse possesses the knowledge to guide the patient and family in making necessary changes. Structural modifications in housing may be secured through the volunteer services of a local construction workers' trade union.

The patient with limited mobility may need transportation to clinics or other health care facilities. Organized community volunteers, the home care program, or ambulance corps can provide this service; or the public health nurse may mobilize some untapped, unorganized resource to meet this need.

The chronically ill patient often needs help with homemaking: cooking, cleaning, shopping, and child care. The community often makes this service available through the visiting homemaker. In the absence of such a community worker the nurse can help the patient plan with friends, family, or domestic help to meet this need. A rehabilitation center or county extension service may teach a disabled individual new ways to handle household activities and so gain independence.

Economic Needs

The economic impact of chronic illness can be overwhelming for patient and family. The costs of medical care, dressings, medication, and equipment are prohibitive for many families. These require the seeking of financial assistance through governmental agencies, voluntary agencies, and service organizations.

Business or industrial homework may be found for the homebound patient. Evaluation of his work potential may be obtained through official or voluntary agency rehabilitation programs. The patient can be encouraged to continue educational pursuits through home instruction and self-study with the aim of economic independence.

The public health nurse helps ensure that the patient and family obtain the services they need expeditiously and without duplication of effort by community workers. The nurse improvises where there are no services, learns to use new resources as they become available, and helps develop needed resources.

Dynamic Quality of Nursing

Chronic illness is dynamic. Nursing care of the chronically ill patient requires an alertness in observing and evaluating the subtle changes that occur. The individualized nursing care plan must be flexible and current to allow for changes in the patient's mental and physical condition, environment, and relationships with family and society. The emotional and physical ability of the family to provide care is dynamic. They may be reluctant to admit increasing difficulty with care which is causing fatigue, stress, and strained relationships, so it is up to the nurse to be alert to the signs of impending problems. She can help the family to prevent these problems through her teaching, support, guidance, and referral to other team members for specialized assistance which she is not equipped to offer.

SUMMARY

Nursing is actively involved in the application of current knowledge to society's major health problem: chronic illness. It accomplishes this through dealing with prevention in its broadest aspects within the framework of the total health program. The public health nurse is the key person who provides comprehensive care. She fosters coordination by facilitating closer interaction between health care facilities, home care units, and other community health and welfare services, thus supplying the thread of continuity essential to comprehensive care. The public health nurse ensures that patient and family receive needed service through the mobilization of their own resources and those of the community. When resources are lacking, the nurse helps stimulate community action to develop services geared to the community's needs. Implicit in the public health nurse's approach to the problem of chronic illness is a willingness to relinquish traditional patterns of service and adopt new modalities of care to meet social changes.

REFERENCES

1. Anderson, E. M.: A continuity of care plan for long-term patients. *Am. J. Pub. Health*, 54:308, 1964.

2. Freeman, R. B.: *Public Health Nursing Practice.* 3rd Ed. Philadelphia, W. B. Saunders Co., 1963.
3. Hilleboe, H. E.: Teamwork in rehabilitation — from fancy to fact. *Am. J. Pub. Health,* 54:751, 1964.
4. James, G.: Emerging trends in public health and possible reactions. *Pub. Health Rep.,* 80:579, 1965.
5. Kottke, F. J., and Anderson, E. M.: Deterioration of the bedfast patient. *Pub. Health Rep.,* 80:437, 1965.
6. Posman, H., Kogan, L. S., LeMat, A. F., and Dahlin, Bernice: Continuity in Care for Impaired Older Persons. Department of Public Affairs, Community Service Society of New York, December 1964.
7. Rothberg, J. S.: An experiment in use of a diagnostic tool. *N.Y. State League for Nursing Brochure* No. 3, 1962.
8. Terry, L. L.: The complex world of modern public health. *Am. J. Pub. Health,* 54:189, 1964.
9. U.S. President's Commission on Heart Disease, Cancer and Stroke. *Report to the President.* Washington, D.C., Government Printing Office, 1964.

6
Community Mental Health Nursing and Consultation

Mildred Mouw
Clarice H. Haylett

How should the community nurse become involved in the area of mental health? At present the nurse's role in this field is developing in several directions. This chapter describes an evolving nurse role, one that includes the entire range of services from prevention to therapy. The authors clearly underscore an important additional element, crucial for community nurses in all settings. The limits of knowledge and skill and when and how to use appropriately the expert consultant must be self-evident to the community nurse.

San Mateo's challenging community mental health adventure has been shared by public health nurses since enactment of the California Short-Doyle Community Mental Health Act in 1957. Although they are not actually psychiatric personnel, these nurses were recognized as care-giving professionals who were concerned with the mental health aspects of their work, and they were considered an appropriate instrumentality for the further extension of mental health into the community.

Public health nurses function in many areas where mental health principles can be practiced: prenatal clinics, schools, child health conferences, and in the family itself. They have entrée to many individuals and families who need help to adjust to the problems of physical illness and emotional stress. In their daily work, they encounter a wide variety of emotional reactions and can refer, for further study and treatment, persons for whom their own counseling and guidance may seem insufficient.

As these nurses engage in case finding and in assisting those who are in need of rehabilitation, they must have a working knowledge of the various mental health facilities in the community. To initiate their acquaintance with community mental health services, a one-and-one-half day orientation visit to the psychiatric inpatient ward and the day hospital is scheduled for all newly employed nurses. In addition to learning something about the philosophy, function, and purposes of these services, the nurses are told that further contacts are welcomed; they are encouraged to discuss patients with physicians, social workers, and staff nurses, to visit patients on the ward and in the day hospital, when appropriate, and to attend case conferences. In particular, the multiphasic staffing conference offers the opportunity for professionals from different disciplines to collaborate, a reciprocal process which may occasion

From H. Richard Lamb, Don Heath, Joseph J. Downing, eds., *Handbook of Community Mental Health Practice,* pp. 188–199, 1969, Jossey-Bass, San Francisco. Reprinted by permission of the publisher.

an expansion of each caregiver's understanding of the patient and his family, as well as an increased appreciation of each other's roles.

In a public health nursing service, nurses have a multitude of opportunities for interventions that may promote and maintain mental health, as well as for activities that expedite recovery and rehabilitation. Guidance and counseling about emotional as well as physical health matters are now a familiar part of the public health nurse's daily work. The nurse's roles as an early identifier of mental disorder and referral-expediter to appropriate community resources also are well established. However, in our community, the public health nurse's role in the management and treatment of diagnosed mentally ill persons was not well defined initially.

As nurses were requested to undertake expanded responsibilities in the after-care of mental patients, many questions of role and function were raised. Physicians from public hospitals and clinics and some in private practice began to ask nurses to make home visits to recently discharged patients. Sometimes the charge was vague: "See how things are going and be supportive." Nurses who had limited experience in psychiatric settings requested both inservice training in the subject area of major mental illnesses and mental health consultation. They needed to know in considerably more detail what was expected of them and what they could do. In the course of the consultative relationship, three roles came to be identified: observer, expediter, and auxiliary therapist.

In the role of observer, the nurse has the responsibility of assessing the patient's adjustment to the home situation. She is especially aware of the quality of his interaction with the family and other important persons in the home. She notes his attitudes toward his drug therapy and his motivation to follow through with aftercare plans. The nurse is also in a key position to determine the family's receptivity to the patient. She considers their understanding of the illness and the aftercare plans as well as their needs for support and counseling. In addition, the nurse is concerned about the general health status of the entire family.

As expediter, she assists the patient or family to follow through on aftercare recommendations. This might involve getting the patient to clinic appointments or expediting referrals to other programs, such as those provided by vocational rehabilitation or social welfare.

The role of auxiliary therapist initially caused the greatest uncertainty and resultant anxiety. Several nurses were concerned that "just visiting and talking" was somehow not as real a service as those nursing arts where there was "laying on of hands." As these nurses came to understand how their interaction with patients could be therapeutic as well as important, however, many began to enjoy the challenge and stimulation of this new dimension in the professional use of self.

In mental illness, as in physical infirmity, the nurse serves as a mothering person who aims to alleviate discomfort, and as a vehicle for the physician's healing instructions. The nurse who comes to the patient's home is, symbolically, one who cares. She becomes available as a model for identification. She may clarify issues, give advice, or suggest environmental changes. Many of these activities are used in supportive psychotherapy. Shared, too, is the professional use of self in an interpersonal transaction.

Nurses have been given administrative sanction to use the nursing hour in an imaginative and creative way. The format of a nursing visit to the home of a recently hospitalized housewife illustrates the nontraditional pattern of inter-action that may be necessary when the assignment calls for socializing and facili-tation of increased social functions. The housewife was having difficulty in mobilizing her energy to buy the food for the family. The nurse and mother studied the grocery ads in the newspaper and made a shopping list. Together they went to the market. When they returned, the mother asked, "Now what do I do the rest of the day?" Together they worked out a step-by-step plan for the remainder of the day. Included were the all-important, albeit prosaic, details involved in cooking the evening meal.

In another instance, a nurse who had been visiting a chronically ill woman for several months arrived one day moments after the patient's husband had died. The nurse assisted the patient in calling her physician and went with her to the hospital where the husband was pronounced dead. Later the nurse accompanied the patient to the funeral home where she gave support while the necessary arrangements were being made.

Patterns of visiting are based on patient and family needs. Visits may vary from as often as once a day or several times a week to once a month. A nurse visited a depressed patient who had been discharged from the state hospital. She found him in his night clothes at two o'clock in the afternoon. The shades were drawn and the atmosphere was one of gloom and despair. He told her he saw no need for her visits. She stated simply that the doctor was concerned and wanted her to come. She indicated that she, too, was concerned and that she would sit with him quietly for a time and would return in two days. The visits continued. Ultimately, the nurse arrived to find the patient dressed and the shades up. One day the nurse accompanied this patient to a neighborhood recreation center. In each of these instances the nurse used her professional self in a series of interpersonal transactions which were rewarding and satisfying to both patient and nurse.

The nurse's psychotherapeutic role technically differs from more formal psychotherapy in several respects. The primary intent and setting are different. The depth of discussion is generally limited to the conscious and current without probing or encouraging free association. Furthermore, as in other home nursing activities, the nurse's self-identification is clearly that of a team member working with medical direction.

As a team member, the nurse is encouraged to assess the nursing needs of patients based on her observations and then to formulate a plan of action. This plan frequently means that the nurse can use her own creativity and ingenuity. As she becomes more secure with that which is nursing, her relationship with the physician becomes more collaborative and reciprocal.

Communication between nurses and doctors is imperative. An interagency referral form has been worked out for use between physicians, hospitals, and service personnel. All orders for public health nursing visits to patients must be renewed every two months. This means that nurses must review and evaluate their services to patients and request renewal of orders from the medical source. Physicians, too, must assess the patient's needs for nursing care, medications, and treatment at these regular intervals. There are times when patients or their families decline to seek the needed medical supervision, despite nurses' attempts to motivate this necessary step. In those instances, nurses must then discontinue service.

That the public health nurse can function comfortably and effectively in the aftercare of patients who have been sick enough to need hospitalization is well documented (Collard, 1966; Donnelly et al., 1962; New Haven V.N.A., 1966; Zolik, Lantz, and Sommers, 1968). She is often able to reach and establish contact with a poorly motivated segment of the population. Because she goes to the patient and has a generally helpful approach, she may be seen as less professionally demanding and more personally caring than others. Furthermore, the public health nurse is frequently viewed by the patient and his family as the least stigmatizing of all public representatives. Not only is she likely to be accorded the easy entrée of a trusted family friend, but, unlike the social visitor, she brings a rich professional armamentarium.

She is a trained observer who sees and hears much but knows the ethics of confidentiality. She knows her community and can help her patient establish new contacts when these are indicated. Increasingly, she individualizes her professional approach, supplementing her intuition with considered interventions. Finally, she knows the importance of keeping communication flowing between herself, her supervisor, and the responsible physician.

It soon became apparent to public health nursing administration that if public health nurses were to contribute to the early detection of mental and emotional disorders as well as to improve their services to patients with diagnoses of mental illness, and their families, a specialist in the field was needed. A request for a mental health nurse consultant was made to the Consultation, Education and Information Service of the Mental Health Services Division in 1961. This request was granted in the division's 1963—64 budget. A mental health nurse consultant, who was intimately acquainted with the system of public health and public health nursing and who had training in the techniques of mental health consultation, was employed and assigned to work primarily with public health nurses.

Goals of the mental health nurse consultant and the consultee group were initially lacking in precision, and methods of working most productively with administration and staff needed to be explored. As nurses were requested to expand their responsibilities in the aftercare of mental patients, roles and functions needed to be identified and clarified. In addition, as the nurse consultant became familiar with the mental health services within the San Mateo County Department of Public Health and Welfare and the state hospital system, it became more clear that a liaison function between these services and public health nursing would serve a useful purpose. Thus, the nurse consultant moved in all of these directions, attempting to improve liaison and to bring greater clarity and structure into consultation transactions.

A great deal has been written about nursing services to the mentally ill person and his family during the hospital interlude and after the patient's return to the community. Such a service has been given various labels: *aftercare, follow-up care,* or *continuity of care.* Perhaps the last term best conveys the idea of the succession and connection of care that presumably will contribute much to the patient's welfare.

Mental health services in San Mateo County are highly complex, and it is difficult to know how or where to "plug in" to this complexity in order to give nursing service to those who might profit from it most. The mental health nurse consultant soon learned that patients moved in a wide variety of ways between services. For example, a patient receiving therapy at the adult psychiatric clinic might be referred to the day hospital or a patient presenting himself at the emergency room might be referred to the inpatient service or to the state hospital. It soon became apparent that by assuming the role of liaison between the mental health units and public health nursing, the nurse consultant could serve to interpret and clarify roles and functions of both.

First, communication between the mental health nurse consultant and the supervising nurses on the inpatient service and the day hospital was established. With administrative sanction, a plan was worked out in which public health nurses are notified daily about new admissions to each of these services. Upon receipt of such notification, the nursing files are checked to learn if this patient is, or was, known to the public health nurse. If he is known, a summary is written and sent to the mental health professionals who are caring for him. Case conferences, telephone conversations, joint conferences bringing together the patient, the public health nurse, and ward personnel, and requests for visits with the family and patient are examples of patterns of service that have resulted from such communication. When a patient has not been known to the public health nursing service, a referral to this service can be initiated by the inpatient or day hospital personnel. Communication has been further facilitated by the planned conferences between the nurse consultant and the supervising nurses on the inpatient service and in the day hospital. The latter two nurses have assisted greatly in the interpretation of public health nursing services to psychiatrists (including residents who may soon be practicing in this or in other communities) and social workers who heretofore were not acquainted with their services.

A modified but similar system of communication has been worked out with the other units of the Mental Health Services Division. These include the adult psychiatric clinic, child guidance clinic, and the regional North County Mental Health Center.

The mental health nurse consultant also serves as liaison between public health nursing and the San Mateo County patients in the regionalized state hospital wards. Regular weekly visits with the state hospital ward personnel are scheduled to discuss discharge plans for patients. Public health nursing aftercare has been extremely helpful for the woman who will be assuming the role of wife, mother, and household manager upon returning home; for the patient who needs encouragement to maintain his drug regime and his appointments at the psychiatric clinic; for the family who refuses to accept the patient as ill and in need of care; or for the patient who needs support to resume his place in the family, in the labor market, or in the community.

The supportive role that the nurse can play by seeing the patient and his family at home is recognized by many psychiatrists, social workers, and psychologists as adding a valuable ingredient, different from those supplied by the traditional clinical disciplines working within clinics or hospitals. Public health nurses are talking with these workers with increasing self-confidence and ease.

As a result of direct channels of communication between nurses and the professional staff at Agnews State Hospital, an understanding of roles and responsibilities has evolved to such a degree that far more comprehensive services are provided to patients and families in the home as well as to patients in the hospital. The public health nurse has frequently enabled the hospital to get better cooperation from family members, thereby contributing to the hospitalized patient's welfare. The assessment and evaluation of the home situation often has led to a more realistic aftercare plan for the patient. Similarly, the public health nurse has been able to formulate her plans with the patient and family more realistically as the result of the assessment and evaluation of the patient in the hospital. Thus, on the part of all workers there is a growing respect for each other and each other's competence.

Another example of mutually helpful cooperation can be found in the relationship with the regional North County Mental Health Center, where each of three team psychiatrists visits the district public health nursing office once a month. At these meetings, the psychiatrists, the supervising nurse, and the staff nurse discuss patients active in both services, with a view of optimum caregiving collaboration.

The numbers of persons with a diagnosis of mental illness referred to public health nurses have increased from 88 in 1962 to 183 in 1968. The number of nursing visits have jumped from 717 in 1962 to 2,105 in 1968. These numbers compare favorably with the statistics from other disease categories such as cardiovascular disease, cerebral-vascular accidents, and cancer. However, when compared with the large numbers of patients discharged from the acute psychiatric ward of the county hospital and Agnews State Hospital, the numbers referred to public health nursing for aftercare are very small indeed. Large numbers of emotionally ill persons present themselves at the emergency room and many are sent back home. Many of these patients could benefit from nursing surveillance to see if they respond to the medications prescribed, to see what further medical or nursing service is indicated, or to give support and guidance to family members as they attempt to cope with the sick person. It is obvious that new methods of closing these gaps of service to people in need are yet to be created.

As experience was gained and shared by consultants from several disciplines, working with many different consultee groups, consultation goals of the mental health nurse consultant became more precise. In general, consultation is now seen as having three aims: (1) helping the visiting nurse with specific work problems, (2) educating the visiting nurse to be more effective in the mental health aspects of her professional role, and (3) educating the mental health nurse consultant, not only in regard to the epidemiology of mental illness, but also in awareness of how she may be more effective in her consulting role.

The public health nurse consultant has proceeded on the premise that a long-term, working relationship with the public health nursing service is a desirable goal. This has provided a variety of indirect services in response to changing interests and needs. In addition to regularly scheduled individual and group consultation, the nurse consultant has been used for emergency consultation, for inservice training, and for collaboration with public health nursing colleagues. As a result of continuing work together, the nurse consultant has been used flexibly and creatively at various levels within the nursing system for consultation about specific cases, administrative policy, and even some aspects of program planning.

Goals for nurse consultees have also become better defined. Our impression is that there have been modifications in performance that we could now consider goals, even though these were not formulated as such in advance. Nurses have become increasingly sensitive to the emotional aspects of their work. Many nurses now consciously listen for "the question behind the question" and systematically consider possible determinants or perplexing behavior. They now tend to individualize each patient in each family, thus lessening the use of stereotypes.

There has been greater acceptance among the nurses of their own strengths and abilities and more tolerance of limitations, both personal and professional. Professional role refinement has occurred, leading to a clearer definition of the nurses' particular contributions to the treatment and rehabilitation of mentally ill patients. This has helped to allay the needless anxiety and guilt that they cannot be all things to all people, and to increase their satisfaction and self-confidence in working with the mentally ill.

In addition to "sanction at all administrative levels," orienting new staff members in detail to the purposes, methods, and process of consultation is especially desirable. In their academic preparation, many nurses have had little exposure to mental health consultants or to the nature of this type of a helping relationship. Thus, careful preparation and structuring of early consultation experience is necessary if both unrealistic expectations and unnecessary fears are to be minimized.

Orientation meetings are now planned with the consultant on a regular basis. A group of newly employed nurses has an opportunity to be a part of a session in which a typical nursing situation is presented and all enter into the problem-solving. Through this demonstration it is hoped that nurses have a beginning understanding of consultation — its values and limitations.

From the outset, the mental health consultants have worked with district office supervisors and nurses as a group. The supervisor generally assumes responsibility for chairing the meeting and for deciding which patients or situations will be discussed. Thus, the consultant is free to interact as a clearly nonadministrative resource person. Usually, one nurse presents a case or situation of current concern and the group participates in clarifying issues and suggesting ways to understand and deal with problems.

The consultant, as well as the supervisor, may facilitate the group process. At the same time, she may make some independent hypotheses about the nature of the problem. She may raise questions that lead to a different conceptualization of the problem or invite group members to share their perceptions and experience with similar cases. In thinking through a problem with her colleagues, the presenting nurse frequently sees its nature in a different context and feels free to proceed with renewed conviction and self-confidence.

Sometimes, the consultant supplements the group's knowledge of child development, personality dynamics, or mental illness. Most often, however, the consultation is a process of shared thinking, which gains strength from the professional relationship with the consultant and from the group interaction.

In addition to regularly scheduled group sessions, individual consultation time is available to district offices. Staff nurses sign up for scheduled time as needed. The supervisor may reserve part of the time to review the problems and concerns she has in developing the potential of staff nurses or to discuss program issues. When early attention is needed, a telephone discussion may suffice or additional consultation time is arranged. It is highly desirable that the consultant have enough flexibility in her schedule to be available for occasional emergency contacts.

Although separating the impact of mental health consultation from many other experiential variables is not possible, shifts in the relationship between the consultant and consultee are noted and are reflected in their communication. In time, a nurse consultee tends to shift her emphasis from what patients say to what she herself says and does, and finally to include how she herself feels about it. Our impression is that a parallel change takes place in many nurse-patient relationships. As the nurse progresses from an intellectual acceptance to an emotional acceptance of a patient's behavior, a more comfortable, warm, individualized transactional pattern results.

Since the initiation of our mental health consultation program, psychiatrists, psychologists, psychiatric social workers, and a mental health nurse have all consulted with the nursing division. Our experience suggests that consultants from various professional disciplines are useful, as each has a special body of knowledge and experience to offer. In practice, however, most of the consultation has been with a psychiatrist or the mental health nurse or both. When both have been simultaneously available to the nursing division, the advantages have been qualitative as well as quantitative. The different disciplines seem to potentiate each other. Each has special assets.

A mental health nurse consultant, for example, already knows nursing as a profession. Although a new nurse consultant must become acquainted with the unique aspects of a particular nursing program, she need not learn a new language or professional philosophy. Her identity is as a nurse. She is not likely, inadvertently, to encourage a nurse consultee toward inappropriate roles. Furthermore, where the nurse consultant can have an office in proximity to the nursing division, she is available for a variety of informal as well as formal consultative activities. On the other hand, a consultant from the same discipline as the consultee does not bring a markedly different knowledge base or perspective. Nor is the potential for interdisciplinary stimulation the same. Although the nurse consultant may not have the advantages or disadvantages of any traditional, interprofessional status differential, staff usually come to associate her with their own supervisory and administrative echelon.

In the San Mateo program, one of the mental health nurse consultant's major contributions has been to bring greater clarity and structure into consultation transactions. She has helped to define roles and functions for supervisors, consultants, and consultee nurses. She also has helped to conceptualize public health nursing roles in mental health.

REFERENCES

Collard, E. J. "Public Health Nurse in Aftercare Program for the Mentally Ill: The Present Status," *American Journal of Public Health*, 1966, 56, 210–217.

Donnelly, E. M., Austin, F. C., Kettle, R. H., Steward, J. R., and Verde, C. W. "A Cooperative Program Between State Hospital and Public Health Nursing Agency for Psychiatric Aftercare," *American Journal of Public Health*, 1962, 52, 1084–1094.

New Haven Visiting Nurse Association, "The Role of Public Health Nursing in the Aftercare of the Psychiatric Patient." A report on the participation of the Visiting Nurse Association of New Haven in the Cooperative Care Project, New Haven, Conn., 1960–1965. New Haven: The Association, 1966.

Zolik, F. S., Lantz, E. M., and Sommers, R. "Hospital Return Rates and Pre-Release Referrals," *Archives of General Psychiatry*, 1968, 18, 712–717.

7

Patient Advocacy or
Fighting the System

Sandra Henry Kosik

The community nurse views patients as parts of families, as members of a community. In addition to giving health care the nurse is often in a strategic position to speak in behalf of the patient's needs and rights. Patient advocacy is basic to comprehensive care and to concern for the whole person. To act as an advocate, the nurse must understand the culture of the group represented. In this selection advocacy encompasses giving support, interceding, and even fighting for the patient.

I work in a large, urban, predominately black ghetto, where just surviving is a resident's daily goal. Poverty and the injustices of our health and social systems have produced here a culture distinct from anything most of us as middle-class health professionals have known.

In this culture there is no faith in the systems we know for in them these people can only struggle to survive. And, when they become patients it is almost impossible for them to fight alone through the maze of public and private agencies for service. They become confused, degraded, and, in the end, largely unaided. It is such people we nurses must serve as patient advocates. Black and other poor people have been called "foreigners" in the sense that their poverty enforces values and life-styles different from those of middle-class health professional workers.[1]

I must disagree in one sense. From my experiences I know that when I work in the poor community I am the foreigner, not they. When we middle-class professionals, black or white, enter a poor community, we are "visiting" a culture foreign to us. Communication and understanding require effort.

I do not envision the objectives, forms of advocacy, and nursing intervention that I espouse in a black urban ghetto to be the same nurses would employ everywhere.

Nevertheless, in general, the philosophy of patient advocacy would remain the same everywhere — humane and just treatment, equality, and an opportunity for all persons to obtain food, clothing, shelter, jobs, health care, and, above all, respect and dignity.

An advocate, according to dictionary definitions, is one who vindicates, or espouses a cause by argument. An advocate is an upholder, a defender, an intercessor, one who pleads for another. These words are not new to us as nurses. Daily we support, defend, and intercede for patients with doctors, peers, supervisors, other agencies, and other professionals. The advocacy I espouse, however, goes further. It involves a deeper commitment. For me, patient advocacy is seeing that the patient knows what to expect and what is his right to have, and then displaying the willingness and courage to see that our system does not prevent his getting it.

The goals of patient advocacy are, first, making a person more independent because he knows the what, why, and how of the system and, second, changing the system to make it more sensitive and relevant by revealing injustices and inadequacies, thereby making complacent continuation of status quo impossible. The nurse may have to make waves. She may have to see that workers and agencies do their jobs and expose the indifference and inhumanity of care givers.

For example, the procedures, treatment, attitudes, waiting time, and red tape in one of our city hospitals that confront children in our PRESCAD [Preschool, School, and Adolescent health care project in Detroit] project and the general population are despicable.

DOCUMENTING INHUMANITY

One opportunity for me to act as a patient advocate came after I took a mother to the emergency room to have her nine-month-old son admitted. The next day she sat in my office relating her story of inadequate, indifferent, and appalling health care. I was so outraged I wrote a verbatim report of this mother's story of the 14-hour delay before her son was admitted to the hospital. I then sent this account, signed by the mother, as "an example of care received by PRESCAD children in the pediatric emergency room" to the director of pediatrics of the hospital, the chairman of Concerned Citizens (PRESCAD's Community Advisory Group), the medical director of my health center, the nursing coordinator of our PRESCAD clinic there, and to PRESCAD's executive director and director of professional services. The results were unexpected and heartwarming.

I received a letter from the director of pediatrics agreeing that the problem was serious and encouraging more such letters. Our chairman of Concerned Citizens, Helen Kelly, who had had several unfortunate experiences there with her own children and complaints from other PRESCAD mothers, began encouraging mothers to write their complaints. Then, after much effort, she arranged a meeting between representatives of Concerned Citizens and the hospital administration to discuss mistreatment, bad attitudes of personnel, and absurd red tape.

Present at the meeting were such notables as the commissioner of the hospital, several of his top administrative assistants, the medical director of the outpatient department, and the director of the outpatient administrative services, just to name a few, plus Ms. Kelly, another PRESCAD staff member, and myself. Unfortunately, several mothers were unable to make it at the last minute. It is interesting to note that the director of nursing was not present.

The meeting was productive in that open discussions between consumers and providers took place in an amicable atmosphere. A decision was made to continue these meetings regularly, and the request to have the director of nurses at future meetings was accepted.

I can't report further progress, as our second meeting held in the director of nurses' office, was interrupted as we were just getting seated by what is now known as the shoot-out at _____ Hospital.

Four PRESCAD mothers, the director and assistant director of nurses, a hospital administrator, five other persons, and I sat huddled on the floor of a tiny cubicle for one-and-one-half hours with gun shots ringing in our ears and tear gas watering our eyes. In this case, the role of patient advocate was far more challenging than I had ever expected.

THE DEPENDENCY BUGBEAR

Although one goal of patient advocacy is patient independence, advocacy many times fosters dependency temporarily. For some reason, nurses seem to avoid or even fear dependency relationships. I can still hear the words of a supervisor saying, "Whatever you do, don't ever let a patient become dependent on you."

Many persons of the ghetto have never really had their dependency needs satisfied. From the toddler stage on, they are taught not to depend on anyone, not to trust anyone, family or friend. They must make it either on their own or not at all. Yet people need to pass through dependency stages at various times.

Dependency upon others is a fundamental human need both during the early developmental periods of life and in critical and stressful periods at any time.[2]

We must face the fact that many people are not capable of fighting the system themselves, emotionally or otherwise. There are also those who have given up, who have no energy left to do even those things they know how to do. We must step in by doing for and fighting for them when necessary.

The patient advocacy I urge does not make the patient permanently dependent, but rather sees that he knows what is available to him, and demonstrates how to get it until he is ready to take over for himself. I have repeatedly watched individuals and families hold their heads higher and assert themselves more in dealing with the system as they began managing their own efforts, an activity previously denied them. They then become advocates for others as they spread what they have learned.

For example, one day during my nursing assessment of the T. family, Ms. T., a tiny, soft-spoken mother of eight children, including two-year-old triplets and a two-month-old infant, casually mentioned that among several other major problems, the plumbing in a house she was buying had been inoperable for the past week. The back yard was full of sewage, and there was no running water as the pipes had frozen and burst a week earlier. She had talked with a real estate company that was trying to find another house for her, and then she had given up, as she did not know what else to do.

I called the emergency welfare shelter, stressed the urgency of the placement, and set it up so that Ms. T. would call and make further arrangements. When Ms. T. called the shelter she was told there was no room or some such nonsense. Again, it took persistent reminders of their responsibilities from a nurse co-worker and me. I called the real estate company. After being informed of the emergency nature of the situation, they were cooperative and agreed to do everything possible to locate Ms. T. in a house they were renovating.

MS. T. MOVES AHEAD

Five days later the construction crew themselves moved Ms. T. and mattresses to the new place. Two teen-age children had to remain at the first house to prevent burglary. If someone did not spend the night in the new residence, the day the windows were put in they would be broken and the house vandalized by the next day. So, Ms. T. and her younger children stayed two days at the new house with no furniture, while her teen-agers remained to guard the old house.

On Saturday, in the snow, my nurse co-worker, her husband, and her brother, who brought his trailer, the janitor at our center, and I moved the T. family, furniture and all, to their new address.

Because the move was an emergency, the quality of the neighborhood had not been evaluated properly. The block, we soon learned, had several dope houses and an apartment house full of transients. Ms. T.'s four-year-old son was shot by ricocheting bullets from a shoot-out in the house next door. Ms. T. again had to relocate.

This time it was Ms. T. who made the decision and all the real estate contacts. She went house hunting on her own, organized a block club on the street to encourage other families to leave the neighborhood, and shared with them her knowledge of house buying and real estate companies. She made arrangements, through the new friends she had made, to move herself to the new house. In this case, one of the goals of advocacy was accomplished, a more independent person.

NEW NURSING PRIORITIES

I believe that advocacy is the responsibility and moral obligation of every person, professional or nonprofessional. However, public health nurses, because they are out where the action is, are conceivably in the best position to be advocates. Far too long, we nurses have been complacent and have been guilty of the same apathy and hopelessness that is seen in the ghetto residents. Perhaps this is because, in the past, we saw no hope for change in our troubled system or perhaps we would not allow our own nursing system to get involved.

If nurses are to be patient advocates, nursing must allow them the time and freedom to become involved in patient and community problems. If manpower is an obstacle, maybe agencies and nursing will have to shift priorities.

Patient advocacy takes time, patience, and perseverance. One example of this occurred when Ms. M. was referred to me by one of our PRESCAD mothers in hope that, although she was not a PRESCAD registrant, I would help her and her husband get back on Medicaid and get an increase in their monthly allotment from Aid to Dependent Children. Mr. M., a patient receiving Social Security disability, had a prescription for seven different medications he had been on continuously since he had a stroke. Ms. M. called because she did not have the $12 necessary to get the latest prescription filled. She had asked her worker several times for help, but with no success.

During my call to their worker, a curt, indifferent woman, she said almost vindictively that Mr. M. had been told to join the job training program or be dropped from assistance. I explained that he was ill on the days of his appointments and that Ms. M. had called her each time to verify it. The worker told me she doubted he was ill and that he would have to get Medicaid somewhere else.

I cannot begin to count how many phone calls Ms. M. and I made to different welfare workers, including supervisors and a division director, over a six-week period before one called me back to admit that they had badly mismanaged this case. The M.'s ADC check was increased to $36 a month and both Mr. and Ms. M. were reinstated for Medicaid, for which they had both been eligible all along.

A ROLE FOR ALL NURSES

Most often we think of staff nurses as patient advocates, but supervisors and administrators must assume the role, too. In many cases their hands are tied, but there are so many little ways in which they can speak out on behalf of patients. For example, there is a director of nursing of a city health department who has the nurses report to her in writing about the injustices, inadequacies, and inhumanity they witness in various local hospital clinics, emergency rooms, and doctors' offices. Then, as specific patterns become evident, she takes these reports personally to the directors of nursing at each of the health care facilities to see if by working together they can improve patient care.

Another example of administrative advocacy is the work of a nursing director of a poverty program with a citizens health council, guiding them in their demands for a voice in managing their health care program. The point of these examples is that nursing administrators also have the opportunity and, thus, the responsibility to be patient advocates.

Staff nurse, supervisor, or administrator, a nurse, if she is truly listening and involved, is exposed to injustice after injustice. She hears, "Food stamps have been cut off," "... did not give me an appointment," "The landlord will not do anything about the inadequate heat," "The doctor did not tell me what was wrong," "They say I am not eligible for Medicaid."

When we allow ourselves to uncover the many seemingly hopeless problems facing low-income families daily, we then *must* also try to do something about them, stepping in whether the issue is health-related or not. It is even more important to step in when the patient cannot express his needs, is not aware his problems can be solved, or when the issues are so involved or frustrating that he gives up. Public health nurses cannot wait around for another person to address himself to the patient's problems, can no longer pass the buck, but, instead, must provide the help themselves. If we refer the patient to six or more different places, what good are we?

A MOTHER'S DESPAIR

If the patient is the center of care, not the agency, institution, or nurse, there is no dilemma. For example, Ms. M. sat at my desk relating her fears of killing her four children, aged six months to eight years, if someone did not get them away from her soon. She had already attempted it twice in the past, but covered it up when the child lived. I verified the urgency of this situation with a protective services worker and, with the three of us working together, the children were removed from the home within four days.

Then we tackled the mother's next problem, her desire for a tubal ligation. She was under the impression that because she was on ADC and had only Medicaid that she could not have a ligation. As her request for a ligation after the birth of her last baby had been denied, she had made no further attempts. Through a call to the clinic nurse, I learned that, because Ms. M. had received no prenatal care and had not established clinic registration, they could not consider her request at the time she made it. Her request could be processed, however, if she would register now as a clinic patient. No one had bothered to tell the mother this.

Ms. M., upon learning it, called the same day for an appointment and regularly kept all scheduled appointments thereafter. One Thursday she called me; she was desperate. Her tubal ligation was scheduled for Tuesday, but her husband still would not sign the necessary papers. She felt sure that he did not object to the ligation itself, but was only concerned that he would be billed and that any papers he signed would get him in financial trouble at a later date. He had not kept two scheduled appointments to sign the papers, and time was running out. She could not get a social worker or nurse from the hospital to call him.

Since he could only be reached at work, we decided I would call him on his break. Mr. M. was quite receptive. After I assured him that his wife's Medicaid would pay the hospital bills and explained to him what paper he had to sign and why, he agreed to go to the hospital emergency room on Saturday morning. He would not have to miss work, and could sign the necessary paper left there by the outpatient nurse. Ms. M. then had a long-wanted tubal ligation.

WHY NURSES? WHY TODAY?

Nurses must become actively involved not only in nurse-patient relationships but also in social-political relationships in order to be a patient advocate.

Far too often, we indict our political environment but do not become involved or share with politicians our concern about the health care delivery system or health issues as we see them. We must learn to work *within* the political environment, perhaps by joining political subgroups or more actively publicizing knowledge gained from our daily exposure to social and health conditions.

Also, we must learn how to work cooperatively with various community groups, for they may be our strongest supporters in our advocacy role and our biggest ally in the fight to change bureaucracies and tradition.

Why is advocacy necessary? In the poor communities it is necessary for many reasons. My community, for example, has a higher death rate and lower levels of health than prosperous communities. Its members depend more on home remedies and folk medicine, since medical care is expensiv :, unavailable, inadequate, and frightening. It is a community where adults go to bed and children to school hungry, where school achievement is low because quality education is unavailable, where verbal skills are inadequate, and where cultural stimulation is almost nonexistent. It is a community where hostility, aggression, and tension are directed more toward its members than at the whole of society and the inadequate system, because usually that is the only way it can be directed.

Another reason why patient advocacy is necessary in the black ghetto is the racism that confronts residents every day. It is there whether we admit it or not. It is evident in the worker who says, "Well he doesn't know any better... you know how they are." It is evident in the winks and facial expressions, in the employment lines, and in hospital wards. I could go on, but the point is that this *is* reality. Are we doing anything about it?

Another reason why patient advocacy is necessary is that the time is right. Herzog pointed out that most people have a dual set of values, those they live by and those they cherish as best.[3] She said the poor largely accept and believe in the standards and values of the middle class, but regard them as a luxury. She said it is possible, without too much discomfort, for people to behave as if these standards did not exist while at the same time preferring them. I disagree with Herzog in one respect. There is indeed a great deal of discomfort, and poor people no longer behave as if middle-class standards did not exist. This discomfort and discontent are being intensified as the poor are told repeatedly nowadays about their rights.

Nursing can expand roles, change names, and develop new settings in which to work. Yet nursing will be of no value unless we also become politically active in changing our deplorable health and welfare systems, constantly demonstrating humane, patient-centered care regardless of traditional and bureaucratic obstacles.

Nursing cannot afford not to allow nurses to become patient advocates.

Advocacy is where the action is. Through patient advocacy we can all begin to address ourselves to the real issues of the day. Patient advocacy is our hope for the future.

REFERENCES

1. Clifford, M. C. Health and the urban poor. *Nurs. Outlook* 17:62–63, Dec. 1969.
2. Hofling, C. K., and Leininger, Madeleine M. *Basic Psychiatric Concepts in Nursing.* 2d ed. Philadelphia, J. B. Lippincott Co., 1967, p. 38.
3. Herzog, Elizabeth G. Some assumptions about the poor. *Soc. Serv. Rev.* 37:389–402, Dec. 1963.

BIBLIOGRAPHY

Clark, K. B. *Dark Ghetto.* New York, Harper and Row, 1965.
Robischon, Paulette. Community nursing in a changing climate. *Nurs. Outlook* 19:410–413, June 1971.

8

Nursing in a Health Maintenance Organization

Barbara Bates

The sphere of community nursing encompasses a wide range of settings: official and voluntary agencies, schools, industries, and clinics, to name a few. However, the influence of community nurses continues to move in ever-widening circles as new patterns of health care are developed and as the nurses themselves assume a higher level of independent decision making. This chapter describes a health maintenance organization that provided the opportunity for fuller development and use of the community nurse's potential.

INTRODUCTION

Competent, comprehensive, personalized, accessible health care services at reasonable cost have long been part of the American dream. They are now becoming national mandate. Recently designated as health maintenance organizations by the federal government,[1] prepaid group practices offer one method of materializing this dream, of fulfilling the mandate. What part can nursing play in this endeavor?

The purpose of the present paper is to stimulate nurses, physicians and health care planners to look closely at this question. It will describe what nurses are doing in one such group practice — the Harvard Community Health Plan — not because it has all the definitive answers but because it is an example of health care innovation from which others may get ideas. Many of the innovations still require rigorous testing, perhaps with new research methods. Some of the changes create philosophic questions; some cause conflict and frustration; some have given insights into the conditions necessary for successful change. Their description may help others faced by similar problems.

THE SETTING

Conceived in 1965, the Harvard Community Health Plan first opened its doors to patients in October, 1969. Its objectives are not only to provide better health care services but also to provide them more efficiently. Like other similar organizations that preceded it, the Harvard Plan provides comprehensive health services including both ambulatory and hospital care; it comprises an organized group of health professionals; and it operates on a prepayment rather than fee-for-service basis. Unlike its predecessors, it is sponsored by a university. A nursing director with a staff of five were present on opening day. By the spring of 1972 this staff had grown to 29 professional nurses, 2 licensed practical nurses,

From *American Journal of Public Health,* Vol. 62, No. 7, pp. 991–993, 1972. Reprinted by permission of the publisher and author.

10 clinic aides, and 2 expediters. In the same time period the participating patient members had jumped from 98 to 23,000 with expectations that the final enrollment would approximate 30,000. Change was inevitable, the time for innovation ripe.

AN APPROACH TO ACCESSIBILITY – THE TELEPHONE TRIAGE

One of the most frequent complaints in health care today centers on inaccessibility. Although the most sophisticated medical machinery in the world may lie within the walls of the modern American medical center, many a patient gropes in confusion for the door. When schedules are busy, he may face many weeks of waiting for an appointment, even though in considerable discomfort.

Could this problem be surmounted and the distress relieved by placing a nurse at the point of first contact for the patient seeking help? Experience to date with a "telephone triage nurse" indicates an affirmative answer. All telephone calls from adult medical patients who are seeking early appointments and who have not yet made their initial medical visits are referred to this nurse. She takes a preliminary history, sometimes in considerable detail, assesses the situation, and makes a judgment as to the appropriate action. Several options are open. Some patients clearly need to see a physician within a short time. For these she can act as patient advocate, making the most appropriate appointment to meet the need. Because of her professional judgment, she can "beat the system" when indicated, arranging a visit even when schedules are full. At the same time, she can give the patient interval advice, a personal contact and a sense of responsiveness.

Other patients have minor problems, e.g., an upper respiratory infection or gastroenteritis, requiring counsel or suggestions. These needs the nurse can meet herself. She can suggest symptomatic therapy and with physician liaison can send out appropriate prescriptions. A few of these patients are undergoing emotional upsets or crises. The nurse's support, perhaps with a short series of calls over a few days, can carry them successfully through.

For a middle group of patients, the best management is less certain or appears to require direct contact for proper assessment. Patients with acute pharyngitis are good examples. These are referred into the health center where nurses see and evaluate them on the same or the following day. Again interim advice is possible and the patient is told what to expect. The subsequent nursing assessment or triage is described in the next section.

Not all nurses thrive in the role of telephone triage, but some do. The position appears to have a unique potential for a nurse with a health problem of her own which precludes more physically active responsibilities. Other qualifications suggested have included sound clinical experience, preferably with some public health, an educational background conducive to a broad perspective and to independent learning, self-confidence and comfort with responsibility, a tolerance of anxiety, sensitivity to people, personal warmth, and a sense of humor. At the health center all of these attributes are put to good use.

PRIMARY ASSESSMENT — NURSING TRIAGE

Telephone triage would be valueless if resources for care were not available. For some patients the nurse appears to be the most appropriate resource. Currently three nurses in the triage area together average over 40 patient visits daily. Most of these patients have been referred by the telephone triage nurse; some are "walk-ins" seeking immediate attention for a variety of complaints. The kinds of problems encountered during one month, November 1971, are listed in Table 1. In addition, there are approximately 1,000 patient-nurse encounters

Table 1. Number of Patient-Nurse Encounters in Triage Area by Primary Presenting Problem during November 1971*

Patient's Presenting Problem	Number of Patient-Nurse Encounters
Trauma	115
Upper respiratory infection	82
Pharyngitis	61
Viral syndrome	60
Muscle pain	55
Dermatitis	45
Urinary tract infection	44
Anxiety	43
Gastroenteritis	38
Vaginitis	28
Allergic rhinitis	18
Gonorrhea	13
Depression	12
Acute bronchitis	10
All other	364
Total patient-nurse encounters	988*

*Including encounters during regular clinic hours, Monday through Friday, only

per month in the triage area during evenings, weekends, and holidays. The nurse interviews the patient and makes a physical and psychosocial assessment within the limits of her training and skill. Statistics show that she herself is able to manage from 70% to 80% of the patients. She requests laboratory tests, makes diagnoses, and implements management. Guidelines drawn up by the medical staff have helped the nurse in her decision-making and, for some specific conditions, she works under standing orders. The guidelines and standing orders appear to have several benefits: (1) they enable the nurse to respond promptly to patient needs; (2) they delineate clearly certain points at which physician consultation is needed; (3) they help to assure interdisciplinary collaboration and high standards of care; (4) they may also have helped the physicians to relinquish more comfortably a portion of their traditional role. The remaining 20% to 30% of the patients currently require medical consultation or judgment. Health center physicians respond readily to this need.

AN APPROACH TO COMPREHENSIVE PERSONALIZED CARE – NURSE-PHYSICIAN TEAMS

In addition to inaccessibility, depersonalization of care is a common complaint against the American system. Pressures on the physician to see large numbers of patients frequently prevent his giving sufficient attention to many of the patient's concerns, to health education and to support, guidance and comfort. As one approach to these problems, the Harvard Community Health Plan has developed collaborative nurse-physician teams which function in major clinical areas including Internal Medicine, Pediatrics, Psychiatry, and Obstetrics-Gynecology.

In Medicine, for example, the physician and nurse frequently confer about patients requiring long-term management and together develop a plan of care. The nurse may explain a diet, review a medication regimen, and help the patient to understand and cope with his illness and treatments. Like the triage nurses, she may respond by telephone or in person when her patients present new problems, coping with some herself, for others acting as liaison with the physician. In Pediatrics, the nurse participates in obtaining an initial health history. On referral from the pediatrician, she conducts some of the well-child visits, assessing the child's development and counseling the parents. She also responds to problems by phone. In Psychiatry, the psychiatric nurse participates in initial patient assessment, in therapy, and in special educational programs dealing for example with sex, drugs, child rearing, and family relationships. In Obstetrics-Gynecology, an analogous educational and therapeutic role is filled by a nurse who provides information and advice in areas such as contraception and pregnancy.

A public health nurse provides comparable services in a community-oriented outreach center.

ARE THESE NURSING ROLES?

Few conversational topics are more successful in provoking a storm within nursing circles than the words "physician's assistant." Although some of the activities described above may suggest this kind of role, nurses in the Harvard Community Health Plan are convinced that they are providing a service qualitatively different from that of medicine. While many physicians concentrate on pathology, because of their training, interests or limitations in time, the nurses feel that they can make important contributions to the psychosocial needs of the patients.

The nurses' role extends beyond the physical problems by filling a caring, expressive function and helping the patient to cope. Physical assessment and management can be a tool not only for their own ends but also to provide access to other patient concerns and to enable the nurse to deal with a larger number of problems more efficiently in a single encounter.

WHAT IS REALLY DIFFERENT?

Simply to describe what nurses do in the Harvard Community Health Plan is to miss the essence of change. As one nurse expresses it, "What we're doing is not really new. We've been doing it in public health for years. A list of what we do looks just like a lot of other lists." When asked then to identify the real difference, a group of nurses responded with the following words: "potential," "freedom," "independence," "decision-making," "confidence in myself as a person and in myself as a nurse that I have something to offer a patient, not just shots, tasks, automaton activities." To an outside observer, the essence of the difference appears to lie in the level of independent decision-making — a level considerably higher than in many other institutional settings — a level that demands a high measure of competence and provides professional satisfaction.

THE CONDITIONS FOR CHANGE

It is impossible to pinpoint or measure all the factors that have created this kind of atmosphere. At least four variables appear, however, to have contributed.

Selection of nursing staff is of course the first and critical step. Most of the nurses at the Harvard Community Health Plan have baccalaureate or master's level education. Most have had previous clinical experience. They were selected for their eagerness to try new methods in their nursing practice, for their ability to tolerate frustration, for their interest in patients and patient care.

Second, the leaders within both nursing and medicine have accepted, supported and expected a high level of independent practice.

Third, the nurses have been involved in planning their own patterns of practice, their own inservice education programs, and new approaches to record-keeping. This involvement has further nurtured the commitment to change and excellence.

Fourth, there are opportunities for learning and feedback. For example, the telephone triage nurse, whose office is immediately adjacent to the nursing triage area, regularly obtains follow-up data on her patients, thus assessing her earlier judgments. In turn the triage nurses can test their opinions against the physicians'. In fact the ready interchange of information and opinions across disciplinary lines may be one of the major advantages of organized group practice over the more isolated situation routinely faced by the public health nurse.

QUESTIONS AND UNSOLVED PROBLEMS

The nurses at the Harvard Community Health Plan would be the first to point out that they have not achieved a utopian ideal. Questions remain, some problems persist, and research is needed to document achievements and costs.

One of the continuing questions — both philosophic and practical — relates to the expanded role of the nurse. How much further into traditional medical practice can the nurse expand her knowledge and skills and still retain the personalized patient caring focus traditional to her profession? Opinions of the staff on this question differ, sometimes varying with the individual's interests, her present skills, her self-confidence, her philosophy and the setting in which she finds herself. We can undoubtedly expect continuing tensions here, between the conflicting forces of science and humanism, both in nursing and in medicine.

Although respect between nurses and physicians is high in the Harvard Plan, not all interdisciplinary problems have been solved. As the nurse acquires her own professional practice, seeing patients by appointment, interviewing and examining them, she faces conflicting expectations from physicians who are accustomed to the assistance she has traditionally provided. Since the space required for patient privacy in taking histories, conducting physical examinations and instructing patients in health care is limited, competition for office space develops. Both nurses and physicians have legitimate needs while medicine has the traditional power. Although not easy, solutions to these problems may take several forms: (1) better articulation by nurses of what nursing is and can do, together with better perception by physicians of these realities and potentials; (2) improved administrative and committee structure to promote interdisciplinary cooperation and representation; and (3) better supporting services so that nurses as well as physicians can be relieved of some technical tasks.

Finally, investigation is required to measure the process of care, its achievements and costs. A prepaid group practice offers unique opportunities for the reallocation of resources so that patients will get the most appropriate services at the most reasonable price. We must assess these efforts by seeking answers to a number of questions. Exactly what activities comprise this new role? Precisely how are they different from traditional roles — of the nurse, of the physician, and now of the physician's assistant?

What is the impact of this nursing role on patients' health and well being? Is the care better? If so, how? How do patients respond? Data in other settings[2, 3] have given some encouraging answers to these questions, indicating such results as improved satisfaction, less disability, fewer symptoms, improved compliance and better understanding of care. Further investigation is needed to find out whether similar results can be obtained in settings that are unprotected by special project and grant support.

What does this kind of care cost? Is it less expensive or more costly than the usual methods of delivering care? What is the relationship of the cost of care to its effectiveness? Does it hold more advantages for some health care settings than for others? A recent theoretical study[4] suggests that a nurse with responsibilities similar to those described above should enhance the economic viability and financial attractiveness of a rural group practice. This hypothesis should be tested, and in a variety of organizations.

Answers to these questions are essential not only for the understanding of new roles but also for the adequate appraisal of health care systems. Data limited to mortality, morbidity and costs are not in themselves enough.

In summary, the Harvard Community Health Plan is pointing toward a new method of delivering care. Its pattern warrants study by others who are planning organized group practices. Final evaluation of these kinds of innovation will be the work of many.

ACKNOWLEDGMENTS

The author's visit to the Harvard Community Health Plan and preparation of this paper were initiated and supported by the Division of Nursing, Bureau of Health Manpower Education, National Institutes of Health. The help given by Doris L. Wagner, R.N., Director of Nursing, by her staff, and by H. Richard Nesson, M.D., Medical Director, is gratefully acknowledged.

REFERENCES

1. Towards a Comprehensive Health Policy for the 1970's. A White Paper. Washington, D.C.: HEW, May 1971.
2. Lewis, C. E.; Resnik, B. A.; and Schmidt, G., et al. Activities, Events and Outcomes in Ambulatory Patient Care. *New Eng. J. Med.,* 280:645–649, 1969.
3. Fink, D.; Malloy, M. J.; and Cohen, M., et al. Effective Patient Care in the Pediatric Ambulatory Setting: A Study of the Acute Care Clinic. *Pediatrics,* 43:927–935, 1969.
4. McCormack, R. C., and Miller, C. W. The Economic Feasibility of Rural Group Practice and Influence of Non-Physician Practitioners in Primary Care. *Medical Care,* 10:73–80, 1972.

9

The School Nurse
and Drug Abusers

Kathryn K. Caskey
Enid V. Blaylock
Beryl M. Wauson

Schools provide another setting for the community nurse to draw upon a background of knowledge and skills in all areas of nursing care — physical, psychological, sociocultural and spiritual. The school nurse's skills in interpersonal communication become particularly important in the following example, a teaching-counseling role in relation to drug abuse.

Seventeen-year-old Jimmy had enrolled in the continuation high school late in the school year. His parents were separated, and he had been living with his father in another state. Now he and his brother Paul, sixteen, had returned to their mother's home.

Jimmy came to the teacher's attention almost immediately because he talked openly about the wide variety of drugs he used. He spoke of "shooting speed" and "dropping LSD." The school nurse was asked to verify these stories and to recommend action.

Jimmy told his story readily under casual questioning in the course of a routine health interview of new students. He said that he had been using many different drugs for several years. He had developed blood clots in the veins of both forearms from "shooting speed," and the physician who had treated him convinced him that these thrombosed areas were endangering his life. So he no longer used "speed," but he was using every other drug he could get hold of, except heroin. He had even tried that drug once on a visit to New York City. But, not being accustomed to it, he had immediately lost consciousness for several hours and concluded that heroin was overrated. Although he had had psychotherapy while in juvenile custody two years previously, he was not now receiving therapy.

Jimmy told the nurse he was worried that drugs might have damaged his brain, and admitted he should stop using them. The nurse explained the effects of "drug wipe-out" — symptoms that Jimmy recognized in himself — and she explained the possibility of nerve pathways being rerouted. She offered, and he accepted, the address and telephone number of a local clinic that counseled drug users.

That night, Jimmy told his mother about the clinic referral and showed her the card on which the address had been jotted. His mother felt the nurse had "really reached him," when no one else could, and the next day she telephoned the nurse to ask her support for her son. She also spoke of her own problems of alcoholism and amphetamine abuse. However, she thought the most pressing problem was Jimmy's indecision about registering for the draft, for he had just passed his eighteenth birthday. His feelings about war were confused and uncertain, she said, but he resisted registering as a conscientious objector because this was evading the issue.

After the discussion with his mother about therapy, Jimmy went on an all-out "trip," taking cocaine, LSD, mescaline, marijuana, Seconal, and red wine. He was treated for drug overdosage at the emergency room of the local hospital, but was not admitted.

When Jimmy did not appear at school the next day, the nurse called at his home. She found the mother and her two sons in their small, but clean, apartment. Mother and Jimmy were sleeping when she arrived; Paul was moving about, unconcerned, preparing lunch, emptying ash trays, whistling, and humming.

Mother's contribution to the conversation that followed consisted mostly of nagging reminders to Jimmy about his draft situation, so the nurse left her out of the discussion. Instead, she talked to Jimmy about how he felt about his drug experience of two nights before. Soon mother and Paul left the apartment, and the nurse could talk to Jimmy alone about his draft registration plans. She offered to get what information she could about obtaining a medical deferment, and he consented.

During the next few days, the nurse conferred with members of an organization of former drug users devoted to rehabilitation of other users, with the draft counseling agencies of local churches and colleges, and with Jimmy's private physician, all of whom gave her valuable information. She was thus able to help Jimmy overcome his indecision and avoidance tactics and register with the local draft board within the deadline.

In later conversations at school and his home, the nurse reinforced his decision to seek help. Jimmy is now receiving therapy at the community counseling clinic and reports at intervals to the nurse on the progress of his rehabilitation. He attends school fairly regularly, and will transfer to standard high school in the fall.

An incidental outcome of this continuing relationship was that Jimmy's mother, referred by the nurse, went to the alcoholic rehabilitation center of the local health department and is now receiving treatment. Paul is also entering therapy.

At their first encounter, the nurse perceived that Paul's mask of unconcern covered a deep well of feeling for his mother and brother. His adjustment problems in school confirmed a source of tension. The nurse's success in establishing a counseling relationship with him was based on his realization of her true interest and concern.

Thus, all three members of this family needed and received much continuing support and encouragement from the school nurse in their efforts toward more effective living.

EXTENT OF THE PROBLEM

Controlling drug abuse among children and young adults is decisive to our whole society, for the stability and progress of a nation depends on the health and vigor of its youth. Although there are no totally reliable data on the extent of nation-wide drug addiction and abuse, recent statistics show that an estimated 0.5 to 1.0 percent of all students admit to having tried heroin. The figure may be as high as 4 percent in certain areas. On the East and West coasts, between 2.5 and 14 percent of students have tried depressants. At the college level, it is estimated that 10 to 27 percent have tried stimulants and, at the high school level, 3.5 to 21.5 percent. While LSD use is estimated at 1 percent at the college level, its use is said to be increasing in high schools.

Marijuana use has increased greatly at all levels, between 5 and 35 percent of all college students having tried it at least once. The nationwide figure for all ages is probably around 15 percent.[1] A San Mateo, California, survey on student use found that "All rates are higher for 1969 than for 1968. Also, the propor-tions of . . . individuals who report using marijuana ten or more times has in-creased consistently over the year."[2]

The list of purported reasons for drug use is extensive and diverse. It includes such factors as boredom, feelings of inadequacy, emotional maladjustment, escape from tensions and frustrations, family disorganization, lack of home discipline, curiosity, experimentation, and belief in the magical power of drugs to solve problems. Today's affluent society, urbanization, and easy access to all sorts of drugs are also frequently cited as reasons. Those closest to the problem are convinced that drug abuse will be overcome only when the underlying social ills of our present society are ameliorated.

The diverse problems associated with the use of drugs among young people call for a multifaceted approach and for close coordination among responsible groups and organizations, including members of the health professions. Until recently no school nurse needed to invest much time or energy in the area of drug abuse. Now, she must try to incorporate a whole new set of ideas and behaviors into her school health activities, and perhaps her most difficult task is defining her role. It is also one of the most important, for the nature of her involvement and the value of her contribution is related to her perception of her role. A school nurse who sees her role as primarily one of detecting and report-ing drug abuse to the administration will behave differently from one who feels a deep responsibility for helping students find healthier ways to self-fulfillment.

The nurse must project her role interpretation and assure its acceptance by administrators, teachers, and others on the health team. Her role has many facets, of which counseling is one not always recognized but of the greatest importance. Besides counseling, other functions include treating and giving follow-up care as well as preventing drug abuse.

PREVENTION OF DRUG ABUSE

Helping children and young people avoid the hazard of drug abuse calls for as much concern and planning as such problems as dental caries and visual defects. The school nurse must incorporate the problem into the broad context of preventive health practice and actively participate in school and community programs concerned with all aspects of drug abuse.

In preventive health practice, education is one of the most effective approaches. Although health educators may assume major responsibility for teaching about drugs, the school nurse provides an important contribution with her medical background, her knowledge of pharmacology, firsthand observations of patients' responses to drugs, study of anatomy and physiology, and her understanding of pathology and psychology. She can talk about drugs with vigor and authority from a broad perspective.

The nurse as educator is pivotal on a teaching team committed to preventive education. She can be a leader, giving impetus to a total drug education program, helping plan curriculum and assisting in implementation, serving as a resource to the classroom teacher, and she can provide inservice education for faculty and staff.

The school nurse should compile and have available relevant literature and information for use by the teaching staff. She should be able to evaluate written professional offerings and recognize that many inaccuracies are in print. She should be able to interpret to the staff the relative usefulness of educational approaches, correct defects in technique, and assist staff in preparing effective programs and lessons. Discussion of drugs should begin early, starting in kindergarten, and can occur naturally in many areas of the curriculum.

Sound mental health, too, is vital to drug abuse prevention. The nurse will emphasize the drug user instead of the drug, and help him fulfill himself in various ways. One approach is through individual and family counseling. She is in contact with a large proportion of pupils and their families. If she is alert and sensitive to the various cues — some quite subtle — which potential drug users and their families often project, many kinds of preventive measures can be instituted. Jimmy's brother, Paul, could have been the forgotten member in a family beset by crises, his reactions overlooked. But his symptoms were recognized by the school nurse, experienced in reading and evaluating the small clues as well as the more evident ones. So Paul, too, shared in the benefits of family counseling.

Dr. Richard E. Carney of United States International University has described the clues by which a potential drug user may be identified before he becomes involved in the drug culture. The pupil may find school work difficult or uninteresting, may experience conflicts with parents and teachers, may be unable to maintain positive relationships with peers or members of the opposite sex, or may experience feelings of inadequacy, any of which could lead to drug abuse as a means of coping with life.[3]

Involvement in community affairs and cooperation with such groups as parent-teacher organizations and school health councils are additional avenues through which the school nurse can work toward drug abuse prevention. Vehicles for active participation include community health planning and coordinating councils, community psychotherapeutic facilities, and educational and inspirational organizations.

COUNSELING

The school nurse is an integral part of the counseling team on drug problems. She is often the first person in whom the student confides his problem, as she cares for his immediate needs. She gives initial understanding and acceptance by helping the student to recognize his needs, and by supporting and encouraging him as he works toward a solution to his problems.

Genuine interest effectively communicated is the key to helping the student develop a feeling of self-worth — an essential first step toward rehabilitation. The nurse must feel and be able to communicate to him her genuine concern, and her desire to help him recognize and solve his problems. If the student can feel strongly the nurse's interest in him as a person, he is more likely to trust and confide in her. This kind of relationship creates a solid foundation for giving real help and for the beginning of real effort on the part of the student. However, if the nurse is required to alert legal authorities to the student's problem, he loses trust in her and confidence in himself. This makes his situation worse than before, because he will be unlikely to confide again, and so will miss the help he so sorely needs. His friends may accept his judgment and so her effectiveness in the school will be lessened.

The nurse must be able and willing to talk with the student on his own level, using the slang terms he is familiar with. This was particularly effective in communicating with Jimmy. The school nurse was able to establish a positive relationship during their first counseling session. The communication aspect of the nurse's counseling role must also extend to the family in order to enlist their support. It was Jimmy's mother who brought his draft registration problem to the attention of the nurse.

Emotional disturbances — sibling rivalry, inconsistent discipline, rejection — are generally associated with family relationships. When the nurse is in intimate contact with students' families and is received in their homes in a positive manner, she can gain valuable understanding of family constellations and relationships. This, plus her knowledge of growth and development, adds to her effectiveness when counseling pupils and their families, whether it is helping a five-year-old develop a good self-concept, a ten-year-old gain recognition through accomplishment, or an adolescent achieve emotional independence.

Differential factors of age, background, family, personality, situational variants, and immediate reactions to the drug make each encounter an individual situation which challenges the nurse's perceptual and interpretive skills. The young girl who has broken up with her boy friend the night before and taken "reds" for the first time presents a therapeutic picture far different from the "pusher" on a tolerance level.

TREATMENT

Since the nurse is frequently the only person available at the school who can make a medical judgment, she is intimately involved with drug abuse problems in students. Her first decision is a medical one, for the physical safety of the student must be the primary concern. In cases of intoxication, she must determine whether the student may be overdosed and in need of emergency medical treatment. For example, if she perceives the situation as a medical emergency, she may decide to call the physician or an ambulance at once. She advises the administrator of her decision and action, dictated by her judgment of the student's condition. The administrator makes any necessary further decisions, including those involving the legal juvenile authorities.

The student under drug influence may not require such dramatic treatment, but he may be uncoordinated and physically incapable of independent movement. He may need protection against losing balance, or falling and injuring himself. He should be put in a secluded area where he can lie down, if this is indicated.

Direct physical contact, such as holding the hand or embracing the student, is a valuable therapeutic tool in caring for the person on hallucinogens and "freaking out." The nurse should understand and appreciate its use, and incorporate it in her treatment method so that it becomes a natural expression of her interaction. The LSD user who is having a "bad trip," and who is losing touch with reality describes his feeling as being "without a body" or "outside his own body." He is consumed by a feeling of terror, of nonbeing, and supportive physical contact such as embracing is an important part of therapy.* The student may be unusually talkative and ready to pour out his problems, concerns, and frustrations; then the nurse may be able to establish a rapport which will continue through months of rehabilitative counseling.

PARENTS' COOPERATION

As soon as feasible, the parents should be advised of the situation so that they may be included in the treatment plan, for they are an integral part of any overall decision. In carrying out these functions, the nurse becomes recognized as an authority and a resource to the community. By her cooperation with

---

First Vibration. Available from Do It Now Foundation, P.O. Box 3573, Hollywood, Calif. 90028.

community agencies in planning and coordinating efforts, she may help to avoid duplication. She systematically bases her decisions and action on the immediate physical and emotional needs of the student, whether or not drug use is an established factor.

However, the extent to which parents can be a positive influence varies with each situation. A plan for treatment may need to begin by helping the parents understand the nature of the problem, because they may initially deny completely the possibility that their child is involved with drugs. In some cases, underlying family conflicts have so separated the family members that the best plan aims at reducing contacts and areas of pressure between family members. On the other hand, mutual family concern may be present and can be utilized. The nurse recognized this family strength in Jimmy's case, and was able to use it effectively in referring the family to appropriate community agencies.

The nurse must be knowledgeable concerning the physical and mental effects of drugs of abuse, and the dangers inherent in their use, so that appropriate treatment can be instituted. The literature in this field is extensive. Workshops and conferences are offered widely and increasingly. Every school nurse should avail herself of these opportunities to update her knowledge about the physiological and psychological effects of the various drugs. It is particularly essential for her to recognize the symptoms produced by the wide spectrum of drugs of abuse that are currently in use.

Stimulants

Symptoms caused by the use of drugs that are designated as stimulants, mostly the amphetamines, include blacking out, extremely restless behavior of any sort, extreme nervousness, tremor of the hands, dilated pupils, dryness of the mouth, heavy perspiration, perhaps delusions and hallucinations, and talkativeness; even dangerous and aggressive behavior with antisocial effects.

Depressants

Symptoms caused by drugs that are designated as depressants and which relieve tension — barbiturates and tranquilizers, for example — include drowsiness or sluggishness, depression, mental and emotional instability, sometimes quarrelsome disposition. The tongue may become thickened and speech slurred and indistinct.

Hallucinogens

Marijuana and LSD are in the group of drugs that are designated as hallucinogens. Marijuana is a mild hallucinogen which causes dilated pupils, glassy bloodshot eyes, slurred speech, sudden sleep, hallucinations, distorted or lost memory, and loss of interest in surroundings. Symptoms associated with the use of LSD include distorted or heightened perception, erratic mental changes, panic, hallucinatory experiences, homicidal behavior, and even behavior dangerous to the self.

Hydrocarbons

Drugs designated as hydrocarbons include airplane glue, gasoline, ether, and lighter fluid. They cause irritation of the nose and mouth, fever blisters, red or watery eyes, nausea, "passing out," an appearance of extreme intoxication, hallucinations, impulsiveness, a tendency to be easily upset and erratic, and an attitude of fear, belligerence, and surliness.

Heroin

This drug affects individuals differently, and no single sign is proof of its use. However, common symptoms of its use include changes in mood and behavior, lack of interest in usual activities such as school or in personal appearance, unusual seclusiveness, loss of appetite, constipation, pinpoint pupils, drowsiness, or intoxication while "high." After he has established a tolerance to the drug, the student may be able to attend classes and converse normally when under its influence. He may appear pale and undernourished, have a poor appetite and persistent constipation. Depending upon his method of taking the drug, marks of injection may be evident.

Follow-up of pupils with problems of drug abuse is difficult and challenging. The school nurse's responsibility does not end when the pupil is referred for treatment. As in the case of Jimmy, continued interest in and concern for the pupil's total rehabilitation are necessary. The nurse needs to remain in a counseling relationship with the student and his family, offering support and encouragement until they have accepted and benefited from treatment, for any of a number of things may go awry. The treatment facility may be inadequate; the pupil may be delinquent in keeping appointments; parents may lack interest or confidence in the treatment process; or the treatment may entail financial burdens that severely limit cooperation. It is very important that the school nurse inquire into these and other problems and help pupils and their parents find solutions. The nature and degree of her concern and commitment, and the persistence, patience, and understanding she brings to bear in her follow-up procedures are important determinants of the outcomes of the rehabilitative process.

SUMMARY

By virtue of her professional preparation and her interest in the health and welfare of children, the school nurse can work effectively in the area of drug abuse prevention and rehabilitation.

Jimmy, Paul, and their mother constitute a microcosm within the drug world. The school nurse in her various roles helped them to shape their lives toward a better future by being a warm and giving friend to these bewildered people and by her professional and personal concern, commitment, and willingness to meet the challenges of drug abuse with vigor and persistence.

REFERENCES

1. Sparatto, G. R.   Toward a rational view of drug abuse.   *J. Sch. Health* 40:192—196, Apr. 1970.
2. Blackford, Lillian F.   Trends in student drug use in San Mateo County.   *Calif. Health* 27:3—6, Nov. 1969.
3. Carney, Richard.   *A Report of the Feasibility of Using Risk-Taking Attitudes as a Basis for Programs to Control and Predict Drug Abuse.*   (E.S.E.A. Title III, Project No. 68-5380, Grant No. 9-8-005380-0064 (056)) Coronado, Calif., Coronado Unified School District, 1970, pp. a-1—a-5.

10

The Occupational Health Nurse and the Patient with Trauma

Hazel L. Gallaher
Ginger M. Wyatt

Effective community nursing includes such basic concepts as prevention, case-finding, positive health teaching, encouraging patient self-direction, continuity of care, total family care and use of the health care team. The full range of these activities are used by the occupational health nurse. In addition, this nurse is often called on to deal with emergencies that require exercising sound judgment and making independent decisions. As in other settings and roles, independent action is one of the defining characteristics of the community nurse.

The occupational health nurse working in an industrial setting is usually the first professional member of the medical team to see the victim of a traumatic accident. As has been shown by the national study of occupational health nurses conducted in 1964 by the United States Public Health Service,[1] two-thirds of all occupational health nurses work alone, without direct medical supervision.

Despite ever improving safety standards enforced by business and industry, and increasing alertness on the part of employees to avoid unsafe practices, all resulting in a downward trend in the number of accidents per employee hour, accidents do occur, and the first line of defense, medical care and treatment, rests with the occupational health nurse. Therefore, this one professional individual must use her own judgment in assessing the degree of severity of the injury.

This paper describes selected types of incidents and actions based on a combined experience of 28 years on the defense line.

INITIAL TREATMENT

The obvious symptoms of shock must be treated immediately at the scene of the accident. In many larger installations, trained first-aid attendants may be in the area and usually initiate this care. When it is known that professional help is on the way, this initial treatment will usually consist of the first three basic steps of first aid: (1) artificial respiration, (2) control of bleeding and (3) treatment for shock.[2]

The occupational health nurse, arriving at the injury site, will not only check these initial ministrations, but initiate further measures. The immediate reassurance of the victim is vitally important. Not only does he have to deal with (usually) intense pain, but also he has to face the realization that this injury

From *Nursing Clinics of North America*, Vol. 5, No. 4, pp. 609–619, 1970. Reprinted by permission of the publisher and authors.

could result in loss of limb, job, and even life. It is therefore essential that the victim be given immediate care, psychologically as well as physiologically.

TRANSPORTATION

Adequate transportation of the injured employee to proper medical facilities is usually left to the supervision of the occupational health nurse. Again, well-trained first-aiders can be utilized to a great advantage. Ambulance service may or may not have trained medical personnel. The nurse must assume the responsibility of seeing that the injured individual is transported in such a way that additional injury does not occur. For example: a puncture wound of the upper, inner thigh causes hemorrhage which has been controlled by digital pressure on the femoral artery in the groin. When this victim is lifted incorrectly, pressure is released and bleeding commences again. Untrained attendants would not know where or how to apply pressure.

In instances in which the injury results in an amputation of a digit or limb, the amputated portion should be transported with the injured person. There is always the possibility that this appendage may be restored to the victim. Although there is seldom any advance preparation of the amputated portion that can be performed at the injury site, a clean, if not sterile, dressing should be used to cover this appendage. Concise instructions to the ambulance attendants regarding these covered appendages must be given prior to leaving with the victim. A transplant is hardly feasible if an appendage is left on the floor of the ambulance.

DETERMINING CAUSE AND EFFECT

With the injured worker on his way to adequate medical care and possible hospitalization, the occupational health nurse has the time and opportunity to assess (1) the cause of the accident, (2) possible remedial measures, and (3) improvement of emergency technique. This may involve counseling with co-workers, safety engineers, hygienists, and top management. If it is determined that the accident was not the result of lax safety standards and/or faulty utilization of safety equipment, then the accident must have been caused by inattention to these safety regulations. This employee, then, will have to be rehabilitated psychologically. In this area, the occupational health nurse will have ample opportunity to practice counseling skills.

EXAMPLES OF OCCUPATIONAL INJURIES

Since traumatic injuries of industrial workers occur in nonmanufacturing as well as manufacturing work locations, we shall attempt to point out some types of injuries occurring in each site and the handling of such emergencies. Mrs. Wyatt's work location is a manufacturing industry; Mrs. Gallaher's, a nonmanufacturing work site.

Injuries in a Manufacturing Industry

This medical division consists of two nurses and a part-time physician who visits the plant twice daily, once in the morning and once in the early afternoon. Both nurses had operating room supervisory experience (not a requirement of employment), which certainly helps. One nurse had had training as an American Red Cross First Aid Training Instructor. She is responsible for the training of the laboratory personnel in the plant, who give first aid in the absence of medical help. Classes are given once a year to four shifts of men, approximately ten men per shift. Two men on each shift are assigned as the ambulance crew each month. During the routine day shift, one nurse will accompany the ambulance crew when the ambulance is needed. There are no nurses in the plant during nights, weekends, or holidays, which places the responsibilities of first aid on these men.

Patients with Burns. In ten years of service, duPont-Beaumont Works has suffered two explosions. The first happened during the day shift, and the nurse accompanied the crew to the area. One man had been burned, and since it was impossible to give a complete estimate of the burns, the nurse and crew took all necessary precautions to prevent shock. The patient was placed on the ambulance stretcher and was on his way to the hospital within three minutes of the injury. While en route to the hospital, the nurse applied KwikKold ice packs to the burned area of the patient's face, hands, and the front of his legs. One of the ambulance crewmen assisted her in placing the packs and making sure the patient was covered sufficiently to maintain body heat. The hospital was only ten miles from the plant, so that a physician was able to see the patient rather promptly. Communication is maintained between the ambulance and the plant medical department through plant radiophones.

The patient's stay in the hospital was short, since the burns suffered were mostly first and second degree and were over a limited area.

The second explosion was more severe, and happened about two o'clock in the morning. The ambulance crewmen had two men to transport to the hospital with second and third degree burns. The burns were so extensive that ice packs were applied only around the faces of the men, and their bodies were wrapped in clean white sheets to help maintain body heat, as well as prevent foreign objects from entering the wounded areas. Both men were kept in a prone position while on their way to the hospital. Nothing was given by mouth.

These men were hospitalized for a period of about three months. The plant physician chose to treat them by the silver nitrate method popularized in 1965 by Dr. Carl A. Moyer and his associates.[3] This treatment involves bandaging the burned areas and saturating them with silver nitrate solution. After three months of treatment, grafting, and physical therapy, the men were allowed to return to the plant on limited duty as specified by the plant physician. Therapy was continued in the medical department for another six weeks before their work load was increased and they were finally restored to their complete jobs some nine months later.

Another incident happened on the 3—11 shift. A mechanic was burned over 55% of his body by a molten chemical substance that ignited his clothing. He suffered second and third degree burns over the left side of his face, neck, arms, both hands, left chest, stomach, pubic area, and both legs. The men in the area with him put him under a safety shower to extinguish the fire. One of them called the ambulance. Arriving on the scene, the ambulance crew assisted the patient onto the stretcher, covering him with a clean sheet and transporting him to the hospital as rapidly as possible. Through radio communication with the plant, the plant physician was contacted and was waiting for the patient in the hospital emergency room. The plant physician's observation included: "The patient's clothing was burned to shreds, but not a piece of skin had been torn. The patient was not in shock, fully conscious and complaining of pain."

This patient, during his hospital stay, also suffered a cardiac arrest in the operating room. Because of this fact and the extent of his burns, he remained in the hospital for five months and at home for another month before being allowed to reenter the plant. Upon return to the plant, he was kept in the medical department for three weeks, assisting in paper work and answering the telephone. This gave the nurses and the plant physician a chance to study his movements, as well as his attitude and reactions. These proved to be satisfactory, and the patient was allowed to return to limited duty in the shop nine months after his injury. He was working in the shop when the first explosion occurred, about a block away from his working area. He sustained no physical injury, but certainly sustained an emotional setback. He was again confined to the medical department, though only for a day this time. The plant physician gave him a sedative to help him sleep that night, and the nurses listened to him talk away many of his anxieties. Here again, first aid was necessary — not the physical first aid that is usually initiated, but the psychologic type. This becomes, perhaps, the greater challenge.

An electrical burn of the right arm and chest has also been among this plant's major injuries. The man was knocked to the floor by the current: however, he did not lose consciousness. His treatment with silver nitrate and his recovery were long but uneventful. He did not require as much therapy because of the location of the burns.

A Lacerated Injury. A mechanic, while working on a crane rigging cable, got his hand caught in the cable gears, resulting in a severe laceration of his right wrist. The ambulance was called. Upon arriving at the shop, the nurse found the 19-year-old boy lying on one of the work tables surrounded by a group of co-workers. One of the men had tied a rag tightly above the laceration to act as a tourniquet. Since this was holding well, the nurse had the men lift the boy to the nearest ambulance stretcher, and the crew placed him in the ambulance.

En route through the plant and to the hospital, the nurse and one of the attendants placed an inflatable splint on the wrist, covered the lacerated area with a sterile 3" X 3" gauze, and applied enough pressure to stop the flow of blood. Then the patient's blood pressure was checked by the nurse and the rest of the time was spent talking to the excited patient to calm him.

Again, the plant physician was contacted by radiophone through the plant medical department. In surgery, the full extent of the injury was disclosed and repairs were made to torn tendons and muscles. The patient spent four days in the hospital, six weeks in a cast, and is still undergoing therapy to promote full use of his wrist. He returned to work after his stay in the hospital and has been on limited duty to this time.

Patients with Cardiac Problems. Although this medical division is not directly responsible for the care of injured construction workers, the nurses in these other areas rely on our plant for ambulance service. Several times workers have been taken to the hospital with suspected coronaries, being treated for shock and receiving oxygen while on the way. One patient was a 62-year-old white male carpenter who had fallen on the job two or three times. This day the ambulance was called and the nurse accompanied the crew. The man appeared ashen and unconscious. He was quickly placed on the stretcher and into the ambulance. The attendant began oxygen as the nurse tried to determine the blood pressure. Vital signs seemed to be absent: no blood pressure, no pulse, no pupil reaction to light, and no pulse in the carotid artery. The oxygen was switched to resuscitation and the nurse began closed cardiac massage. This was continued until the hospital emergency room was reached. The plant doctor was waiting as was the patient's private physician, who had been contacted by the construction company nurse from information on the patient's medical chart. These men worked with the patient for some time, using drugs and the defibrillator twice in an attempt to maintain and increase the faint heart beat. The physicians finally could no longer maintain any response from the heart, and the patient was pronounced dead by his own doctor.

Last year one of the plant mechanics came to the medical department complaining of indigestion. Ordinarily a jovial man, he was extremely quiet and pale. His blood pressure was normal and his pulse very regular. The nurse, however, did not like the appearance he gave. She kept the man in the medical department, sitting down, until she could contact his private physician, who suggested he be brought to his office immediately. Still not trusting the situation, the nurse called the ambulance crew and took the man, lying on the stretcher, to his doctor's office. The doctor was not satisfied with the man's appearance even though he was in no distress. His stretcher was again placed in the ambulance and he was taken to a nearby hospital. Five minutes after he was left at the hospital, the man suffered a massive myocardial infarction, but was close enough to the coronary care unit to be helped immediately.

The man has recovered now and returned to light duty in the plant. His physician told the nurse that without such action on the part of the plant nurse, the man would have expired in the plant before help could be obtained. This was an example of a different type of "first aid" that faces occupational health nurses.

Shipping chemicals by barges created another situation for the medical department about a year ago. A call was received on the ship-to-shore phone stating that one of the crewmen on a tow boat was having a heart attack. Another crewman, a known cardiac, had some nitroglycerin tablets with him and had given one to the stricken man. Other members of the crew had assisted the stricken man to his bunk, but he was having difficulty breathing. The captain was instructed by phone to elevate the man's head and open the windows to give him as much air as possible, then proceed to the plant dock area about a quarter mile from their location. When the boat docked, the ambulance was waiting at the dock. However, one of the barges had to be crossed to get to the tow boat. There was no way to get a stretcher to the man because of the pipes on the barge.

When we arrived in the man's quarters, he was propped up in bed, still having some difficulty breathing and appearing very pale. His blood pressure was slightly elevated and his pulse was slightly irregular. The man kept insisting he could walk, so with the aid of the ambulance crew he was led to the dock side of the barge. Here he was placed on the ambulance stretcher, strapped into place and lifted over the side to the dock below. He was then placed in the ambulance and taken to the hospital coronary unit. He was hospitalized for about three weeks.

Special Problems. Sometimes construction men fall from structures. With these cases, no chance can be taken. The Dr. Greene Safety Litter* is used to lift these men in case there is back damage. Luckily, so far there have been no back fractures, but we cannot afford to take risks.

In a chemical plant, sometimes there are fume releases. Scott Air Paks are used to get the men out of the contaminated areas and to the medical department or the ambulance where Pneolators, free-flow oxygen, and/or resuscitators are available.

Family Problems. Other emergency care consists of talking out problems that arise at the employee's home. Many calls are received from members of an employee's family for advice on what to do for chicken pox, measles, coughing, infected cuts, and, very often, quieting a hysterical mother. One employee's wife drove up to the plant gate one morning with a two-year-old baby and a five-year-old boy. The woman was almost hysterical and was trying to get the patrolman at the gate to find her husband. On quick investigation, the patrolman found that the two-year-old had stepped on a Coca Cola bottle and severely lacerated the bottom of her foot. The baby appeared white and quite limp to the patrolman, and the towel around her foot was soaked with blood. The

*Manufactured by Allendon Industries, P.O. Box 5406, Beaumont, Texas 77706.

patrolman brought the family into the medical department for aid and then returned to locate the father. Both nurses worked with the baby, applying a pressure dressing to the foot to stop the bleeding, making sure the baby was still breathing. When the father came to the medical department, about three or four minutes later, one of the nurses took the baby and the parents to the hospital in the ambulance. Oxygen was given to the baby on the way and by the time the hospital was reached, she had regained consciousness.

Injuries in Nonmanufacturing Industries

Nonmanufacturing sites in industry such as banks, department stores, office settings, etc., have fewer and usually less severe injuries than do the manufacturing industries. The majority of these injuries can be cared for at the work location. However, there are occasions when severe traumatic injuries are sustained: falls down stairways resulting in fractures; digital amputations caused by office machinery; lacerations resulting in severe hemorrhage and extensive tendon damage; crushing injuries due to falling objects (file cabinets, shipping crates, etc.). The occupational health nurse in a nonmanufacturing company may have occasion to see and care for any of these injuries.

Fractures. The immediate care of an obvious fracture is learned in basic first aid. However, what about the nonobvious and/or questionable? A fall down a flight of stairs can result in a fractured vertebra. This may not be so obvious. It is essential that this type of injury be seen immediately by a physician who, hopefully, will do complete radiologic studies to determine the extent of damage. Even with no apparent injury to the back, this employee should be lifted carefully by *two* (at least) or more individuals and placed on a hard, flat surface. Care must be taken to transport this individual as quickly as possible to the proper facility for evaluation of the injury.

Most nonmanufacturing companies, where traumatic injuries are fairly uncommon, rely on local commercial ambulance service when such service is needed. The occupational health nurse, in this situation, is well advised to supervise the lifting and transfer of the injured employee and, whenever possible, to accompany him to the hospital and/or doctor's office. Few commercial ambulance attendants are trained first-aid attendants. Severe and permanent damage can be sustained by the injured person if adequate precautions are not observed during transportation.

Other "nonobvious" fractures are sometimes excused by the injured person as "just a bad sprain." The occupational health nurse may very well insist that this type of injury be checked by a physician, particularly when the accident occurs on the work site. Example: A small, slight-framed, female employee jumped down three steps on a stairway when she felt herself falling. After landing flat on both feet she insisted she was "fine," although she could not bear weight on her left leg. X-ray revealed a linear fracture of the left tibia, and she walked on crutches for three weeks, after having to stay off her feet completely for two weeks.

In this instance, the nurse had to more or less "pull rank" and insist that this employee see a physician, who diagnosed the fracture and prescribed proper care and treatment.

Amputations. Digital amputations can and do occur in the nonmanufacturing industrial setting. Many companies large enough to employ an occupational health nurse and initiate an employee health program also have office machinery on the premises for printing, binding, heavy stapling, cutting, etc. These machines can and do "bite." In most instances, this type of injury is due to improperly used safety devices and/or negligence of the employee-operator.

Excessive bleeding is the major concern in this type of injury and usually digital pressure will control hemorrhage until proper medical attention can be obtained. Use of tourniquets, of course, should be avoided whenever possible. Surprisingly, many experienced operators of such machinery can adequately control their own bleeding until the nurse reaches their work site or they arrive at the health unit. Example: A printing machine operator amputated his left forefinger at the proximal phalanx. Using a piece of rough (but clean) "waste" held tightly over the stump, he calmly walked into the unit stating, "I cut my finger off. Maybe you'd better look at it."

A sterile dressing was placed over the stump and pressure applied at the wrist by the nurse, who accompanied this employee to the doctor's office. It was only at this point that the employee-patient seemed even a little apprehensive because "the end was smashed so I know you can't sew it back on, Doc." The pain was his least concern; disfigurement was much more important.

Crushing Injuries. Crushing injuries are rare, fortunately, in most industries, manufacturing as well as nonmanufacturing. Safety of the employed worker is vital to any profit-making organization, and therefore safety measures are of prime concern to industry. Seldom does a crushing injury in a nonmanufacturing setting result in a fatality as there is very little heavy equipment in such a setting. However, injuries of this nature can be sustained, and the usual cause is carelessness. File cabinets not bolted to wall or floor can topple when two or more drawers are pulled out at the same time. When this occurs, the unfortunate employee can sustain a crushing injury of any part of the body that happens to be caught under the fallen cabinet.

Fractures may occur in such a situation and rib fractures are not uncommon. This type of injury leads readily to apprehension and hysteria, both of which must be controlled at the work site, not only for the victim's welfare, but for that of fellow workers.

Immediate treatment for the victim may consist mostly of reassurance by the nurse. When the nurse is notified, usually by telephone, of such an occurrence, she should take with her to the injury site spirits of ammonia and oxygen. A *portable* oxygen container should be standard equipment in the health unit of any industry. With a few quietly spoken words of reassurance, the nurse can usually assist the injured employee in taking a few deep breaths of oxygen. This serves two purposes: it reassures and quiets the victim and it will definitely indicate to the nurse whether there is damage to the chest. The injured person will certainly tell you if it hurts or causes any discomfort to take that deep breath. The ammonia, of course, can be used in the event of faintness.

Once the extent of possible damage is determined, the nurse again will supervise the transporting of this individual to either the doctor's office or the emergency room of a local hospital. In the event there *appears* to be no injury, the employee should be taken to the health unit and observed for a short period of time. Internal hemorrhage is not uncommon in such instances.

The Use of Drug Therapy. There may be a question in the mind of the reader as to why there is no mention of the use of any drugs in the nonmanufacturing setting for the initial care of the traumatically injured employee. As was mentioned earlier, many occupational health nurses work alone without direct medical supervision. This is especially true in a nonmanufacturing site or office setting. Therefore, emergency care, as outlined above, must be administered without drug therapy, in compliance with state laws and the ethics of professional nursing practice.

CONCLUSIONS

True, much of the occupational health nurse's work is paper work, patching minor scratches and burns, ice-packing and hot-soaking strained ankles, and doing routine physical examinations. But a traumatic accident offers a definite challenge, and it must be met.

REFERENCES

1. Brown, Mary Louise, and Bauer, M. L.: *Occupational Health Nurses: An Initial Survey.* Washington, D.C., U.S. Department of Health, Education and Welfare, Public Health Service, Division of Occupational Health, 1966.
2. *First Aid Training Guide:* API Publication #2017. New York, American Petroleum Institute, 1965.
3. Moyer, C. A.: Progress Report on a New Treatment for Burns. *Medical Tribune,* Weekend Edition, January 8–9, 1966.

11

Working in a
Nonhealth-Oriented Setting

Janice Hitchcock

If primary prevention means working to keep people well, community nurses
may be expected to work frequently outside of health care agencies. But what
kind of activities will this involve and are they considered part of nursing
practice? The community nurse has an increasing responsibility to move into
the community, outside the security of health care institutions, and outside
the defined nurse role. In this capacity the nurse will interact with others
first as a person and second as a health professional. This chapter describes
a legitimate setting for the community nurse, but one that is outside the
usual health care agency.

The recent trend for members of the health professions to focus on more
effective ways to meet the health needs of communities has brought to the forefront a group of people in great need of health care but not identified as
"patients." They are found in many environments but predominantly among
the low-income and minority groups. For years, these people have been largely
alienated from and have lived in ignorance or fear of most community service
agencies. Some have learned the system well enough for use on a crisis basis,
but seldom for what we might term a mental health problem.

As nurses, we are well equipped to develop programs to reach these people.
Our orientation tends toward the kinds of day-to-day issues that concern this
group. More than that of any other discipline, our educational background has
prepared us to work comfortably in homes and a community environment as
well as within the walls of institutions.

If we accept community outreach as necessary to the development of more
effective health services, our community contacts must become much more
numerous and varied. Since the indigenous community organization frequently
has already established a relationship with community members, we must learn
to work through these agencies and their workers to reach the community.

This paper describes one such arrangement wherein I worked as a consultant
in an indigenous Spanish-speaking agency. First, I will briefly describe the
environment in which this experience took place, followed by an account of my
involvement as consultant to the agency, and concluding with an exploration of
the implications for nursing that arose from my consultant experience.

THE AGENCY SETTING

The setting is a community-action project, staffed by indigenous workers, designed to serve the needs of both urban and rural Spanish-speaking people

From *Nursing Clinics of North America*, Vol. 5, No. 2, pp. 251–259, 1970. Reprinted by
permission of the publisher and author.

throughout a mid-California county. Offices are in operation in two locations to accommodate these diverse needs. The statistics gathered by the agency indicate economic and social deprivation and a paucity of marketable skills among the majority of Spanish-speaking persons in this county. These problems tend to alienate them from the larger society, in turn contributing to their inability to communicate with the institutions that exist in the community to meet human needs.

The overall purpose of the agency is to help the Spanish-speaking population develop those abilities necessary to relate effectively to the community institutions. It addresses itself to four major areas of need: (1) interpretation and translation services to help those who are monolingual in Spanish to utilize community resources; (2) education in all areas but with particular emphasis on learning English and maintaining Spanish; (3) development of leadership abilities in the community members; and (4) orientation of the Spanish-speaking community to the availability and utilization of community resources. Services offered to meet these needs include information and referral, advocating the interests and rights of the Spanish-speaking with respect to other agencies, specific services and training programs, and community organization for collective social action in their own behalf.

The staff now consists of a director (A.A. degree in business administration and recent experience as community organizer in a community-action program), an administrative director, two secretaries, seven community workers, and a community organizer assigned to the rural area (all low-income people). Several of the staff members have not completed high school and none has had previous community experience other than incidental volunteering, interpreting, or church-related activities.

In addition to this staff, an important group of people influential to the project is its sponsoring agent — a council made up of representatives of many of the Spanish-speaking organizations within the county. This council is responsible for developing personnel policies and for hiring staff members, but decisions are usually made in conjunction with the recommendations of the director. The council members are nonprofessional people with varying degrees of organizational ability. Most are primarily oriented to and concerned with the problems of the Spanish-speaking community; a few have shown considerable vision with respect to total community involvement.

THE WORK SITUATION

My position as mental health consultant can only be discussed in relation to the events that have led to my present status. Initially, neither the staff nor I was at all clear about what my role should be. What puzzled them (and — I soon found out — other professionals, too) was the fact that I deviated from their stereotype of a nurse. Nurses are expected to work with sick people in a hospital. Since this agency did not deal directly with illness, what could I possibly offer?

I decided at the outset not to force any suggestions on the staff members. It took me a while to cease thinking in terms of "health," which was my orientation and thus the easiest subject for me to talk about. With conscious effort, I followed the leads of staff for conversational topics, only offering my opinions when asked.

The staff was unfamiliar with the intricacies of rendering community service, and they quickly encountered many situations with which they were unprepared to cope. One community worker did not know how to ask her client to control her children so they would not jump around in the car on the way to the health center. Another worker found herself in the midst of a family fight and was asked to take sides. When asked questions particularly related to health and family relationships, the workers felt completely unprepared to respond. I soon discovered the most comfortable way to share my knowledge was during informal conversations in which staff members might just happen to bring up some of their problems. My suggestions offered in conversations were accepted much more readily than they would have been in a more formal situation.

As the staff members became acquainted with me through coffee and dinner exchanges and general office conversation, or when we worked together with a client, they began to ask me for more formal classes.

Since the project had asked for but had not received funds for an inservice trainer, staff training was lacking. By this time the needs of the workers were becoming clearer, and since they were asking for help, inservice training seemed an obvious area for me to develop.

Consultation via Inservice Education

Although teaching seemed a good idea in theory, in practice I felt somewhat unprepared. My teaching experience in the past had been with student nurses and graduate students. Now I must plan classes for a group of highly motivated but uneducated people whose culture was still to a large degree unfamiliar to me. My questions were many. What kinds of materials would be meaningful? What issues should have high priority? Would they accept me as instructor once classes began? I would only know by trying!

I began by planning classes around their expressed concerns — consumer education, sex information, how to talk with clients, and information about other community agencies. A variety of teaching techniques were used. Least effective was the use of films, as few films were current and none dealt with the low-income Spanish-speaking community. It was very difficult for the community workers to apply the ideas expressed in the films, for they didn't believe that the approach depicted could be utilized with their clients. Rather, discussions wherein they could relate their own experiences proved more meaningful.

A very effective approach was to arrange trips to other agencies or have an agency representative come to a meeting with the community worker. Although most of the workers had had personal experiences with many agencies, these had been mostly as clients themselves or when helping another client. They had little knowledge or understanding of the inner functioning of these systems. Now the community workers were expected to negotiate as colleagues with many people in these agencies, and were very uneasy about how to approach them. In many instances, they had prejudices and distortions as well as unpleasant personal experiences that led them to mistrust the establishment with whom they must work.

These field trips helped to dispel many wrong assumptions and offered more accurate information about the agencies. This form of practice teaching was well accepted; abstract ideas and theories were beyond the readiness of the group. At this point, they needed practical solutions and suggestions to help them deal effectively with tangible problems.

Relationship with the Director

My relationship with the community workers was primarily through group inter-action; my association with both the original and present director has been on a one-to-one basis. The first director felt that his needs were of a different type from those of the community workers. He viewed me as helpful to his staff and supported my educational programs but did not at first seek self-consultation with me. Rather than try to force my ideas, I waited for him to ask offhand questions whereupon I endeavored to be available for discussion. Gradually, our relationship became more solid and our conversations lengthened, always con-sisting of a discussion of issues. He seldom solicited direct advice but frequently I found ideas I had previously mentioned were being put into effect, especially those concerning personnel relationships.

A change of directors has necessitated a partial change in my method of oper-ating in the agency. This shift seems related primarily to two main facts — the difference in interests and personalities of the two men, and the shifting priorities of the agency itself. The past director felt competent in administration of the agency rather than inservice education. Since the project was newly formed, this was an appropriate emphasis, encouraging my move into education. Because the new director came into an organization that had become administratively sound, he could channel his energies into other areas. One of his interests was education, so he chose to develop the inservice program himself, using me as a consultant rather than asking me to prepare the actual classes.

This change fitted my immediate needs because I now had less time available to commit to this project. It also harmonized with my philosophy of consultation — to move from a more to a less active role as the consultee is able to work on his own. Had the first director remained, I would have considered a similar move but perhaps over a longer period of time.

Present Consultant Role

With a change of directors, there has been a large turnover in staff since I first began, so my role is constantly undergoing revision, at least as perceived by the staff members. Each new member tends to stereotype me as one who deals with "mental illness." Since most of their clients are not "mentally ill," the community workers see little need for me initially, but gradually they begin to see that I can help with many of their interpersonal problems with clients. Several of the staff members have asked for advice about personal problems also, including one worker whom I see informally in a continuing supportive role.

I felt at first that I should have a clear and precise definition of my role, and thus was not sure what to respond when questioned as to why I was there. But with further thought, I realized that my role would become mutually clear through discussions in which I could show how I could help. The more I was available and showed a willingness to talk with the staff members about their clients or accompany them to a client's home, the more easily they turned to me for consultation. Upon recognizing the process evolving, I ceased to be concerned about my role or how to explain it to others. In addition to meeting with community workers at the office, at times I have gone with them to visit a client. I have found that when they have seen me in action with a client and know that I am aware first-hand of the problems, they subsequently may request discussion.

A Case Example. One community worker, Mr. A., was assigned to Mrs. B., a woman from a South American country who had come to the office seeking help to get a divorce. She complained that her husband was away a great deal because of his work, and when at home, he expected her to wait on him as well as care for their three children and the house. He became angry every time she wanted to go out with friends or do anything independent of his wishes. She claimed she had taken all she could and wanted to get him out of the house and start divorce proceedings.

Because Mr. A. did not believe in divorce, he found it unpleasant to discuss the issue with her and was making every effort to persuade Mrs. B. not to take legal action. During conversation one day, Mr. A. brought up the case and indicated frustration over Mrs. B.'s unwillingness to accept his point of view. He asked if perhaps I could talk with her and help her to see the importance of keeping her family together.

When I asked for more information, I discovered that Mr. A. had not seen Mrs. B.'s husband but suspected that the husband did not know Mrs. B. was planning divorce. I knew that the male was usually the authority in a South American family such as this one, and that it would be highly disruptive to both Mr. B. and the family to proceed without including Mr. B.

I sympathized with Mr. A.'s frustration and suggested that probably little could be accomplished without the inclusion of his client's husband in the discussion. Mr. A. said he recognized the importance of this but had not known how to bring about such a meeting. I agreed to meet with Mr. A. and Mrs. B. to help him arrange such a meeting, if possible. Mr. A. was still primarily interested in saving the family. I intended to use the joint interview to demonstrate techniques of obtaining data about both sides of the issue, and to consider with him alternatives for this family if reconciliation did not seem best.

This situation presented two major areas of learning for the community worker: first, an opportunity to explore his own feelings and to separate them from those of his client; second, a chance to learn more about how to arrange and conduct family meetings and to work with the total family unit when the issue involves all members.

Mrs. B. agreed to meet with us and her husband in their home. Mr. B. was willing to have us come to talk with him. Neither expected anything to be accomplished by this move. As Mrs. B. had predicted, Mr. B. felt his wife should obey him and saw no reason for divorce. She, on the other hand, pointed out that he virtually kept her a prisoner at home and she was learning that it was possible for women in America to be much freer than the customs of their native country had permitted. There was much argument, bitterness and resentment were expressed, and voices were raised in anger most of the time.

As a result of the interview, it became clear that the problem would require professional services beyond the ability of the community worker or the services offered by the agency. I was able to demonstrate the complexity of the problem to Mr. A. and help him to recognize that reconciliation would not be a simple matter, if possible at all. Mr. A., however, was not yet convinced of this, for his own attitudes about the need to preserve marriage clouded his thinking. My attempt to help him consider referral for this family did not take immediate hold because of Mr. A.'s attitude and the paucity of referral agencies for Spanish-speaking clients. Gradually, Mr. A. recognized that his own feelings were preventing him from aiding his client and was able to turn the family over to another worker who began to investigate referral possibilities. During the time he was sorting out his ideas about the case, he was able to ask me for help because he knew I had first-hand knowledge of the situation and he felt that what I had to say would be relevant.

This case example illustrates several points. As a nurse, I felt comfortable working with Mr. A. in the client's home. My background in psychiatric nursing, family therapy, and community health experience helped me to assess the family situation and to use the interview as a demonstration for Mr. A. Had I sat in the office spouting suggestions about how he should proceed, my ideas would not have been accepted by this community worker no matter how valuable they might have been. As a result of the visit, I could use illustrations of family interaction that we had both observed, thus giving authenticity to my observations. He could watch and listen to my interventions in the actual setting rather than only hearing what I might suggest from the sterile environment of the office.

My nursing background has helped me to feel an easiness about dealing with the day-to-day problems of the clients as described by the community workers and a comfortableness about conducting business in the home. These are necessary tools that precede effective consultation. The armamentarium of psychiatric and interpersonal skills may be useless if the personal and actual involvement in client and community worker problems is omitted.

I often bring up client problems to discuss with the worker even though I do not visit or meet the client. After looking at the records, I can ask pertinent questions about areas the workers may have overlooked as they have worked with their clients. My concern is presented as a question regarding a client about whom I'm curious. From the exchange that follows, I can point out similarities to other client situations, or the workers tell me of others to whom the suggestion is applicable.

In addition to my new status as consultant to the inservice program and my continuation as consultant to the community workers about their client concerns, I have also acted as a mediator in staff meetings when the occasion demanded.

Staff meetings were deliberately scheduled at times when I was in the agency. From time to time, there were conflicts between the administration and staff and among the community workers which needed to be resolved through open group discussion. Although not part of the conflict situation, I was accepted as someone knowledgeable about the problem whose opinion could be respected. In this capacity, I acted much as a group leader, using many techniques of family therapy. Many of the relationships were similar to those seen in families, such as the information of coalitions among members, defective communication leading to misunderstood actions, and game playing. My neutral stance helped to reduce tension within the group, thus allowing them to look more objectively at the issues needing to be solved.

A final function has been as consultant to the sponsoring agency. This group of men and women have been given the responsibility of developing agency policy and hiring and firing staff. They are also caught up in many interpersonal and agency conflicts, with very little experience on which to draw. At first I joined in their meetings as an observer. After about four months they began to ask for my opinion. Now they ask for my ideas on given issues and have requested me to be on policy-making committees. As this group learns how to work as administrators, they are also learning a great deal about all relationships and about the larger social world. The knowledge they gain here can be integrated into their life activities and communicated to the larger community.

The trial and error process that has gone on as I have become a part of a new and developing organization has been satisfying. It has been challenging to find new ways to reach the community and learn how to relate to community workers as intermediaries as well as members of the community. This type of work is an exhilarating and stimulating experience which offers many rewards, often from unexpected sources.

IMPLICATIONS FOR NURSING

This experience has illustrated that without ever having to work directly with a labeled patient, the nurse can intervene effectively in promoting health and preventing illness. This kind of involvement, however, raises many issues that must be answered.

Our present modes of relating to the community-at-large are challenged. The concept of meeting the client's need as *he* requests our help, rather than telling him what *we* think he needs, is an approach unfamiliar to most of us. We must spend time learning to understand those with whom we have been working and must consider this an important and necessary part of our working time. We are often so busy giving services that *we* think are needed by others that we do not hear them telling us that the way in which we offer our service makes it irrelevant to their needs.

It has never been proper for a professional relationship to become a personal one. Yet the community, particularly those who have not accepted *our* approaches, are telling us that we must first meet on a person-to-person basis. Only as we become accepted as individuals will our professional skills be given credence and utilized. This approach is alien to our present mode of operation; many of us have forgotten or have never learned how to relate on any basis other than as professional to client. There is much to change in our own relationships.

In working with people who are not familiar with mental health issues, consultation must be coupled with education. But first we must learn what is needed and wanted by the particular group with whom we are working. We cannot assume we know, and expect a group to accept our ideas unquestioningly. The traditional role of a consultant as "one who sits back without comment and listens to a client" is not acceptable to those who are demanding that we be real people rather than shadows hiding behind our professional identities. We must be prepared to function without a defined role or acknowledged profession. The acceptance of such a vague and changing role is being resisted by all professional groups, but is a position which *must be taken.*

To work with the person not labeled as a patient is to move into primary preventive work. Nursing has talked for years about primary prevention but, as with other health disciplines, in practice has continued to focus on more tangible secondary and tertiary prevention. It is more difficult to justify our nursing role in this nebulous world of the nonpatient — one who is not yet and may never be a sick person. But if we really wish to do more than continue simply to put our finger in the dike of the world's ills, we *must* turn our efforts toward reducing the flow of illness rather than repairing those already ill.

CONCLUSIONS

In summary, the role of the nurse must change. She must become involved in her community and community-action activities, as a person first and then as a professional. She must be prepared to modify or relinquish her previously established professional role and become more flexible in her approach to people. Working with the nonpatient will require a larger percentage of her time than does clinic work.

Above all, the nurse must move outside the medical facility and learn to operate in an environment that does not use the medical model. This move may lead to a change in legislation that would allow her greater freedom from traditional medical supervision. Frequently, this relationship is unnecessary.

Finally, it is important that while operating from an independent base, she must do so in cooperation with other disciplines both inside and outside of medicine.

Where will nursing go? What commitment will we make to change? It is up to us to decide. And we should to it with utmost speed!

III

The Expanded Nurse Role and Team Relationships

Changes in patterns of health care delivery and concepts of public health are widening the dimensions of the community nurse's role and functions. If nurses are committed to assisting people maintain a high degree of wellness, they cannot wait until some illness sends people to a physician for diagnosis and treatment. If health care is a right of community members, it becomes a powerful reason to redefine the boundaries of what nurses should be doing. And so, increasingly, community nurses function in primary health care roles. They take responsibility for nursing diagnosis; they are involved in independent and higher level decision making; they assume leadership functions in the health care team.

The expanded role of nursing is not a new concept. It has been evolving for many years and community nurses have been at the forefront of its development. Independent nursing judgment, decision making and physical assessment have been hallmarks of public health nursing practice. However, as health care grows so must the role of the community nurse. Increased scientific knowledge plus the demand for improved quality of health care require expanding the knowledge and skills on which nursing practice is based. This is the challenge faced by community nursing. The chapters that follow present some recent thinking on the nature of this expanding role of community nurses as well as specific examples of such changes.

But the role of community nurses is not expanding in a vacuum. These changes mean that the nurse is now doing things that previously were the sole responsibility of other professionals. New relationships between community nurses and physicians, counselors, social workers and others must be developed. This calls for frequent communication and joint efforts at redefining the roles of all members of the health care team. It also requires a conscious aware-ness of the traditional ways that nurses and other health personnel have worked out their relationships. These traditional roles are often undefined. They are taken for granted as accepted ways of dividing up the work of decision making, diagnosis, treatment and education. The following chapters identify some of these customary team relationships as well as suggesting new directions for nurses and other professionals to work together.

12

Extending the Scope
of Nursing Practice

As nursing roles expand, the changes affect other areas of nursing in ever-widening circles. In 1971 the secretary of Health, Education and Welfare brought together a group of leaders from the nursing and medical professions and from hospital administration and allied health professions to discuss and delineate the new responsibilities and relationships of nurses in expanded roles. This chapter represents the major portion of their report and recommendations. It is an excellent overview of the expanded role of nursing and its relationship to such things as education, legal considerations and team relations.

Over the centuries nursing and medicine have joined in varied but often poorly defined relationships ranging from close collaboration to outright independence. The rapid advance of biomedical knowledge in the last three decades has created much broader horizons for all health professionals and increased expectations for the people they serve. The assumption by nurses of extended responsibilities for patient care makes possible a wider professional opportunity for both professions and clearly implies, and has in fact demonstrated, increased effectiveness and efficiency in the delivery of health services. As such changes take place, however, both nurse and physician feel threatened and are troubled by ambiguities, uncertainties, and misconceptions of their symbiotic roles.

There is growing recognition of the importance of physician-nurse collaboration in extending health care services to meet increasing demand. The nurse is a provider of personal health care services, working interdependently with physicians and others to keep people well and to care for them when they are sick. The role of the nurse cannot remain static; it must change along with that of all other health professionals, which means that the knowledge and skills of nurses need to be broadened. A basic problem is that many nurses are not practicing at their highest potential nor receiving training and experience that would enable them to extend the scope of their practice and thereby extend the availability of health services

While an exhaustive discussion of the scope of nursing could not be encompassed in this brief report, it is essential to survey the extending outlines of professional nursing practice as a prelude to recommendations for extending the role of nursing in the provision of health services.

Nursing practice — that is the provision of nursing services directly to patients*

From *Extending the Scope of Nursing Practice: A Report of the Secretary's Committee to Study Extended Roles for Nurses,* November 1971. United States Department of Health, Education, and Welfare Publication No. (HSM) 73-2037. The full report including preface, appendix and the names of the committee members is available from the U.S. Government Printing Office, Washington, D.C.
*The word "patient" as used in this report means any person, well or sick, who is receiving the services of a professional provider of health care for the purpose of promoting, maintaining, or restoring health, or minimizing the consequences of illness.

and members of their families, may be compartmentalized under three broad headings: primary care, acute care, and long-term care. These categories are not mutually exclusive — a patient may in fact have his initial need for nursing services in connection with long-term care at home or in a medical facility. It is helpful, however, to approach the subject of extending the roles of nurses in terms of the potential for increasing the availability and effectiveness of care in each of the major segments of the delivery system.

Many elements of nursing practice are, of course, common to primary, acute, and long-term care. Among these are: maintaining or restoring normal life functions — respiration, elimination, nutrition, circulation, rest and sleep, locomotion, and communication; observing and reporting signs of actual or potential change in a patient's status; assessing his physical and emotional state and immediate environment; and both formulating and carrying out a plan for the provision of nursing care based on medical regimens, the factors affecting the patient and his family, and the need for integrating the skills and resources of other health personnel.

In order to provide these services as effective members of a health care team, nurses are called upon to carry out an enormously wide range of tasks often under close supervision by a physician, but frequently without such supervision and with the assistance of other health professionals who look to the nurse for guidance.

For example, nurses are responsible for the safe and prudent administration of medicines and the execution of treatments prescribed by physicians. They are responsible for preparing patients for diagnostic procedures, surgery, and other kinds of care and for monitoring the condition of patients. They have a major part in the interpretation of treatment and rehabilitation regimens, in the provision of emergency care, and in the creation of the patient's record.

Nurses in every area of health care are called upon to render effective and appropriate counseling so that patients and their families will know where they may turn for other health-related services, essential elements of comprehensive health care.

In short, the professional nurse is expected to function as a responsible member of a health care team by interpreting and carrying out the instructions of others — chiefly physicians, by collaborating with professional colleagues in the planning and delivery of health services, and by acting independently when the needs of the patient and the standards and principles of nursing practice so warrant.

The present role of nurses covers a span from simple tasks to the most expert professional techniques necessary in acute life-threatening situations. It embraces teaching people about themselves and about how to maintain and promote health. And it affords an opportunity for significant and necessary extension of the part professional nurses can play in making health care accessible to a population whose demands and expectations, and whose acknowledged right to health care, impose an increasingly heavy burden on the present health care delivery system.

The path toward extending roles for nurses is hindered by obstacles of several kinds, some quite real, others of exaggerated significance that must be bridged. To do this will require the collaborative efforts of the various health professions, the schools and centers of health teaching, the public and private institutions and organizations involved in the delivery of care, and the consumers themselves who will gain most from an orderly and effective extension of the roles of professional nurses. There is also an important obligation for the Federal Government, especially the Department of Health, Education, and Welfare, to bring about certain of the changes needed to facilitate extension of these roles.

The Secretary's Committee has arrived at certain conclusions and recommends some broad courses of action as guides to all who seek and have responsibility for achieving improvement in the availability and effectiveness of health care for the American people.

CONCLUSIONS AND RECOMMENDATIONS

There is much concern about the implementation of expanded roles for the nurses: many nurses, graduates of hospital diploma schools, or of associate degree, or baccalaureate programs, are *not* now prepared to assume this expanded role, and some are reluctant to accept it; many believe that present nursing school curricula do not prepare the nurse to function in an expanded role; rising costs of nursing services and the economic rewards for the nursing profession are of concern to many; and still others believe that there are legal barriers which prohibit nurses from assuming expanded roles.

The Committee considered these concerns at length. In accordance with its charge, the following conclusions and recommendations are aimed at those areas which the Committee believes are significant in achieving extended roles for nurses.

Education

Conclusion. Much of the training received by health professionals, including nurses and physicians, neither prepares nurses for extended roles in patient care nor equips their co-workers to collaborate effectively with nurses who are or could be trained to function in an extended role. Barriers that inhibit extension of the scope of nursing and result in a reluctance of physicians to delegate significant responsibilities and of nurses to accept them, must be bridged through education and training.

Recommendation. Health education centers should undertake curricular innovations that demonstrate the physician-nurse team concept in the delivery of care in a variety of settings under conditions that provide optimum opportunity for both professions to seek the highest levels of competence. Financial support should be made available for programs of continuing nurse education that could prepare the present pool of over one million active and inactive nurses to function in extended roles. The continuing education of nurses should be structured to encourage professional advancement among and through all nursing education programs and to encourage the use of equivalency examinations to evaluate competence, knowledge, and experience.

Legal Considerations

Conclusion. State licensure laws affecting nursing present no perceived obstacles to extending roles for nursing as envisioned in this report. Medical and nursing services are complementary but they are not interchangeable either in authority or accountability. An orderly transfer of responsibilities between medicine and nursing has proceeded over many years and there is no reason to assume that questions of law might impede this process.

Recommendation. Increased attention should be paid to the commonality of nursing licensure and certification and to the development and acceptance of a model law of nursing practice suitable for national application through the states. The nursing profession should undertake a thorough study of recertification as a possible means of documenting new or changed skills among practicing nurses.

INTERPROFESSIONAL RELATIONSHIPS
BETWEEN PHYSICIANS AND NURSES

Conclusion. An extension of nursing practice will be realized only as physicians and nurses collaborate to achieve this objective. Expanded roles for nurses will require major adjustments in the orientation and practice of both professions. A redefinition of the functional interaction of medicine and nursing is essential; it must be couched in terms of their respective roles in the provision of health services rather than in terms of professional boundaries and rigid lines of responsibility. While the formal educational process will necessarily be a prime vehicle for formulating and inculcating a new definition of the interaction of medicine and nursing, the critical test of any such concept will come in its practical application.

Recommendation. Collaborative efforts involving schools of medicine and nursing should be encouraged to undertake programs to demonstrate effective functional interaction of physicians and nurses in the provision of health services and the extension of those services to the widest possible range of the population. The transfer of functions and responsibilities between physicians and nurses should be sought through an orderly process recognizing the capacity and desire of both professions to participate in additional training activities intended to augment the potential scope of nursing practice. A determined and continuing effort should be made to attain a high degree of flexibility in the interprofessional relationships of physicians and nurses. Jurisdictional concerns *per se* should not be permitted to interfere with efforts to meet patient needs.

Impact on Health Care Delivery

Conclusion. A fundamental extension of the scope of nursing practice will have a profound impact on the health care delivery system sensitive not only to health providers but to consumers as well. To the extent that nurses are able and encouraged to accept a greater share of responsibility for the provision of health services, they will contribute to a corresponding increase in the ability of physicians and other health professionals to meet the demands upon them. While it is reasonable to assume that nurses who function in extended roles will be able to command more earnings than their more narrowly utilized colleagues, this shift should not represent an inflationary factor since it would reflect increased productivity for the entire health care system.

Recommendation. Cost-benefit analyses and similar economic studies should be undertaken in a variety of geographic and institutional settings to assess the impact on the health care delivery system of extended nursing practice.* Toward the same objective, attitudinal surveys of health care providers and consumers should be conducted to assess the significance of factors that might affect the acceptance of nurses in extended care roles which they do not now normally occupy.

EXTENDED ROLES FOR NURSES

To attempt a definitive statement on the nature and scope of extended roles for nurses would go beyond the function of the Committee and, moreover, may not even be possible. Professional nursing, as suggested here and elsewhere, is in a period of rapid and progressive change in response to the growth of biomedical knowledge, changes in patterns of demand for health services, and the evolution of professional relationships among nurses, physicians, and other health professions.

The following pages represent the Committee's attempt to delineate elements of nursing practice in primary, acute, and long-term care and to indicate, for purposes of illustration, those elements for which nurses now generally have primary responsibility, those for which responsibility is exercised by either physicians or nurses or by a member of one of the allied health professions, and those responsibilities that generally fall outside the practice of nurses who are not now utilized or prepared to practice in extended roles as envisioned by the Committee. The groupings in each of these categories are by no means all-inclusive.

* The appendix to this paper lists more than 30 locations in which nurses are being prepared for or are practicing in extended roles.

... In Primary Care

One of the most important opportunities for change in the current system of health care involves altering the practice of nurses and physicians so that nurses assume considerably greater responsibility for delivering primary health care services. *The term Primary Care as used in this paper has two dimensions: (a) a person's first contact in any given episode of illness with the health care system that leads to a decision of what must be done to help resolve his problem; and (b) the responsibility for the continuum of care, i.e., maintenance of health, evaluation and management of symptoms, and appropriate referrals.*

In present practice the utilization of nurses varies extensively. Some are responsible for institutional areas of management and communication, such as inventory and supply, making requisitions for laboratory and other diagnostic and treatment services, routine charting and managing the flow of charts, and making appointments. A study reported by Yankauer, Connelly, and Feldman (*Pediatrics* 45:No. 3, Part II, March 1970) reveals that in pediatric practices nurses engage primarily in technical and clerical tasks along with such patient care activities as giving minor medical advice and information and interpreting instructions.

In contrast, nurses in public health agencies have traditionally functioned relatively independently, but with physician collaboration, in patients' homes, in remote, isolated rural and ghetto areas, and more recently in clinics, hospitals, and community care centers where they have: assessed problems of individuals and families; treated minor illnesses; referred patients for differential medical diagnosis; arranged for referrals to social service agencies and organizations; given advice and counsel to promote health and prevent illness; supervised health regimens of normal pregnant women and of children; and worked with health-related community action programs. Such functions, however, have not been institutionalized by common agreement of nurses and physicians or by medical and nursing educators.

As health care becomes increasingly valued in our society, nurses will be expected to take more responsibility for the delivery of primary health and nursing care, for coordinating preventive services, for initiating or participating in diagnostic screening, and for referring patients who require differential medical diagnoses and medical therapies.

*Primary Care Functions for Which Many Nurses
Are Now Generally Responsible:*

Case finding and medical referral. These activities usually are carried out by nurses who function in patients' homes, in community clinics, in schools, and in industrial settings. Identification of ills, actual and impending, is expected of all nurses.

Case finding and social agency referral. Generally this function is carried out in patients' homes, in community clinics, in schools, and in industry, although hospital nurses increasingly assess social and economic circumstances of patients and seek to prevent problems and complications that are related to social and economic factors.

Primary Care Functions for Which Nurses and
Physicians Share Responsibility:
Health surveillance of pregnant and postpartum women, well babies and children, patients discharged from therapeutic regimens, homebound invalids, and persons in rest and nursing homes.
Identification of the need for, and assisting in the planning and implementation of, changes in living arrangements affecting the health of individuals.
Evaluation of deviations from "normal" in patients who present themselves for treatment.
Assessment of the responses of patients to illness and of their compliance with and response to prescribed treatment.
Performance of selected diagnostic and therapeutic procedures, e.g., laboratory tests, wound care.
Prescription of modifications needed by patients coping with illness or maintaining health, such as in diet, exercise, relief from pain, and adaptation to handicaps or impairments.
Making referrals to appropriate agencies.

Primary Care Functions for Which Many Nurses
Are Now Prepared and Others Could Be Prepared:
Routine assessment of the health status of individuals and families.
Institution of care during normal pregnancies and normal deliveries, provision of family planning services, and supervision of health care of normal children.
Management of care for selected patients within protocols mutually agreed upon by nursing and medical personnel, including prescribing and providing care and making referrals as appropriate.
Screening patients having problems requiring differential medical diagnosis and medical therapy. The recommendation resulting from such screening activities is based on data gathered and evaluated jointly by physicians and nurses.
Consultation and collaboration with physicians, other health professionals, and the public in planning and instituting health care programs.

Assumption of these responsibilities requires that nurses so engaged have knowledge and requisite skills for:
Eliciting and recording a health history;
Making physical and psychosocial assessments, recognizing the range of "normal" and the manifestations of common abnormalities;
Assessing family relationships and home, school, and work environments;
Interpreting selected laboratory findings;

Making diagnoses, choosing, initiating, and modifying selected therapies;
Assessing community resources and needs for health care;
Providing emergency treatment as appropriate, such as in cardiac arrest, shock,
   or hemorrhage; and
Providing appropriate information to the patient and his family about a diagnosis
   or plan of therapy.

...In Acute Care

The role of the nurse in acute care is in many ways more clearly defined than it
is in other areas of health care. *Acute care consists of those services that treat
the acute phase of illness or disability and has as its purpose the restoration of
normal life processes and functions.* The nurse's role in acute care has, by tradition, been somewhat restrictive in many clinical settings, perhaps by virtue of
the fact that the physician is recognized as the chief health care practitioner in
these settings. It should be anticipated that nurses, and head nurses in particular,
will become increasingly free of managerial functions. This will provide opportunity for nurses to assume added responsibility for the clinical management
of patients.

Acute Care Functions for Which Nurses
Are Now Generally Responsible:
Recognizing "cue complexes" or syndromes — such as pulmonary embolism,
   acute renal failure, insulin shock, and hemorrhage — and the making of
   clinical inferences.
Provision of emergency treatment as appropriate, e.g., in cardiac arrest, shock,
   hemorrhage, convulsions, and poisoning.
Provision of appropriate information to the patient and his family about diagnosis or plan of therapy following physician-nurse appraisal.

Acute Care Functions for Which Nurses
and Physicians Share Responsibility:
   Such responsibilities are now being shared in some settings on the basis of
mutually agreed upon protocols by physicians and nurses:
Carrying out selected diagnostic and therapeutic procedures and interpreting
   information such as biochemical reports.
Translating research findings into practice, e.g., previous research conclusions
   concerning the causes of postcardiotomy delirium can be used to minimize
   sensory monotony and sleep deprivation in intensive care units.

Acute Care Functions for Which Many Nurses Are
Now Prepared and Others Could Be Prepared:
Securing and recording a health and developmental history and making a crit-
   ical evaluation of such records as an adjunct to planning and carrying out a

health care regimen in collaboration with medical and other health professionals.

Performing basic physical and psychosocial assessments and translating the findings into appropriate nursing actions.

Discriminating between normal and abnormal findings on physical and psychosocial assessments and reporting findings when appropriate.

Making prospective decisions about treatment in collaboration with physicians, e.g., prescribing symptomatic treatment for coryza, pain, headache, nausea, etc.

Initiating actions within a protocol developed by medical and nursing personnel, such as making adjustments in medication, ordering and interpreting certain laboratory tests, and prescribing certain rehabilitative and restorative measures. Two examples of these actions are: (1) a coronary care nurse recognizes sino-atrial arrest or block, discontinues the maintenance dose of digitalis according to standing orders, notifies the physician, and prepares to assist with such measures as transvenous pacing or Isoproterenol drug therapy, and (2) a nurse administers postural drainage, clapping, and vibrating as a part of the treatment cycle for patients with chronic pulmonary problems caused by bronchiectasis, emphysema, or fibrocystic disease.

...In Long-Term Care

The increasing numbers of people affected by long-term illness make it imperative to reshape and extend the roles of physicians and nurses in providing for their care. Nurses involved in long-term care often function at less than the level for which they are prepared and less effectively than society has a right to expect. As nurses assume broadened responsibility for continuing care of the chronically ill in all age groups, we can expect positive changes in this increasingly important area of health care.

Long-term care consists of those services designed to provide symptomatic treatment, maintenance, and rehabilitative services for patients of all age groups in a variety of health care settings. Provision of this care should be the result of mutual agreement between medical and nursing staffs, and should be based upon the needs and resources of the patient and the readiness of the family to participate in the plan of care.

Many experimental efforts relating to extended roles of the nurse are now in progress (see appendix). It is likely that all of the activities described below are now being practiced in a few settings. Their relative rarity, however, warrants pointing to them as areas in which nurses discharge or could be prepared to assume further responsibility.

The nurse's responsibility in long-term care varies greatly according to the practice setting, the viewpoints of both physicians and nurses, the educational preparation of the nurse, and the extent of her competence and experience.

Long-Term Care Functions for Which Nurses
Are Now Generally Responsible:

Giving treatments, rehabilitative exercises, and medications as prescribed by the physician.

Teaching the patient, members of his family, or both to give treatments or medications when indicated.

Teaching patients and family members to carry out the medical plan for special diet, taking into consideration cultural background, personal preferences, and financial status.

Observing and evaluating patients' physical and emotional condition and reaction to drugs or treatments.

Calling new signs or symptoms to the attention of the physician and arranging for medical attention when the patient's condition appears to warrant it.

Recommending appropriate measures regarding physical and social factors in the environment that affect patient care.

Instituting immediate life-saving measures in the absence of a physician.

Assisting the patient and family to identify resources which will be helpful in maintaining him in the best possible state of health.

Long-Term Functions for Which Nurses
and Physicians Share Responsibility:

Making necessary changes in a treatment plan in light of changes of the patient's physical or emotional tolerance and in accordance with an established treatment plan.

Giving families information and encouragement which may help them to adopt attitudes and practices that promote health and reduce anxiety, tension, and fatigue.

Providing continuous health guidance for mentally ill patients and their families until all practicable rehabilitation of patient and family has been achieved with a joint decision of therapists involved.

Making appropriate referral for continuity of care.

Long-Term Care Functions for Which Many Nurses
Are Now Prepared and Others Could Be Prepared:

Assessing physical status of patients at a more sophisticated level than is now common in nursing practice.

Securing and maintaining a health history.

Within protocols mutually agreed upon by medical and nursing staff — make adjustments in medications; initiate requests for certain laboratory tests and interpret them; make judgments about the use of accepted pharmaceutical agents as standard treatments in diagnosed conditions; assume primary responsibility for determining possible alternative for care settings (institution or home) and for initiating referral.

Conducting nurse clinics for continuing care of selected patients.

Conducting community clinics for case findings and screening for health problems.

Assessing community needs in long-term care and participating in the development of resources to meet them.

Assuming continuing responsibility for acquainting selected patients and families with implications of health status, treatment, and prognosis.

Assuming responsibility for the environment of the care setting as it affects the quality and effectiveness of care.

13

An Approach to Role Expansion — The Elaborate Network

Margaret L. Shetland

Expanding the community nurse's role requires readjustments not only for the nurse but also for physicians, other health professionals and patients. The change contributes to new role definitions, perceptions and utilization by all persons involved. Dr. Shetland uses role theory to explore the problems this change creates and proposes strategies that nurses can employ to effect successful role expansion.

One of the inevitable concomitants of social change is disequilibrium among the various groups contributing to the organization and workings of the system undergoing change. As knowledge increases and values shift, stronger forces emerge which require drastic accommodations in the organization of social structure. The significance of its consequent modification of role is generally oversimplified among those contributing to the delivery of health services. Structure and function are defined by the system and are frequently based upon cultural role rather than individual or group competencies. It is the purpose of this paper to present a descriptive model of role expansion as a function of social change and to present some strategies for effecting change within the system.

In developing my model I wish to differentiate among operational definitions of activity, function, and role. Dictionaries provide little clarification of the differences I wish to advance, but with a reasonable amount of liberty it is justifiable to assign differential definitions for the purpose of this discussion. *Activity* can be defined as a single action or pursuit. *Function,* then, can be thought of as a set of normal characteristic actions. *Role* is more complex deriving from its original use in relation to a character or a part performed by an actor in a drama. Although somewhat specified, role allows enough latitude to allow individual interpretation by each actor. One of the barriers interfering with role expansion of any group within a system derives from the tendency to use activity, function, and role interchangeably. It seems obvious that transferring an activity from one group to another, or even modifying functions is much less complex than the disequilibrium inherent in role expansion of any group within a social system. When the social system has as its purpose services to society, the adjustments and accommodations are enormously increased, as are the numbers of social groups and individuals involved in the process, since the recipients of the services as well as those providing the service also contribute to the role definition and perception.

At this point further exploration of role theory may be useful. The following

From *American Journal of Public Health,* Vol. 61, No. 10, pp. 1959–1964, 1971. Reprinted by permission of the publisher and the author.

definitions and concepts are based upon those presented in Sargent's *Social Psychology*.[1]

Social scientists use the term "role" in a variety of ways, depending upon their particular orientation. For example, "role" or "social role" is frequently used by social psychologists although with some disagreement as to its precise definition, function, and scope. In general, however, they use "role" to refer to social functioning of individuals in the group or larger society which may be considered a phase of personality in the sense that a person learns his social roles as he learns other habits. Group members occupy positions implying roles, whether these are formally prescribed or merely implied. Sex, occupational, or other roles assigned to groups imply decision-making privileges. Nursing in a sense is in a position of double jeopardy because it is predominantly female.

Anthropologists speak of roles in describing behavior of persons belonging to different age, sex, and occupational groups. In this context, role is defined by Linton as the dynamic aspect of status, a special position in society involving the rights and duties constituting particular status.[2]

These views of role are, indeed, multifaceted bringing out many variations. Particularly significant for the purpose of this paper is the distinction between assigned and achieved roles; those assigned by society and those achieved by an individual or group. Ascribed roles tend to pertain to age, sex, or class status. Parsons' conception has great significance as we consider expanded roles for nursing within the health care system. He views the social system as a pattern of institutionalized roles through which varied human potentialities "dovetail into a single integrated system capable of meeting the situational exigencies with which society and its members are faced."[3]

Becker, in dealing with the nature of professions, suggests a sociological view which regards professions "which have been fortunate enough in the politics of today's world to gain and maintain possession of that honorific title."[4] This view insists that profession is not a scientific concept, but rather what Turner has called a "folk concept."[5] The symbol of professional autonomy conferred upon medicine may not, as it implies, invest the profession with a monopoly over the total health care system and all of the related knowledge acquired by research and logical analysis. The fact is that the professional role assigned to medicine by society, supported by legal and other institutional panoply, (and unquestioned by many members of the profession) constitutes a formidable barrier to role expansion by other health occupations.

By this time the enormous complexity of role change requiring significant perceptual and set changes by many groups within the health care system is obvious. The health care system with its monolithic structure monopolized by one profession, generally oriented in its education and its practice to care of acutely ill hospitalized individuals, is not entirely the result of the self-perception of organized medicine, but is supported by society itself although increasingly less firmly. The system in general as well as the medical profession fails to recognize and reward disciplines other than medicine which responds by seeing the competencies of other disciplines as extensions of medicine, encompassed and limited by medical knowledge. An obvious evidence of this is the tendency — even within such agencies as comprehensive health planning — to use health care and medical care interchangeably. The concept of health care in the true sense of encompassing preventive measures, promotion of health, economics of health care, community and family planning for health promotion and maintenance requires the knowledge and talents of several disciplines, knowledge and talents that are not usually possessed by the practitioners of medicine since they are not formalized within their educational system. Obvious to us, this fact is not recognized by the public any more than it is by organized medicine. An amusing encounter with an appropriations committee of a state senate illustrates this point. An attempt was being made to demonstrate that medicine, although extremely important, is only one of the many disciplines required to deal with the health needs of the people. "Do you mean nurses have knowledge and skills physicians do not possess?" (This in incredulous tones.)

"Yes!"

"Do you mean that physicians are not knowledgeable?"

"No, I am saying that health care is enormously complex, that no one discipline can possibly have all of the knowledge needed to deal with all of the problems." This was followed by illustrations of competencies and contributions of several disciplines, including nursing.

"Oh, I think I understand that nurses have different knowledge and skill, but did you say pharmacists know something physicians do not?"

"Yes."

And again, "Well, did you say that physicians are not knowledgeable?"

"No!" More illustrations requiring a painful readjustment of the concept of the all-knowing father figure followed.

Nurses attempting to meet health and sickness needs of the people find that it is not difficult to add new activities or even functions when these are subordinated to medical approval, especially when the recipients are those disadvantaged by poverty or geography. The point of conflict arises when nurses insist upon using their knowledge and competencies in mature and responsible decision-making. Anxiety, frustration, denial, and withdrawal are inevitable when authority derives from cultural role rather than knowledge and competence. Because the role group — medicine — defines its own values in a system, interrole transactions are not encouraged and sometimes not allowed. Various medical groups are presently engaged in redefining the nurse role — with or without nursing collaboration. Doctor Gershenson, Acting Director, Research Division, Maternal and Child Health Service, Health Services and Mental Health Administration, Public Health Service, has this to say.

> But everybody wants to meet the health manpower shortages by redesigning the role of the nurse. The pediatrician wants to use and train her for his needs.... The role of the nurse is the battleground for job definition within the health delivery system.[6]

The American Medical Association's Committee on Nursing Position Paper, "Medicine and Nursing in the 1970s," illustrates a positive effort on the part of organized medicine to deal with health manpower shortages. But the failure to recognize a broader role for nurses is obvious. Objective 2 is supported by the statement: "Professional nurses, by the nature of their education, are equipped to assume greater medical service responsibility under the supervision of physicians."[7] The "expanded" role is to be achieved by "translating medical services into nursing functions."[8] The objective on nursing education ignores all of the forces that have been at work over the last several years and which change not only nursing, but all types of education. I shall not recount these forces here — all of you are aware of them. The point is that this group feels itself competent to make judgments, revealing colossal ignorance in supporting what is being demonstrated as an anachronistic system. The paper also reveals the preoccupation of the writers with hospital care of acutely ill patients. It is essential that steps be taken by both medical and nursing organizations to achieve a joint position which recognizes nursing as a responsible, mature profession and which also recognizes that no one profession, no matter how well-meaning, has the right to make unilateral judgments out of its own area of competency. Nurses operating within the system in which one role group defines and limits the role of all other participants find themselves blocked in their attempts to perform in a manner consistent with their own role expectations.

Another strong force influencing nurse role is described by Kramer in a recent issue of *Nursing Research* in which she deals with effects of professional-bureaucratic conflict on graduates of baccalaureate programs in nursing.[9] Studies are cited that indicate higher susceptibility to role deprivation among graduates of these programs than among graduates of diploma programs. The researchers explain this finding in terms of the level of professional role conception. The bureaucratic structure with its division of patient care into component tasks with its hierarchal control structure is in conflict with the internalized norms and ethics promulgated by the professional system. The conflict between professional and bureaucratic systems is obviously not unique to nurses, but is experienced by other occupational groups. In some instances physicians are exposed, although they tend to maintain control over the bureaucracy through hospital staff organizations and other mechanisms.

Another barrier to role fulfillment by nurses is the position of multiple subordination occupied by nurse practitioners within the bureaucracy. Nurses themselves contribute to this limiting of other nurses through their own hierarchal supervisory system which tends to deny professional judgment to the practitioner. In a course I once taught in public health nursing administration, we dramatized the dilemma of multiple subordination by attempting to draw on a blackboard the individuals who by their positions were empowered to give orders to a staff public health nurse. Our blackboard was too small. It is no wonder that nurses should respond in terms of their own preservation and choose the alternatives that make them the least anxious. The recipient of patient care seldom holds the threat inherent in the other actors in this drama. Nurses' notes show where nurses give up, as does the retreat to the desk and the equipment.

Another barrier to role satisfaction — expanded or otherwise — lies in the questionable validity of role expectations as presented to nursing students. Nursing must learn to limit its claims in terms of reality and reasonable expectations. Students are imbued with the notion that they can, in a four-year program, acquire a broad and specific set of knowledge and competencies probably beyond the attainment of any one human being in a lifetime. They are expected to be knowledgeable about nutrition, child guidance, marital and spiritual counseling, physiology, psychology, anthropology, and more besides. In addition, they are expected to achieve the aims of general education in culture and personal development — and, of course, good citizenship plus the arts. They usually are told in the schools that they will need to perfect the more technical nursing skills in practice, but find themselves in conflict with employer's expectations. Then they are told to be "change agents" which places an unbearable burden on the young and inexperienced to achieve a goal in which their elders have failed. In public health we go even further by labeling individuals who lack preparation as public health nurses and sending them out with the symbolic paraphernalia. Then we wonder why the public and our colleagues in other disciplines have some difficulty in recognizing what public health nursing is. Professional nursing must face the reality that few people — those served and colleagues — have experienced the type of nursing we envision.

I am convinced that the health care system is in need of the contribution that can be made by professional nurses. "Expanded," or, as I would prefer to think of it, "new" role is a part of this. We have heard and will hear more about new roles requiring a higher level of decision-making. But I am also convinced that we must validate the more general role for professional nursing by less global claims, by assuring preparation consistent with the claims, and by restructuring the system so that the practitioners are able to function in a manner consistent with their role expectations.

Another strategy that nurses could employ in order to effect the changes in role modification needed to provide necessary health care is the abandonment of the doctor-nurse game. Doctor Leonard Stein, in describing the maneuvers familiar to all of us in this elaborate game, has this to say:

> The major disadvantage of a doctor-nurse-like game is its inhibitory effect on open dialogue which is stifling and anti-intellectual. The game is basically a transactional neurosis, and both professions would enhance themselves by taking steps to change the attitudes which breed the game.[10]

Until nurses can learn to view themselves as responsible, mature professionals with a significant identifiable contribution to make, others will not view them as such. Defensiveness regarding territorial or jurisdictional rights has no place for nurses or for physicians if the health care system is to be reformed.

The problem of changes in role which affect deeply valued privileges of one group, which seem to be threatened when another group claims similar privileges, cannot be solved by directing hostility against each other. In discussing the problems of inclusion of the American Negro into full citizenship, Parsons identifies some of the same forces which operate in the health care system. He points out that we have been "witnessing major steps in the extension and consolidation of the societal community."[11] A significant observation is the fact that "By being included in larger community structure, the individual does not cease to be a member of smaller ones, but the latter must relinquish certain of the controls over him which they previously exercised . . . the basic demands for full inclusion, not for domination or for equality on the basis of separateness."[12] There are indications that medicine, at least physicians in significant numbers, are also thinking in terms of involvement of other disciplines based upon health care needed and diverse competencies.

It is up to nurses to continue to constantly reappraise the congruity between the health needs of the people and their legitimate contributions. Successful strategies for role expansion must be based on analysis of changing health needs and firmly backed by demonstrations of the effectiveness of new role in dealing with the needs.

REFERENCES

1. Sargent, S. Stanfeld, and Williamson, Robert C. *Social Psychology*. 3rd ed. New York: The Ronald Press Company, 1966.
2. Ibid., p. 384, citing Linton, R. *The Study of Man*. New York: D. Appleton-Century Company, Inc., 1936, pp. 113—14.
3. Ibid., citing Parsons, Talcott. "Systematic Theory in Sociology." *Essays in Sociological Theory*. New York: The Free Press, 1949, p. 35.
4. Henry, Nelson B., ed. *Education for the Professions*. Chicago: The National Society for the Study of Education, 1962, p. 33.
5. Ibid., citing Turner, Ralph H. "The Normative Coherence of Folk Concepts." Research Studies of State College of Washington, 25:127—136, 1957.
6. Gershenson, Charles. "Trends in Health Care: An Interview." *Maternal and Child Health Information*, 4:2 (Mar., 1970).
7. Committee on Nursing, AMA. "Medicine and Nursing in the 1970s: A Position Statement." *J.A.M.A.*, 213,11:1181—83 (Sept., 1970).
8. Ibid.
9. Kramer, Marlene. "Role Conceptions of Baccalaureate Nurses and Success in Hospital Nursing." *Nursing Research*, 19,5:428—439 (Sept.-Oct., 1970).
10. Stein, Leonard I. "The Doctor-Nurse Game." *Arch. Gen. Psych.* 16:699—703 (June, 1967).
11. Parsons, Talcott. *Politics and Social Structure*. New York: The Free Press, 1966, p. 280.
12. Ibid.

14

The Doctor-Nurse Game

Leonard I. Stein

Although the following description of nurse-physician relationships is more typical of the past than the present, many vestiges of the "game" still remain. Community nurses often find it difficult to communicate directly with physicians about patients the nurse sees at home. The physician may not be willing to accept diagnostic statements and recommendations from a nurse, or the nurse may be fearful of making them. If the expanded nurse role is to become a reality and patients more effectively served, such inhibited dialogue must cease. Leonard Stein describes the reasons behind this behavior and challenges both professions to reexamine their roles and move toward a system of open communication.

The relationship between the doctor and the nurse is a very special one. There are few professions where the degree of mutual respect and cooperation between co-workers is as intense as that between the doctor and nurse. Superficially, the stereotype of this relationship has been dramatized in many novels and television serials. When, however, it is observed carefully in an interactional framework, the relationship takes on a new dimension and has a special quality which fits a game model. The underlying attitudes which demand that this game be played are unfortunate. These attitudes create serious obstacles in the path of meaningful communications between physicians and nonmedical professional groups.

The physician traditionally and appropriately has total responsibility for making the decisions regarding the management of his patients' treatment. To guide his decisions he considers data gleaned from several sources. He acquires a complete medical history, performs a thorough physical examination, interprets laboratory findings, and at times, obtains recommendations from physician-consultants. Another important factor in his decision-making are the recommendations he receives from the nurse. The interaction between doctor and nurse through which these recommendations are communicated and received is unique and interesting.

THE GAME

One rarely hears a nurse say, "Doctor I would recommend that you order a retention enema for Mrs. Brown." A physician, upon hearing a recommendation of that nature, would gape in amazement at the effrontery of the nurse. The nurse, upon hearing the statement, would look over her shoulder to see who said it, hardly believing the words actually came from her own mouth. Nevertheless,

From *Archives of General Psychiatry*, Vol. 16, pp. 699–703, June 1967. Copyright © 1967, American Medical Association. Reprinted by permission of the publisher and the author.

if one observes closely, nurses make recommendations of more import every hour and physicians willingly and respectfully consider them. If the nurse is to make a suggestion without appearing insolent and the doctor is to seriously consider that suggestion, their interaction must not violate the rules of the game.

Object of the Game

The object of the game is as follows: the nurse is to be bold, have initiative, and be responsible for making significant recommendations, while at the same time she must appear passive. This must be done in such a manner so as to make her recommendations appear to be initiated by the physician.

Both participants must be acutely sensitive to each other's nonverbal and cryptic verbal communications. A slight lowering of the head, a minor shifting of position in the chair, or a seemingly nonrelevant comment concerning an event which occurred eight months ago must be interpreted as a powerful message. The game requires the nimbleness of a high wire acrobat, and if either participant slips the game can be shattered; the penalties for frequent failure are apt to be severe.

Rules of the Game

The cardinal rule of the game is that open disagreement between the players must be avoided at all costs. Thus, the nurse must communicate her recommendations without appearing to be making a recommendation statement. The physician, in requesting a recommendation from a nurse, must do so without appearing to be asking for it. Utilization of this technique keeps anyone from committing themselves to a position before a sub rosa agreement on that position has already been established. In that way open disagreement is avoided. The greater the significance of the recommendation, the more subtly the game must be played.

To convey a subtle example of the game with all its nuances would require the talents of a literary artist. Lacking these talents, let me give you the following example which is unsubtle, but happens frequently. The medical resident on hospital call is awakened by telephone at 1:00 a.m. because a patient on a ward, not his own, has not been able to fall asleep. Dr. Jones answers the telephone and the dialogue goes like this:

This is Dr. Jones.
(An open and direct communication.)
Dr. Jones, this is Miss Smith on 2W — Mrs. Brown, who learned today of her father's death, is unable to fall asleep.
(This message has two levels. Openly, it describes a set of circumstances, a woman who is unable to sleep and who that morning received word of her father's death. Less openly, but just as directly, it is a diagnostic and recommendation statement; i.e., Mrs. Brown is unable to sleep because of her grief, and she should be given a sedative. Dr. Jones, accepting the diagnostic statement and replying to the recommendation statement, answers.)
What sleeping medication has been helpful to Mrs. Brown in the past?
(Dr. Jones, not knowing the patient, is asking for a recommendation from the nurse, who does know the patient, about what sleeping medication should be prescribed. Note,

however, his question does not appear to be asking her for a recommendation. Miss Smith replies.)

Pentobarbital mg 100 was quite effective night before last.

(A disguised recommendation statement. Dr. Jones replies with a note of authority in his voice.)

Pentobarbital mg 100 before bedtime as needed for sleep; got it?

(Miss Smith ends the conversation with the tone of a grateful supplicant.)

Yes, I have, and thank you very much, doctor.

The above is an example of a successfully played doctor-nurse game. The nurse made appropriate recommendations which were accepted by the physician and were helpful to the patient. The game was successful because the cardinal rule was not violated. The nurse was able to make her recommendation without appearing to, and the physician was able to ask for recommendations without conspicuously asking for them.

The Scoring System

Inherent in any game are penalties and rewards for the players. In game theory, the doctor-nurse game fits the nonzero sum game model. It is not like chess, where the players compete with each other and whatever one player loses the other wins. Rather, it is the kind of game in which the rewards and punishments are shared by both players. If they play the game successfully they both win rewards, and if they are unskilled and the game is played badly, they both suffer the penalty.

The most obvious reward from the well-played game is a doctor-nurse team that operates efficiently. The physician is able to utilize the nurse as a valuable consultant, and the nurse gains self-esteem and professional satisfaction from her job. The less obvious rewards are no less important. A successful game creates a doctor-nurse alliance; through this alliance the physician gains the respect and admiration of the nursing service. He can be confident that his nursing staff will smooth the path for getting his work done. His charts will be organized and waiting for him when he arrives, the ruffled feathers of patients and relatives will have been smoothed down, and his pet routines will be happily followed, and he will be helped in a thousand and one other ways.

The doctor-nurse alliance sheds its light on the nurse as well. She gains a reputation for being a "damn good nurse." She is respected by everyone and appropriately enjoys her position. When physicians discuss the nursing staff it would not be unusual for her name to be mentioned with respect and admiration. Their esteem for a good nurse is no less than their esteem for a good doctor.

The penalties for a game failure, on the other hand, can be severe. The physician who is an unskilled gamesman and fails to recognize the nurses' subtle recommendation messages is tolerated as a "clod." If, however, he interprets these messages as insolence and strongly indicates he does not wish to tolerate suggestions from nurses, he creates a rocky path for his travels. The old truism "If the nurse is your ally you've got it made, and if she has it in for you, be prepared for misery" takes on life-sized proportions. He receives three times as many phone calls after midnight than his colleagues. Nurses will not accept his telephone orders because "telephone orders are against the rules." Somehow, this rule gets suspended for the skilled players. Soon he becomes like Joe Bfstplk in the "Li'l Abner" comic strip. No matter where he goes, a black cloud constantly hovers over his head.

The unskilled gamesman nurse also pays heavily. The nurse who does not view her role as that of consultant, and therefore does not attempt to communicate recommendations, is perceived as a dullard and is mercifully allowed to fade into the woodwork.

The nurse who does see herself as a consultant but refuses to follow the rules of the game in making her recommendations has hell to pay. The outspoken nurse is labeled a "bitch" by the surgeon. The psychiatrist describes her as unconsciously suffering from penis envy and her behavior is the acting out of her hostility towards men. Loosely translated, the psychiatrist is saying she is a bitch. The employment of the unbright outspoken nurse is soon terminated. The outspoken bright nurse whose recommendations are worthwhile remains employed. She is, however, constantly reminded in a hundred ways that she is not loved.

GENESIS OF THE GAME

To understand how the game evolved, we must comprehend the nature of the doctors' and nurses' training which shaped the attitudes necessary for the game.

Medical Student Training

The medical student in his freshman year studies as if possessed. In the anatomy class he learns every groove and prominence on the bones of the skeleton as if life depended on it. As a matter of fact, he literally believes just that. He not infrequently says, "I've got to learn it exactly; a life may depend on me knowing that." A consequence of this attitude, which is carefully nurtured throughout medical school, is the development of a phobia: the overdetermined fear of making a mistake. The development of this fear is quite understandable. The burden the physician must carry is at times almost unbearable. He feels responsible in a very personal way for the lives of his patients. When a man dies leaving young children and a widow, the doctor carries some of her grief and despair inside himself; and when a child dies, some of him dies too. He sees himself as a warrior against death and disease. When he loses a battle, through no fault of his own, he nevertheless feels pangs of guilt, and he relentlessly searches himself to see if there might have been a way to alter the outcome. For the physician a mistake leading to a serious consequence is intolerable, and any mistake reminds him of his vulnerability. There is little wonder that he becomes phobic. The classical way in which phobias are managed is to avoid the source of the fear. Since it is impossible to avoid making some mistakes in an active practice of medicine, a substitute defensive maneuver is employed. The physician develops the belief that he is omnipotent and omniscient, and therefore incapable of making mistakes. This belief allows the phobic physician to actively engage in his practice rather than avoid it. The fear of committing an error in a critical field like medicine is unavoidable and appropriately realistic. The physician, however, must learn to live with the fear rather than handle it defensively through a posture of omnipotence. This defense markedly interferes with his interpersonal professional relationships.

Physicians, of course, deny feelings of omnipotence. The evidence, however, renders their denials to whispers in the wind. The slightest mistake inflicts a large narcissistic wound. Depending on his underlying personality structure the physician may obsess for days about it, quickly rationalize it away, or deny it. The guilt produced is unusually exaggerated and the incident is handled defensively. The ways in which physicians enhance and support each other's defenses when an error is made could be the topic of another paper. The feeling of omnipotence becomes generalized to other areas of his life. A report of the Federal Aviation Agency (FAA), as quoted in *Time Magazine* [sic] (August 5, 1966), states that in 1964 and 1965 physicians had a fatal-accident rate four times as high as the average for all other private pilots. Major causes of the high death rate were risk-taking attitudes and judgments. Almost all of the accidents occurred on pleasure trips, and were therefore not necessary risks to get to a patient needing emergency care. The trouble, suggested an FAA official, is that too many doctors fly with "the feeling that they are omnipotent." Thus, the extremes to which the physician may go in preserving his self-concept of omnipotence may threaten his own life. This overdetermined preservation of omnipotence is indicative of its brittleness and its underlying foundation of fear or failure.

The physician finds himself trapped in a paradox. He fervently wants to give his patient the best possible medical care, and being open to the nurses' recommendations helps him accomplish this. On the other hand, accepting advice from nonphysicians is highly threatening to his omnipotence. The solution for the paradox is to receive sub rosa recommendations and make them appear to be initiated by himself. In short, he must learn to play the doctor-nurse game.

Some physicians never learn to play the game. Most learn in their internship, and a perceptive few learn during their clerkships in medical school. Medical students frequently complain that the nursing staff treats them as if they had just completed a junior Red Cross first-aid class instead of two years of intensive medical training. Interviewing nurses in a training hospital sheds considerable light on this phenomenon. In their words they said,

A few students just seem to be with it, they are able to understand what you are trying to tell them, and they are a pleasure to work with; most, however, pretend to know everything and refuse to listen to anything we have to say and I guess we do give them a rough time.

In essence, they are saying that those students who quickly learn the game are rewarded, and those that do not are punished.

Most physicians learn to play the game after they have weathered a few experiences like the one described below. On the first day of his internship, the physician and nurse were making rounds. They stopped at the bed of a fifty-two-year-old woman who, after complimenting the young doctor on his appearance, complained to him of her problem with constipation. After several minutes of listening to her detailed description of peculiar diets, family home remedies, and special exercises that have helped her constipation in the past, the nurse politely interrupted the patient. She told her the doctor would take care of the problem and that he had to move on because there were other patients waiting to see him. The young doctor gave the nurse a stern look, turned toward the patient, and kindly told her he would order an enema for her that very afternoon. As they left the bedside, the nurse told him the patient has had a normal bowel movement every day for the past week and that in the twenty-three days the patient has been in the hospital she has never once passed up an opportunity to complain of her constipation. She quickly added that *if* the doctor wanted to order an enema, the patient would certainly receive one. After hearing this report the intern's mouth fell open and the wheels began turning in his head. He remembered the nurse's comment to the patient that "the doctor had to move on," and it occurred to him that perhaps she was really giving him a message. This experience and a few more like it, and the young doctor learns to listen for the subtle recommendations the nurses make.

Nursing Student Training

Unlike the medical student who usually learns to play the game after he finishes medical school, the nursing student begins to learn it early in her training. Throughout her education she is trained to play the doctor-nurse game.

Student nurses are taught how to relate to physicians. They are told he has infinitely more knowledge than they, and thus he should be shown the utmost respect. In addition, it was not many years ago when nurses were instructed to stand whenever a physician entered a room. When he would come in for a conference the nurse was expected to offer him her chair, and when both entered a room the nurse would open the door for him and allow him to enter first. Although these practices are no longer rigidly adhered to, the premise upon which they were based is still promulgated. One nurse described that premise as, "He's God almighty and your job is to wait on him."

To inculcate subservience and inhibit deviancy, nursing schools, for the most part, are tightly run, disciplined institutions. Certainly there is great variation among nursing schools, and there is little question that the trend is toward giving students more autonomy. However, in too many schools this trend has not gone far enough, and the climate remains restrictive. The student's schedule is firmly controlled and there is very little free time. Classroom hours, study hours, mealtime, and bedtime with lights out are rigidly enforced. In some schools meaning-less chores are assigned, such as cleaning bedsprings with cotton applicators. The relationship between student and instructor continues this military flavor. Often their relationship is more like that between recruit and drill sergeant than between student and teacher. Open dialogue is inhibited by attitudes of strict black and white, with few, if any, shades of gray. Straying from the rigidly outlined path is sure to result in disciplinary action.

The inevitable result of these practices is to instill in the student nurse a fear of independent action. This inhibition of independent action is most marked when relating to physicians. One of the students' greatest fears is making a blunder while assisting a physician and being publicly ridiculed by him. This is really more a reflection of the nature of their training than the prevalence of abusive physicians. The fear of being humiliated for a blunder while assisting in a procedure is generalized to the fear of humiliation for making any independent act in relating to a physician, especially the act of making a direct recommen-dation. Every nurse interviewed felt that making a suggestion to a physician was equivalent to insulting and belittling him. It was tantamount to questioning his medical knowledge and insinuating he did not know his business. In light of her image of the physician as an omniscient and punitive figure, the questioning of his knowledge would be unthinkable.

The student, however, is also given messages quite contrary to the ones de-scribed above. She is continually told that she is an invaluable aid to the physi-cian in the treatment of the patient. She is told that she must help him in every way possible, and she is imbued with a strong sense of responsibility for the care of her patient. Thus she, like the physician, is caught in a paradox. The first set of messages implies that the physician is omniscient and that any recommen-dation she might make would be insulting to him and leave her open to ridicule. The second set of messages implies that she is an important asset to him, has much to contribute, and is duty-bound to make those contributions. Thus, when her good sense tells her a recommendation would be helpful to him she is not allowed to communicate it directly, nor is she allowed not to communicate it. The way out of the bind is to use the doctor-nurse game and communicate the recommendation without appearing to do so.

FORCES PRESERVING THE GAME

Upon observing the indirect interactional system which is the heart of the doctor-nurse game, one must ask the question, "Why does this inefficient mode of com-munication continue to exist?" The forces mitigating against change are powerful.

Rewards and Punishments

The doctor-nurse game has a powerful innate self-perpetuating force — its system of rewards and punishments. One potent method of shaping behavior is to reward one set of behavioral patterns and to punish patterns which deviate from it. As described earlier, the rewards given for a well-played game and the punishments meted out to unskilled players are impressive. This system alone would be sufficient to keep the game flourishing. The game, however, has additional forces.

The Strength of the Set

It is well recognized that sets are hard to break. A powerful attitudinal set is the nurse's perception that making a suggestion to a physician is equivalent to insulting and belittling him. An example of where attempts are regularly made to break this set is seen on psychiatric treatment wards operating on a therapeutic community model. This model requires open and direct communication between members of the team. Psychiatrists working in these settings expend a great deal of energy in urging for and rewarding openness before direct patterns of communication become established. The rigidity of the resistance to break this set is impressive. If the physician himself is a prisoner of a set and therefore does not actively try to destroy it, change is near impossible.

The Need for Leadership

Lack of leadership and structure in any organization produces anxiety in its members. As the importance of the organization's mission increases, the demand by its members for leadership commensurately increases. In our culture human life is near the top of our hierarchy of values, and organizations which deal with human lives, such as law and medicine, are very rigidly structured. Certainly some of this is necessary for the systematic management of the task. The excessive degree of rigidity, however, is demanded by its members for their own psychic comfort rather than for its utility in efficiently carrying out its mission. The game lends support to this thesis. Indirect communication is an inefficient mode of transmitting information. However, it effectively supports and protects a rigid organizational structure with the physician in clear authority. Maintaining an omnipotent leader provides the other members with a great sense of security.

Sexual Roles

Another influence perpetuating the doctor-nurse game is the sexual identity of the players. Doctors are predominately men and nurses are almost exclusively women. There are elements of the game which reinforce the stereotyped roles of male dominance and female passivity. Some nursing instructors explicitly tell their students that their femininity is an important asset to be used when relating to physicians.

COMMENT

The doctor and nurse have a shared history and thus have been able to work out their game so that it operates more efficiently than one would expect in an indirect system. Major difficulty arises, however, when the physician works closely with other disciplines which are not normally considered part of the medical sphere. With expanding medical horizons encompassing cooperation with sociologists, engineers, anthropologists, computer analysts, etc., continued expectation of a doctor-nurselike interaction by the physician is disastrous. The sociologist, for example, is not willing to play that kind of game. When his direct communications are rebuffed the relationship breaks down.

The major disadvantage of a doctor-nurselike game is its inhibitory effect on open dialogue which is stifling and anti-intellectual. The game is basically a transactional neurosis, and both professions would enhance themselves by taking steps to change the attitudes which breed the game.

15

The Primary Care Nurse —
The Generalist in a Structured
Health Care Team

Eleanor Brunetto
Peter Birk

The expanded nurse role takes a variety of forms and has several titles. The role of primary care nurse, described in this chapter, is that of a generalist or family nurse—clinician. The nurse is a primary care giver with a family-centered focus. Such nurses work interdependently with a team of health professionals "in a system which facilitates communication." A strong case is made for nurse-physician collaboration and mutual respect at both the training and the practice levels. The authors describe the preparation of nurses for this expanded role, identify their function with the other primary care team members and discuss why they are the most appropriate professionals for this role.

INTRODUCTION

Planners and organizers of new health service programs are challenged by serious national problems relating to the provision of primary care, especially by their local manifestations. Nationwide shortages, maldistribution and inappropriate utilization of family physicians, general internists and pediatricians result in difficulties recruiting staff for such programs. The need for primary health services of far greater scope than can be provided by physicians alone virtually mandates using multidisciplinary teams for maintaining health and treating illness.[1] Increasing pressures for greater efficiency and lower costs necessitate trials of new methods and careful monitoring of quality.

During the past three years, the authors collaborated with an organized group of consumers in Albany, N.Y., to help correct deficiencies in health services experienced by large numbers of economically disadvantaged people in the northside neighborhood of the city. Working jointly, the Northside (Health) Advisory Council (the consumer group) and the staff of the Albany Medical College-Community Medical Care Program established the Whitney M. Young, Jr., Community Health Center, which initiated services in July, 1971. For demonstration purposes, they designed a model primary care unit which is now operational and being evaluated. The objectives were to create an organizational structure, professional roles and procedures which would: provide effective, efficient and highly personalized primary care; be generally applicable in terms of existing or achievable levels of manpower, money and knowledge; provide highly satisfying career choices for professionals by utilizing their skills most appropriately; be acceptable to patients from several socioeconomic strata;

From *American Journal of Public Health*, Vol. 62, No. 6, pp. 785–794, 1972. Reprinted by permission of the publisher and the authors.

be sufficiently flexible for adaptation to a variety of practice patterns and financing arrangements; and maintain high quality care.

The model was called the *Primary Care Team,* a highly organized multidisciplinary group of professionals and lay health workers. It was designed with the *Primary Care Nurse* or nurse-clinician generalist coordinating services and functioning in the key role of primary health care trustee* for individuals and families in the ambulatory setting.

The major aim of this paper is to define Primary Care Nurses and to describe their functions, qualifications and training. We also describe in detail the Primary Care Team because how Primary Care Nurses function and how their roles differ from other similar nursing roles cannot be appreciated thoroughly without an understanding of the context in which they work. In the discussion, we demonstrate that, were most primary care to be provided by multidisciplinary teams staffed by physicians and physicians' associates, the number of primary care physicians practicing in the United States could actually represent a surplus, rather than the currently perceived shortage. Finally, we explain why nurses were selected as the associated providers of care and discuss our views about the educational implications of this model.

THE PRIMARY CARE NURSE

The title, *Primary Care Nurse* (P.C.N.), was selected to identify the profession and the task. P.C.N.s are registered nurses specially trained to share with primary care physicians health trusteeship for adults and children in ambulatory settings. They maintain health, define problems, evaluate needs, implement and coordinate health action, educate patients and co-workers and assess outcomes. Working in association with physicians and other members of multidisciplinary primary care teams, they function as family health care generalists and team leaders. They perform many of the tasks traditionally carried out only by primary care physicians, social workers and nutritionists, as well as those for which they have been trained as nurses. Relating to their patients on an ongoing one-to-one basis, they assume major responsibility for providing or securing all required primary health services.

Although P.C.N. functions will vary somewhat with the needs of a particular primary care working situation, they can be classified conveniently under three headings: Independent, Interdependent and Dependent.[2]

Independent functions are those which the P.C.N. can perform legally without a physician's or other professional's immediate supervision. Guidelines, policies

---

*We define a health care trustee as a licensed health professional who is responsible for providing health care in a one-to-one provider-patient relationship; exercising independent decision-making and judgmental authority within the limits of his training, knowledge and skill; and seeking consultation or participation from other professionals where appropriate to the patient's needs.

and limitations are established for each function in consultation with the appropriate team colleagues. Examples include: (1) health care coordination and implementation (e.g., stable chronic illness, home care); (2) complete histories and physical examinations for well babies and adults; (3) responsibility for coordinating and monitoring a health maintenance and prevention program for each patient; (4) emergency triage; (5) uncomplicated pre- and postnatal care; (6) family planning, health education and patient counseling; (7) initial mental health assessment and triage; (8) laboratory and other diagnostic test selection in illness situations for which they have been trained; (9) telephone advice and referrals; (10) responsibility for the quality and content of problem-oriented records; (11) teaching and supervision of paraprofessionals and clerical staff; (12) performance or delegation to paraprofessionals of a variety of tests including, but not limited to venipuncture, simple clinical laboratory procedures, audiometry, electrocardiography, tonometry (without anesthetic), visual acuity, perimetry, obtaining specimens for cultures, cytological examinations, etc.

Interdependent functions are performed together with other professionals (physicians, social worker, nutritionist, physical therapist and others) whose competences complement those of the P.C.N. Examples include: (1) decisions regarding disposition, i.e., home care, nursing home placement, etc.; (2) joint patient care planning with physicians; (3) dietary planning; (4) support and counseling for families with parent-child conflicts, adolescent, mental health or fiscal problems and referrals (combined skills of nurse, social worker, and mental health team are required).

Dependent functions are performed by P.C.N.s under the immediate supervision and guidance of physicians or other professionals. Examples include: (1) determination of etiological labels for illnesses (medical diagnosis); (2) histories and physical examinations on acutely ill or unstable chronically ill patients; (3) therapeutic decisions involving drugs, physical agents, or minor surgical procedures; (4) selection of laboratory tests or other diagnostic procedures in illness situations for which they have not received specific training, i.e., standing orders or consultation; (5) psychotherapy and counseling for patients with emotional or behavioral disorders; (6) performance of minor surgical procedures (e.g., uncomplicated suturing, etc.); (7) referrals for diagnostic evaluations or specialty care outside of health center; (8) admission of patients to hospitals, extended care facilities, etc.; (9) tonometry (requiring anesthetic).

QUALIFICATIONS AND SELECTION PROCESS

The prerequisite qualifications for the first group of nurses selected to receive training were established at a high level because of the program's experimental character. To qualify, a candidate was required to be a registered nurse; to have earned a baccalaureate degree; and to have had responsibilities for patient care outside of the in-hospital setting, e.g., ambulatory care, public health nursing, home care, employee health or school nursing. Each candidate's past record was investigated for evidence of demonstrated ability to learn independently; to discharge responsibility consistently without undue supervision; to communicate effectively with patients and co-workers; to write competently; and to function reliably when fatigued or under stress.

In the setting of in-depth interviews, judgments were made of the candidate's degree of understanding of the new role and enthusiasm about assuming the responsibilities of the Primary Care Nurse; their maturity; their motivation for service; and the level of their comprehension of the health problems and needs of poor people. No candidate was accepted without a consensus among the Director of Nursing, a physician and a committee of consumers. Seven nurses were selected for the first Primary Care Team.

Although the initial group was limited to registered nurses with baccalaureate degrees, subsequent groups selected for training will probably include graduates of three-year programs. Their performance will be evaluated comparatively to determine whether the baccalaureate degree should continue to be required.

TRAINING

Training for the first team was provided by the faculty of the Albany Medical College and the Russell Sage College, Department of Nursing, and certificates were awarded jointly. A two-part program was designed, consisting of: (1) four and one-half months of intensive, full-time lecture, seminar, demonstration and practice sessions — approximately four hundred hours of formal classroom instruction supplemented by clinical practice and guided study of selected readings; and (2) six months of on-the-job training in actual patient care and continuing part-time formal teaching.

The first portion of the program was planned to be organized into eight general categories:

1. Information management
   a. History-taking
   b. Interviewing technique
   c. Problem-oriented records
2. Pediatrics
   a. Well-child assessment and health maintenance
   b. Physical diagnosis
   c. Diagnosis and management of common conditions
   d. Triage and management of common emergencies
   e. Common learning and behavior problems of childhood and adolescence
3. Adult medicine
   a. Assessment of the well adult and health maintenance
   b. Physical diagnosis

    c. Diagnosis and management of common conditions
      (1) Acute
      (2) Chronic
    d. Triage and management of common emergencies
4. Obstetrics and gynecology
    a. Family planning
    b. Routine prenatal care
      (1) Assessment
      (2) Diagnosis and management of common problems
      (3) Counseling
      (4) Triage and management of common emergencies
      (5) The unmarried mother
    c. Diagnosis and management of venereal disease
    d. Diagnosis and management of common gynecological problems
5. Specialties (otolaryngology, ophthalmology, dermatology, surgery, neurology)
    a. Routine diagnostic techniques and screening methods
    b. Diagnosis and management of common problems
    c. Standard pre-referral evaluation
      (1) Indications
      (2) Data-base
      (3) Available resources and referral procedures
6. Mental health
    a. Case finding
    b. Evaluation and initial management of common problems
    c. Counseling techniques
    d. Relationships with on-site mental health team
    e. Team building
7. Nursing seminars
    a. Role changes
    b. Health teaching
    c. General principles of nutrition
8. Social and economic issues
    a. Family structure and function
    b. Economic factors in health and illness
    c. Health related attitudes and behavior by social class
    d. Familiarization with the community to be served

The first course was held in the spring of 1971. Because the training activity took place in the urgent atmosphere of a newly developing health care program, many schedule changes were necessary and the curriculum continued to evolve. All of the trainees accepted their positions with enthusiasm concerning the expanded responsibilities they would assume, but most of them experienced a moderate degree of anxiety during the formal portion of the training. Although fears were expressed about insufficient time to develop confidence in newly learned skills, medical staff and other observers have noted the enthusiasm and clinical competence of the Primary Care Nurses.

Disciplined evaluation of the training could not be achieved, but informal and subjective assessment indicates that training nurse practitioner generalists in such a short time creates anxiety and provides too little opportunity for concurrent clinical practice and observation. Accordingly, we suggest that future programs be offered in two semesters, involving approximately seventeen credit hours each.

THE PRIMARY CARE TEAM

As stated in the introduction, we believe that understanding completely the Primary Care Nurse's role requires familiarity with the *Primary Care Team's* setting, staffing, organization and service program.

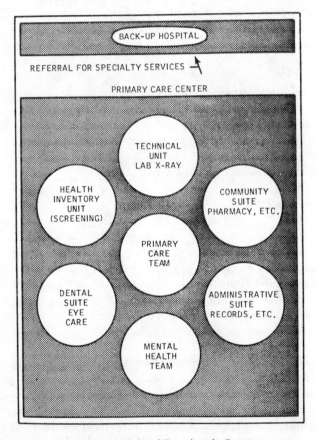

Figure 1. Relation of Team and Associated Functions in Center

As shown in Figure 1, the Team is the central functional unit in a *Primary Care Center* which relates to a back-up hospital for specialty services and inpatient care and includes other patient service functions such as dental care, eye care, pharmacy and mental health. Also present are activities which support the Primary Care Team such as a technical unit with laboratory and x-ray, a Health Inventory or screening unit and administration, including records, purchasing, billing, facility maintenance and other related activities. Depending on the size of the population served, several *Primary Care Teams* could be housed and supported in a Center. Although the organization described in this paper is an O.E.O. funded neighborhood health program, a Center could be operated by any organized health care service program. (See Appendix for our definition of the full service program of an "ideal" Primary Care Center.)

Figure 2 illustrates a *Primary Care Team's* organization and staff, which includes a full-time internist and pediatrician and a part-time obstetrician; six Primary Care Nurses; six Primary Care Assistants; three Health Assistants; social worker; nutritionist; part-time physical therapist; and clerical staff.

The physicians teach, consult and collaborate with all team members, but mainly with Primary Care Nurses. They retain ultimate responsibility and authority for clinical decisions; supervise quality of medical care; design standing orders and clinical paradigms for the nurses; perform all clinical functions beyond the P.C.N.'s competence; and participate as continuing education faculty for P.C.N.s and other team members. The degree of physicians' participation in a patient-nurse encounter varies directly with the seriousness and complexity of the patient's problems and inversely with the nurse's training and competence in performing a particular task.

The relationship between nurses and physicians in this model merits explanation because it illustrates a difference between P.C.N.s and some other versions of nurse-practitioner function. P.C.N.s are neither physician-assistants nor surrogate physicians. In some situations in the U.S., such as several wilderness programs, nurses must make medical diagnostic and therapeutic decisions while wholly out of contact with physicians. In the Primary Care Team, physicians and nurses work together in one facility and consult with each other whenever they deem it necessary. Conversely, P.C.N.s do not depend on physicians or other professionals for *all* their decisions. The Team's working style can be described as a continuously varying degree of interdependence among a group of professionals relating to each other in a system which facilitates communication.

The Primary Care Assistants (P.C.A.) are trained indigenous outreach workers assigned to and supervised by individual Primary Care Nurses. The P.C.A. meets daily with the nurse and team to formulate plans for home visits and share pertinent information. Home visits are made to check on patient's compliance with medication orders or other health-related advice; explore causes for broken appointments; reinforce health teaching; make simple clinical observations; assist families to cope with sanitation, social welfare and mental health problems;

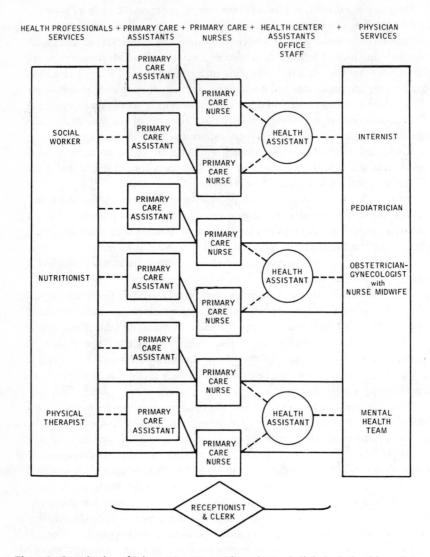

HEALTH PROFESSIONALS + PRIMARY CARE + PRIMARY CARE + HEALTH CENTER + PHYSICIAN
SERVICES   ASSISTANTS   NURSES   ASSISTANTS   SERVICES
                                                   OFFICE
                                                   STAFF

Figure 2. Organization of Primary Care Team (shows internal clinical relationships only)

discover new problems; perform accident hazard appraisals; and administer simple first aid. The Primary Care Assistants also function as social work, nutrition and mental health aides and serve to bridge cultural gaps between patients and professionals.

Health Assistants are indigenous workers who function as aides to P.C.N.s and physicians in the health center. They are trained to prepare examination and treatment rooms; measure vital signs; collect specimens; complete routine paperwork; perform electrocardiograms; and assist with administrative and communication tasks.

Figure 3 illustrates the patient's view of his relationship with those members of the Team who work most closely with him and the members of his family. It also indicates the predominant communication patterns between a particular P.C.N. and the other members of the Team with whom he or she works most immediately. Assigning each of the members of a family to the same P.C.N. facilities the "family medicine" concept by assuring that one care provider remains constantly in tune with how the health problems and service needs of each patient relate to those of the other members of his family.

Figure 4 is a flow chart of the steps involved in a new patient's entry into the program and the Primary Care Nurse's procedures in initiating and implementing a program of required health action. Patients may register whether they are well or have an acute health problem. In either case, they and their families are assigned to a P.C.N. If the patient's initial encounter is for an acute problem, the P.C.N. begins the process of care immediately. In the absence of an acute problem, well or worried well patients undergo a health assessment procedure in which an age- and sex-related standard data-base is acquired by the *Health Inventory Unit,* a group of trained paraprofessionals called *Health Inventory Technicians.* Figure 4 outlines P.C.N.'s responsibilities for evaluating and treating an initial acute problem and describes how they utilize information supplied by the

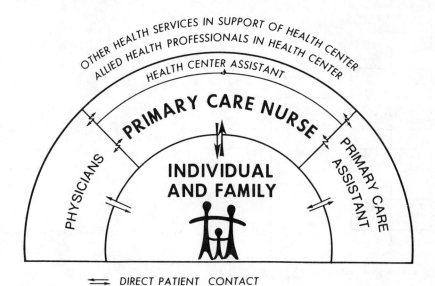

Figure 3. Patient View of Relationship to Primary Care Team

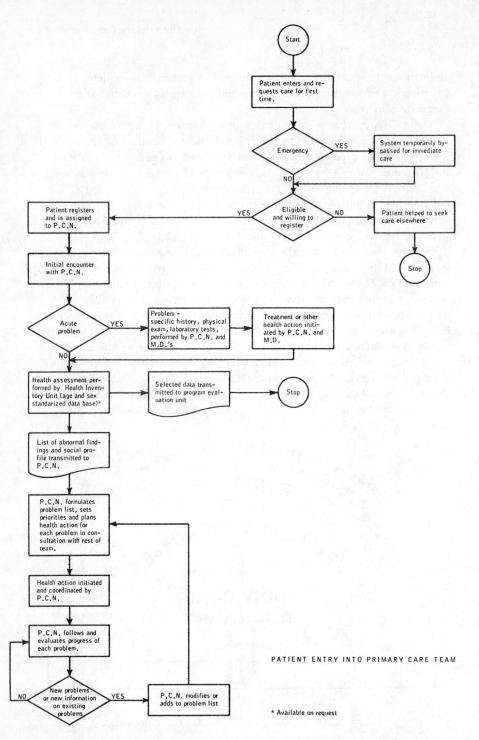

Figure 4. Patient Entry into Primary Care Team and P.C.N.'s Role in Health Action

Health Inventory Unit (and knowledge acquired directly) to formulate a complete list of problems, establish priorities and plan health action for each problem in consultation with other members of the Team. The figure illustrates P.C.N.s' duties to initiate and coordinate health action, and to follow and evaluate the progress of each problem.

The Team's appointment system is designed to reinforce the P.C.N.'s function as the predominant primary care provider. All medical appointments for registered patients are made or requested by the P.C.N.s. No direct appointments are booked for the physicians, who maintain an open schedule, seeing patients jointly with the P.C.N.s on an "as needed" basis. During the program's initial operational period, as required by the extension of the P.C.N. curriculum into an "on-the-job" training phase, physicians see all patients, if only briefly, and confer with the nurse. Nonmedical appointments (social work, nutrition, etc.) may be scheduled by the appropriate professional in coordination with the patient's nurse. Patients may telephone their P.C.N.s for advice. To discuss complex problems requiring group decisions, daily team conferences are held.

All members of the Team were trained to use the Problem Oriented Record System,[3,4] and this form of record-keeping was mandated to help meet the staff members' needs for accurate and timely information about patients and for effective intramural communication. The system's advantages have been observed to include: (1) Facilitation of coordinated action in the multidisciplinary team setting. (2) Heightened team awareness of the full scope and changing nature of a patient's problems and how each relates to the others. (3) Rapid and efficient access to all plans, actions, symptoms, observations, laboratory information and results concerning any single problem. (4) Compatibility with the requirements of formal record audit and evaluation of individual, team and program performance.[5]

DISCUSSION

Effect of Primary Care Team on National Physician Manpower Needs

Consensus exists that, without successful solutions of the related problems of maldistribution and inappropriate untilization of manpower, training larger numbers of physicians is unlikely to alleviate the crisis in health care.[6] In its report to the President in 1967, the National Advisory Commission on Health Manpower cited a crisis caused by manpower being channeled into "inefficient and inappropriate activities," resulting in difficulties for patients in gaining entry into the medical care system.[7]

Widespread use of multidisciplinary teams similar to the model described in this paper could contribute significantly towards alleviating primary care physician shortages. Were such models in general use, primary care of adequate scope and economy could be provided nationally with existing numbers of physicians and attainable numbers of nurses. To illustrate this point, we have compared the number of primary care physicians working alone, which would be needed to provide every American five primary care visits a year, with the number needed if they all worked in teams like the Primary Care Team.

Were all people to receive only from physicians the scope of primary services described in the Appendix, sufficient numbers of internists, pediatricians, obstetricians and family physicians are not likely to be available soon. This can be demonstrated by comparing the number of primary care physicians presently in practice with how many would be required (Table 1). Currently, we estimate that slightly more than 125,000 primary care physicians practice actively in the United States.[8]

Table 1. Estimate of Primary Physicians Practicing Currently in U.S.A.

80,894	M.D.s in General Practice
+19,129	Internists providing primary care. (Estimate based on ½ of 38,258 total internists in all subspecialties)*
+17,926	Pediatricians
+ 9,042	Obstetricians and gynecologists. (Estimate based on ½ of 18,084 total obstetricians)*
126,991	Total M.D.s active in primary care

*(Assuming that no more than half the work of all internists and obstetricians is primary medical care.)

If each physician's service capability were 20 encounters per day or 5,000 per year (250 working days) and the average number of primary care visits were five per person annually, we would need a primary care physician-population ratio of 1:1000 or more than 200,000 primary care physicians nationally. Therefore, our estimated deficit of primary care physicians is at least 75,000 and more than that if inappropriate geographic distribution continues.

Were all primary care to be provided by multidisciplinary teams similar to the Primary Care Team, the present number of 125,000 practicing primary physicians would be adequate to meet the national need. Estimating that each P.C.N. could manage 20 encounters per day, and that there were 250 working days a year, we predicted a potential of 5,000 encounters per nurse annually and 30,000 encounters for the group of six P.C.N.s. By assuming a utilization rate of five medical visits per patient per year, we calculated the capacity of a total of 6,000 patients or 1,000 per P.C.N. Should P.C.N.s be able to see more than 20 patients a day or should the average utilization rate be closer to the national average of 4.3 visits per patient per year, the Team's patient service capacity could be correspondingly higher. Therefore, it was projected that one Primary Care Team with 2 to 2¼ full-time physicians' equivalents (1 internist, 1 pediatrician and

¼ of a full-time obstetrician) could provide comprehensive primary health services for at least 6,000 registered patients. Based on a physician-population ratio of at least 1 : 2667 derived from these estimates, the national need for primary care physicians would be less than 76,000 (75,499), a number well below the 125,000 practicing currently. It should be noted that such teams could be staffed either by family physicians or by internists and pediatricians.

WHY NURSES?

Nurses were selected to be the physicians' associates on the Primary Care Team because they can assist with appropriate technical tasks to increase efficiency and also assume independent authority for a variety of activities beyond the scope of traditional diagnostic or curative care, including shared responsibility for trusteeship. By utilizing skills and knowledge already inherent in their background, nurses can function as generalist clinicians in ambulatory settings with limited additional training. Nurses have traditionally worked with physicians; been broadly trained in team, psycho-social, family and multidisciplinary approaches; and are legally free to accept responsibility. As with medicine, appropriateness of function seems also to be a current and critical issue for nursing.

Because the nurse-patient ratio of the Primary Care Team is 1 : 1000, a maximum of 200,000 P.C.N.s would be required to serve the present American population. To recruit and educate 200,000 additional nurses would, of course, demand a tremendous effort, but perhaps one of no greater magnitude than training 75,000 additional physicians.

Nursing represents a tremendously large manpower pool. It is not only likely that additional people might eventually enter nursing were this role accepted nationally, but also the field currently represents the "single largest licensed and well-trained health manpower pool in the nation."[9] In 1970, there were over 700,000 employed nurses in the United States.[10] With its existing educational establishment, nursing could produce large additional numbers of nurse physician-associates.

Nurse practitioner programs,[11-13] now proliferating across the country, are based on assumptions of nursing competence; patient acceptance; acceptance by nursing education institutions and organized nursing; recognition of nursing services in primary care by third-party payers; that liability issues will ultimately be settled satisfactorily; and that medicine and nursing are sufficiently flexible to create and tolerate change. The National League of Nursing Ad Hoc Committee, formed in 1969 to study the nurse's role, reported that "the traditional use which has been made of the ability of the professionally prepared nurse has been shortsighted and wasteful of talent and manpower..." and that "professional nurses must accept large and more significant responsibilities...."[14]

Although many programs train nurse clinician specialists (e.g., Pediatric Nurse Practitioners), the Albany Medical College-Community Medical Care Program trained nurses to function as generalists or family clinicians on the assumption that primary care should be family-centered. Whether family physicians or teams of several types of physicians provide the care, we felt that the nurse should work with all family members. The well-trained nurse generalist should be able to function adaptably in solo practice pediatric or adult medicine settings as well.

Nurse clinicians participating in primary care on a nationwide scale could contribute significantly toward resolving problems relating to currently inadequate numbers of relevant types of manpower. Of equal importance, primary care itself could become a far more comprehensive and effective service, especially in the areas of health maintenance, mental health, chronic illness management and health education. Physicians might find greater attractions in this career area than they do now because their skills would be more appropriately exercised. No longer forced to work alone, primary care physicians would function as colleagues, teachers and consultants. By working in teams, such as the model described in this paper, they could devote a large proportion of their time to managing complex and difficult health problems, thereby maintaining higher levels of competence in diagnosis and therapy.

The effect of Primary Care Teams staffed by physicians and P.C.N.s on quality and effectiveness of care remains to be evaluated. Whether greater scope of service, continuity of care and the involvement of a wider range of professional skills in primary care eventually will result in lower costs and better health outcomes for patients has yet to be established. The authors believe that urgent need exists for the experiment to be undertaken on a wide and adequately supported scale, not only in health centers, but also in group and private practice settings and outpatient clinics.

IMPLICATIONS FOR NURSING AND MEDICAL EDUCATION

Currently, almost all programs for training nurse-clinicians exist separately from the mainstream of nursing education. They are special enterprises administered by nurses and physicians which function in a variety of educational contexts, such as medical colleges, schools of public health and service projects. Granting master's degrees or certificates, they recruit relatively limited numbers of interested nurses who have finished their basic training and worked in a variety of nursing positions.

If nursing is to assume a leading role in primary health care trusteeship, sufficient numbers of professionals who can exercise primary care nursing responsibilities must be graduated by schools of nursing, creating a nationally available manpower pool. Service programs cannot be expected to educate all new staff members. Even if many primary care providers desire to use multidisciplinary teams analogous to the Primary Care Team described in this paper, few will be able to function in this manner if they must muster the faculty resources and money necessary for a continuing basic educational effort.

The authors suggest that nursing schools provide to candidates for the B.S. degree the option of preparing themselves for the field of primary care at the undergraduate level. We propose a senior year elective curriculum combining didactic teaching and supervised practical experience. It seems likely that many students, who might not have previously selected nursing, would be motivated to enter the field, were this career option available. A few colleges in the U.S. have already implemented new programs, but have not yet graduated their first students.

Medical colleges must share in designing educational programs for nurses in the primary care field, and their faculty should participate in teaching wherever their knowledge or skills are needed. Practical experience should be offered in appropriate clinical settings with physician and nurse educators in joint supervisory roles. Since nursing functions in primary care must mesh with those of physicians, the educational effort must be as closely collaborative as subsequent clinical operations in which physicians and nurses will be associated.

The success of the proposed model depends upon mutual respect by physicians and nurses and their understanding of each other's functions. *We share Adamson's viewpoint that nursing and medical students should be trained together in team situations.*[15] Hopefully, primary care nurse and primary care physician training programs, collaboratively administered by nursing and medical colleges, might become the predominant national pattern.

Primary care nursing personnel are needed at several levels of sophistication and training. The largest proportion would function clinically and should be trained at the baccalaureate level. For those who must discharge administrative responsibilities or serve as junior faculty in nursing or medical colleges, several varieties of postgraduate programs should be designed. Some might emphasize supervision and administrative skills and others focus on educational methods and higher levels of professional competence. For students with appropriate ability and interest, research-oriented Ph.D. or M.D. options could be provided. Indeed, collegiate nursing programs could provide baccalaureate students with opportunities to select courses required for admission to medical or graduate schools. As a result, several "career ladders" could be made available to Primary Care Nurses, including a "bridge" to medicine and medical education.

SUMMARY

This paper described a model multidisciplinary primary health services unit now operating at the Whitney M. Young, Jr., Community Health Center in Albany, New York. It explained how *Primary Care Nurses* function in the setting of the *Primary Care Team* as family health care generalists; share with primary care physicians health trusteeship for adults and children; and implement or coordinate all health action for patients on the basis of a continuing nurse-patient relationship.

Team structure and function, including each member's role, was outlined;

and procedures, patient-flow patterns, the record system and the training program were described. Program planning was discussed in terms of the scope of
an ideal primary care service and current health manpower realities. The authors'
viewpoint about the model's implications for nursing and medical education was
presented.

Appendix

Ideal Primary Care Service Defined

In the absence of a generally accepted functional description of primary care,
no new model should be designed without an explicitly documented definition
of the intended scope of services. The literature abounds with brief, general
statements, but none seem sufficiently specific to serve adequately as a basis for
model design.

For example, the Working Party on Primary Medical Care of the British Medical Association defined it as "the work of the doctor whom the patient first
approaches when he wants advice or medical treatment."[16] Dr. Kerr L. White
equated primary care to "first contact" care.[17] The U.S. Public Health Service
emphasizes that it should be the "range of services adequate for meeting the
great majority of daily personal health needs," the entry point into a comprehensive health care system linking primary with secondary and tertiary services.[18]
Collins and Bonnyman specify the primary care provider as "the agent of first
contact who provides entry into the health care system and serves as the primary
medical resource and counselor to an individual or family in all their health
needs."[19]

For our purposes, we defined an ideal primary care unit as one which should:

1. Directly provide preventive or health maintenance, acute and chronic illness
   and rehabilitation services in general adult medicine, pediatrics and obstetrics-
   gynecology; minor surgery; preventive and first-level mental health care;
   general dental services; and resources for working with health related social,
   economic, legal and environmental problems.
2. Have a systematic and formalized mechanism for identifying all patients'
   important health problems prospectively, i.e., prior to acute crises where
   practical.
3. Offer the individual and family a long-term, personal relationship with one or
   a very small number of providers who are aware, so far as possible, of the full
   scope of his health problems; and who would plan, provide and coordinate all
   necessary services, establishing priorities in consultation with the recipient.
4. Secure and coordinate fully comprehensive services for patients and continuing
   education for staff by linking formally with services not provided on-site, i.e.,
   psychiatry, operative dentistry, all other medical and surgical specialties and
   health-related community-based agencies and programs.

5. Minimize access problems for patients and providers by locating conveniently to patients' homes and a community hospital; including staff members who are congruent culturally with patients; providing as many services as possible in one facility or on one campus; and operating at times of day compatible with patient's life styles, offering 24-hour availability for emergent problems.
6. Share program planning with consumer groups through one of several mechanisms for consumer participation.
7. Be replicable in terms of currently available or easily recruited and trained health manpower.

REFERENCES

1. Beloff, Jerome S. and Willet, Marion. Yale Studies in Family Health Care: III. The Health Care Team. *J.A.M.A.* 205:663—669 (Sept. 2, 1968).
2. Hallstrom, Betty and Osterman, Karen. *Independent, Dependent and Collaborative Functioning and The Nursing Role.* Systems Development Project. Minneapolis, Minnesota: University of Minnesota, No. 9:2(13).
3. Weed, Lawrence L. Medical Records That Guide and Teach. *New Eng. J. Med.* 278: 593—600, 652—657 (March 14, 21, 1968).
4. Weed, Lawrence L. *Medical Records, Medical Education and Patient Care.* Cleveland, Ohio: The Press of Case Western Reserve University, 1970.
5. Birk, Peter; Ward, Thomas; and Dutton, Cynthia. Problem Oriented Analysis of Medical Care Episodes — A New Evaluation Model. Presented before APHA, 99th Annual Meeting, Minneapolis, Minn., Medical Care Section, 1971.
6. The Carnegie Commission on Higher Education. *Higher Education and the Nation's Health, Policies for Medical and Dental Education.* A special Report and Recommendations. McGraw-Hill Book Company, (Oct. 1970).
7. *Report* of the National Advisory Commission on Health Manpower, Volume I. (Nov., 1967.)
8. *Health Resources Statistics, Health Manpower and Health Facilities, 1970.* Public Health Service Publication No. 1509, 1970 Edition. Rockville, Maryland. Public Health Service, Health Services and Mental Health Administration, National Center for Health Statistics, U.S. Department of Health, Education, and Welfare. (Feb., 1971), p. 139.
9. *National Commission for the Study of Nursing and Nursing Education.* McGraw-Hill, Inc., U.S., 1970.
10. Op. cit., Health Resources Statistics, Health Manpower and Health Facilities, 1970, p. 149.
11. Collins, M. C. and Bonnyman, G. G. *Physician's Assistants and Nurse Associates: A Review.* Washington, D.C.: The Institute for the Study of Health and Society, (Jan., 1971).
12. *Selected Training Programs for Physician Support Personnel.* Bethesda, Maryland. National Institutes of Health, Bureau of Health Professions Education and Manpower Training. U.S. Department of Health, Education, and Welfare (June, 1970).
13. Silver, H. K. and Hecher, J. A. The Pediatric Nurse Practitioner and the Child Health Associate: New types of health professionals. *J. Med. Ed.* 45:171—176, 1970.
14. Ad Hoc Committee to study the Nurse's Role In The Delivery of Health Services. Statement and Recommendations: Council of Baccalaureate and Higher Degree Programs. Exhibit I — National League for Nursing, New York, N.Y., (Sept. 11—12, 1969).
15. Adamson, T. Elaine. Critical Issues In The Use of Physician Associates and Physicians. *A.J.P.H.* 61:1765—1779 (Sept., 1971).
16. British Medical Association Planning Unit Report No. 4. *Report* on the Working Party on Primary Medical Care. London, W.C.I.: B.M.A. House (May, 1970).

17. White, Kerr L. Primary Medical Care for Families — Organization and Evaluation. *New Eng. J. Med.* 277:847—52 (Oct. 19, 1967).
18. *A Conceptual Model of Organized Primary Care and Comprehensive Community Health Services.* Rockville, Maryland. Public Health Service, Health Services and Mental Health Administration, Community Health Service, Division of Health Care Services, U.S. Department of Health, Education and Welfare, 1970.
19. Op. cit., Collins, M. C. and Bonnyman, G. G.

16

The Nurse as Family Practitioner

Jo Ellen Murata

How is the expanded role different from the traditional public health nurse role? The author of this chapter describes her responsibilities as a family nurse practitioner, illustrating the application of new skills as she intervenes in a family situation.

The efficient use of medical care facilities is often thwarted by poor coordination of clinic and community resources and little knowledge about the consumer and his home environment. As a result, I felt frustrated working as a public health nurse with patients attending a county outpatient clinic. But county clinics are not alone in this regard. The same problems occurred in a large prepaid medical group where I was a consumer. Much of my nursing knowledge was required to coordinate the health services offered and obtain access to the facilities.

As the size of my own family increased, I became even more aware of consumers' problems. Our individuality seemed lost in a maze of specialty clinics and red tape. My neighbor's plaintive remark, "*I* have to make the diagnosis before I know where to call!" increased my own doubt that people with little medical sophistication could secure good health care from our present system of health care delivery.

As a result, when I learned that a unique pilot educational program was starting in Berkeley, California, I enrolled. In this program, the traditional skills of six experienced public health nurses in evaluation, referral, and counseling were deepened and their responsibilities broadened by knowledge and skill in community medicine, physical diagnosis, and clinical management. The goal was to learn to facilitate a person's entry into the existing health care system and coordinate available health care resources so that better care could be obtained.

The nurses in this program worked in an ambulatory care setting in a new role — family nurse practitioner — to bridge the gap between home and clinic, coordinate services, and assist with the care of all age groups.

The application of new skills and some steps taken in an expanded role are discussed here to demonstrate a recurring and vexing health care situation — the management of the multiproblem family or, from the consumer's vantage point, the client's management of the multiproblem clinic.

FAMILY STUDY

Fifteen-year-old Robert was a cooperative, taciturn, Caucasian boy who held his head habitually hunched over his right shoulder as though he were constantly flinching. His mother had brought him to the county hospital medical clinic because a teacher asked that he be examined for thyroid trouble or anemia. The teacher said Robert seemed tired all the time and had frequent infections. Robert's mother thought that he slept more than usual. Robert said he felt nervous and irritable.

As a student family nurse practitioner, I examined Robert with the instructor, a family physician, and observed the history-taking process. Robert's mother, an obese, garrulous woman, answered all questions. We learned that Robert had had encopresis until he was eight years old and enuresis until age 14, and that he had been placed in an educationally handicapped class at school the preceding year because of "disagreement with a teacher." Ms. S. said Robert's grades were "O.K. — Bs and Cs."

Robert was the youngest of five children born in a 15-year span. All the children now "had trouble," Ms. S. said. Apparently the problems were psychosocial. All except Robert were married and lived away from home. Ms. S. had divorced Robert's father because of alcoholism and sexual deviance when Robert was seven. Two years later, she married a man whom Robert liked and respected, but who was 17 years older than Ms. S.

Robert's most recent elicited problem, during a brief review of systems, was school-associated temper outbursts that had ended one year before. However, Ms. S. had many of the symptoms about which we inquired of Robert. She cheerfully described her "bad disposition," which she believed had led to a hysterectomy and hiatal herniorrhaphy. In addition, she had had persistent diarrhea for years, epigastric pain, shortness of breath, hypertension, swelling of her legs, back pain, and numerous other symptoms. She seemed an anxious woman who had no medical supervision for her chronic ailments. She completely eclipsed her son throughout the visit.

Robert's physical and intellectual development seemed within normal limits for his age, and no abnormalities were noted during physical examination. Robert was reassured that the physical findings were normal.

An X-ray of his neck and chest were ordered to rule out disease related to his habitual hunched posture; a complete blood count, urinalysis, and repeat protein bound iodine (PBI) were requested, and the reasons and technique explained to Robert and his mother. During Robert's initial drop-in visit to the medical clinic two weeks earlier, a physician had ordered a heterophile antibody titer to detect infectious mononucleosis and a PBI to study thyroid function. The heterophile antibody titer had been normal, but the PBI had been slightly elevated and was now to be repeated. Robert was given a trial prescription of methylphenidate hydrochloride (Ritalin), a drug used in some childhood school disturbances and adult depressions.

Ms. S. was urged to make an appointment with the family nurse practitioner for evaluation of her many symptoms and continued health supervision. Ms. S. hesitantly said, "Maybe I will." I hoped to coordinate health care for the S.

family, evaluate physical findings, and refer them to appropriate resources while providing continuity of care.

As the visit ended, Ms. S. collapsed into Robert's arms. Stolidly lowering her large body to the floor, he explained apologetically, "Momma is having another attack." She had painful muscle cramps which caused hyperextension of her feet, legs, and hips. She was conscious. No unusual respiratory or cardiovascular findings were noted except a blood pressure of 170/100 during the obviously painful muscle spasms. When Ms. S. had recovered spontaneously, she said she had had this type of attack for 30 years, but no abnormalities had ever been found nor treatment suggested.

Robert was solicitous of his mother during and after her attack. His anxiety lessened as we urged her to return for an examination.

During my discussion of the visit with the family physician, who was my instructor, the psychosocial aspects of this family's health problems became apparent. Ms. S.'s attacks suggested either hysterical conversion symptoms or a hyperventilation syndrome. We suspected that the emotional impact of these dramatic attacks on the family probably caused some of Robert's apathetic and anxious behavior.

At the next visit, I interviewed Robert after a reminder to Ms. S., who insisted on accompanying him to the examining room, that it was important to hear directly from him. Laboratory results and X-rays were normal except for a trace of albumin and three to five white blood cells per high-powered field in the urine specimen. Robert said he had nocturia twice nightly, urinated 10 to 12 times a day, and had tenderness in his back. He pointed to the costovertebral angle. As Robert voiced each symptom, Ms. S. scoffed, "Oh, you do not!"

I reviewed the few abnormal physical and laboratory findings with the physician. We agreed that Robert's frequency of urination, nocturia, costovertebral angle tenderness, pyuria, and albuminuria suggested a urinary tract infection. These symptoms and his enuresis until recently suggested a chronic renal disorder — perhaps a congenital anomaly or a chronic infection. However, the urinalysis abnormalities could also have resulted from poor technique in collecting the urine specimen. Or, since occasional albuminuria is found in adolescents after periods of standing, it could have occurred because Robert stood in line so long at the laboratory. Of course, chronic psychological problems resulting from inadequate parent-child relationships could have produced enuresis or malingering. But regardless of cause, the urinary tract infection needed treatment. I suggested tetracycline and increased fluid intake as indicated therapy and the physician signed the prescription. However, a urine culture with antibiotic sensitivities testing was to be done before drug therapy was initiated.

The laboratory results, reasons for the urine culture and sensitivity tests, drug therapy, and need for increased fluids were discussed with Robert and his mother, and he was given an appointment to return in two weeks.

During the visit, I had discovered that Robert's sister had an acute problem with drug abuse and concurrent mental illness. The moral implications of her behavior disturbed Robert and Ms. S., whose religious background was strongly evangelical. They saw legal sanctions as punishment to effect behavior change. The concept of drug abuse as a symptom of illness was suggested and alternatives to the authoritarian judgment-punishment method of dealing with the sister's disturbing behavior were discussed.

A second family problem was Mr. S.'s ill health. He had severe emphysema for which medication and home treatment had been ordered. However, he insisted that his health was "good" and largely ignored his doctor's advice. The family arguments about his medication and treatment led Ms. S. to ask me to see her husband. His visit was subsequently approved by his physician.

During the interval between Robert's appointments, Ms. S. had her initial visit with me. I did a physical examination, ordered multiple laboratory tests, and referred her to the cardiology, neuromedical, and peripheral vascular clinics. Her primary problems were obesity, varicose veins, and a neuromuscular disorder, discovered by electromyogram. Overlying these were anxiety about family relationships and concern that Robert was developing a pattern of deviant behavior like his natural father and sister, in that Robert had been stealing money from her purse to play pinball machines. In her anxiety about the repetitive pattern of deviance in the family, she had reacted so punitively that communication between her and Robert was disrupted even more.

The next time Robert came, I insisted on seeing him alone. I wondered whether his stealing was a result of his hostility and anxiety so I explored his feelings about his parents. This interview was difficult. Robert, although friendly, was taciturn and replied in monosyllables until I asked, "How do you think we can help you, Robert?" With great emotion, he said, "Help my mom stop having her attacks!" I assured him that she was having many tests and consultations to find the cause of her disorder.

Robert then spoke tersely, but with feeling, of his home, his school, and his hope of finding a part-time job to improve his life. It seemed possible that a job might prevent Robert's pilfering, increase his self-esteem, and allow him to contribute in an adult way to the family's welfare. They lived on the social security payments of Mr. S., a retired laborer.

Robert's laboratory tests of the preceding visit, all normal, were discussed. His drug therapy was reviewed and the Ritalin discontinued since Robert reported that it had little effect on his school and home behavior. The use of illicit drugs at school was discussed and the pharmacological effects and common misconceptions of these drugs were emphasized. With the incidence of drug abuse in Robert's peer group, it seemed unwise to continue his psychotropic drug therapy.

Robert reported feeling a "little better" with no costovertebral angle tenderness since taking the tetracycline. However, his urine had shown a bacteria count of slightly less than 10,000 per milliliter, the decisive point at the clinic for proceeding with a bacterial culture. For this reason, no urine culture had

been done. A repeat urinalysis was requested; it showed clearing of the albuminuria, but 2—3 white blood cells per high power field remained. A consultation
with the urologist was requested to determine the presence or absence of disease.
Robert was to return to me in one month with his stepfather.

I asked Robert's permission to discuss the results of his health assessment
with the teacher who had originally referred him to the clinic. He quickly agreed
as had his mother during her visit.

In a telephone conference the teacher verified Robert's report of his school
behavior. Ritalin had made no difference in his classroom behavior and there
had been only slight improvement in his play activity.

Robert had seen a psychologist before he was placed in the educationally
handicapped class, and the teacher agreed to talk with the psychologist about
additional help for the family.

I told the teacher about Robert's hopes for a job and my concern about the
unavailability of employment in the depressed economy of his community,
already overloaded with unskilled workers. He shared my concern.

The conference ended on a bleak note. The problems Robert identified —
his parents' ill health, the family's lack of money, and his inability to find a job
— were matters for which the community's economic, psychological, and medical
support were very limited.

The most effective treatment for Robert seemed to be supportive therapy for
his mother; continuity of family care was provided through visits with her. Ms. S.
kept her multiple laboratory, X-ray, and specialty clinic appointments. Conferences between the family physician and me continued at each of her visits to
interpret physical examination results and laboratory and consultation reports.
These teaching-supervisory conferences included frequent chart reviews as the
interpretation of her problems became more complex.

The clinic staff, even though accustomed to giving less personalized care,
became involved in helping to plan Ms. S.'s multiple appointments. The S. family lived far from the clinic and transportation was difficult.

Then, tragically, another stress was added. Mr. S. died suddenly at home
shortly before he was to visit the family nurse practitioner clinic.

When Ms. S., in her distress, called the clinic for advice about her medication
during my absence, the family physician provided information and some much
needed emotional support. In a return telephone call, I arranged to visit Ms. S.
and Robert at home.

During my visit, I learned that Ms. S. had kept Robert home from school
because her "attacks" had grown worse since her husband's death. She was
afraid to be alone. I emphasized the importance of outside social activities for
both of them and urged Ms. S. to return to her church activities as soon as
possible.

Ms. S. said Robert had been having nightmares which she attributed to "his
not crying about Dad." She believed, and Robert affirmed, that he did not want

to express emotion because it was "unmanly." Despite encouragement to express his feelings, Robert remained steadfastly impassive. He said: "I wouldn't want to talk to anyone about how I feel."

However, Ms. S. was interested in psychological counseling. Her grief was acutely painful and she hoped to find a counseling service for herself and Robert, whom she intended to convince to attend.

I gave Ms. S. the names of two counseling clinics near her home. She was refused an appointment at the first clinic because she was judged to need long-term supportive therapy which the clinic did not provide; at the second clinic she was seen four times and referred back to me for the same reason.

In the interim, Robert told his teacher that his stepfather had died and that money was now crucial for him and his mother. The teacher arranged for a summer job cleaning and refurbishing the school. Robert worked under the supervision of a vigorous, expressive man who presented a sharp contrast to his ailing, taciturn stepfather.

Robert's job interfered with his return to the family nurse practitioner clinic. However, he did see a urologist who found no urinary tract disease. Ms. S. faithfully kept her appointments. The brief psychological counseling increased her decision-making ability and understanding of her own needs.

After help from classroom lectures and discussions of supportive psychiatric counseling, I assumed the responsibility for independent supportive counseling with the S. family to prevent further problems.

The absence of definitive mental health evaluation and treatment methods, the lack of a psychiatric consulting clinic, and my inappropriate undergraduate education in institutional psychiatric treatment provided a weak foundation for long-term supportive counseling.

However, with a sociological view of the family as a mediator between the individual and society and my belief that the actions of each family member as well as external social and ecological conditions affect family function over time, some of the S.'s family problems have been defined — lack of a father and husband, low income, low educational level, chronic ill health, recurrent social deviation, inadequate parent-child communication, and poorly accessible care and recreation resources. In my counsel, I have attempted to support Ms. S.'s efforts toward self-reliance and independent decision making. I have listened sympathetically to her accounts of struggles with the welfare and health care bureaucracy and I have encouraged her to understand Robert's feelings and his need for independence. Ms. S. now is finding interests and activities outside her family and is trying to reintroduce Robert to his estranged father. Robert continues his job and relishes his new-found independent life; there is no current indication of pilfering. Ms. S. continues to seek comprehensive coordinated care for her complex health problems at the county clinic where the staff now know her, her family, and their problems.

With care by the family nurse practitioner, Ms. S.'s anxiety and physical complaints are no longer intensified by brief specialty clinic visits in which tradition and economics dictate a hurried 15-minute visit oriented to physical evaluation and drug therapy. Instead, pertinent data and necessary screening-tests obtained by the family nurse practitioner during a supportive visit are available to the specialist for his expert evaluation and treatment. Continued visits with the family nurse practitioner after specialty clinic appointments for interpretation of treatment, personalized health teaching and supportive counseling — all areas of nursing expertise — benefit Ms. S., Robert, and the county clinic budget since complications secondary to misunderstandings are prevented, revisits and drop-in visits are reduced, and nurses are less expensive than physicians. The information gathered during repeated visits with the family helps the staff to understand how the family and social milieu affect Robert's health and his mother's.

The free communication necessary to maintain the S.'s current level of health is being facilitated by the continuity of care provided by the family nurse practitioner.

Sensitive nurses have never limited their roles to the dictates of job specifications and the status quo when human integrity and the limitations of the system have demanded a change in role. Nursing is contributing significantly to improved health care by expanding its efforts to keep pace with changes in health care delivery needs.

17
Community Nurse Practitioners — A Partnership

Jocelyn Greenidge
Ann Zimmern
Mary Kohnke

When nurses find it difficult within the institutional framework to provide the quality and continuity of care to patients that they desire, what can they do? Three community nurses found an answer by forming an independent group nursing practice. They considered their services to be "the fulfillment of the basic role of the nurse — providing services directly to the client."

The idea of starting our own private nursing group practice did not strike us with the speed of lightning. Rather it developed over time and became crystallized in the many discussions we had with each other and with our colleagues.

Like other nurses, we knew the frustrations of trying to practice as professionals in the present institutional framework of the health delivery system. We felt our lack of influence on policies that govern the delivery of nursing care in these facilities, and we were aware of the many roadblocks that kept us from expressing ourselves as knowledgeable practitioners in a creative or innovative way.

At the same time, we were concerned with our inability to provide continuity of care for our patients within the hospital, or when that care was extended into the community. We were also aware of the lack of nursing service for groups not being reached through the present system — the very young, the very old, and those with chronic and long-term illnesses.

We often talked about these problems and tried to figure out solutions to them. Because we were concerned with health care as well as sick care, we wished to help people maintain their health or, if they were sick, to help them return to a maximum level of independence within their limitations. We believed that patients and their families should be involved in their care, and that our role should be a collaborative one with other professionals in all aspects of the delivery of health services. All of these considerations led us to the conclusion that there was a real need to try a new way to deliver nursing care — as independent nurse practitioners in group practice.

We liked this idea. We realized that instead of practicing individually, it would be in the best interests of potential patients and ourselves to pool our combined knowledge and experience. This effort would also enable us to provide continuity of care on a 24-hour, 7-day-a-week basis. Patients would be able then to reach us at any time should the need arise.

NEIGHBORHOOD SERVICE

Once we had decided to open an independent practice and had established our major goals, we faced the question of where to locate the practice. This answer seemed easy, since we all lived in the Stuyvesant Town-Peter Cooper Village of New York City. This is a middle-income community, with a population of approximately 33,000 people, enclosed within a three by nine city block area. In general, people who live in the housing complex fit into the present health economic category of "too rich to qualify, but too poor to afford."

We already knew quite a bit about the population in the area from the results of a community health survey conducted by one of us during a college course. For example, we knew that (1) approximately 45 percent of the population are 45 years of age or over (of these, many are of retirement age and live alone); (2) in the remaining 55 percent are many married couples with young children and adolescents; (3) the median income of the total population is approximately $9,600 per year; and (4) while there are numerous hospitals, clinics, and private physicians around the area, most of the people are too rich to qualify for the clinics, and, therefore, must use private physicians or delay seeking medical care until a crisis develops.

These characteristics indicated to us that there would be a sufficient variety of health care needs to warrant our opening a private nursing group practice in the area, so the 27 blocks became the nucleus of our practice. We have since extended our service to a limited number of blocks surrounding this housing complex.

PRACTICALITIES IN GETTING STARTED

The next step facing us was how to start our practice. The three of us had other commitments, not only to our work, but also to our ongoing education. Our financial assets were limited, so we chose to practice in the most economical way possible.

Incorporation or Partnership?

We consulted our own lawyers and the New York City Business Advisory Board (this is a free service offered by the city to people opening small businesses). The consensus was in favor of a partnership, rather than a corporation, primarily because of the expense involved in incorporating — $500 to $600. The chief value of incorporating is that only the assets of the corporation are then liable to a legal suit. This means that should the corporation have any outstanding debts, it can be sued only for debts to the extent of the corporation's assets. Since our debts would be negligible, this was not a primary concern.

Furthermore, corporations are doubly taxed, whereas there is only a single federal tax for partnerships. Although there was the possibility of lawsuits, these would most probably be in the area of malpractice. But, since we were individually covered for malpractice, the legal consensus was that this would be sufficient protection for the present time.

After we decided to form a partnership, we were informed by the advisory board that a name should be chosen for the partnership. So forms setting forth this name had to be bought at a local stationery store and then completed, notarized, and filed at the county clerk's office.

After much deliberation we arrived at the name "Community Nurse Practitioners." We believe this title describes not only the setting but also the nature of the practice.

We then opened a checking account in the name of the partnership and were required by the bank to produce a notarized stamped copy of the partnership papers that we had filed at the county clerk's office. We discovered that the county clerk's office will not let anyone use the name "nurse" unless one can prove by licensure that one is a registered nurse.

Office Versus Answering Service

Although our first desire was to convert one of our apartments into an office for our practice, we were informed that under the terms of our respective leases this was not possible. Therefore, we decided to establish our practice through an answering service. We soon discovered that to establish a service of this kind, we had to first arrange with the telephone company to put in our own answering line. This guaranteed that the line would be answered by the exclusive name of our service.

We had this line put into the answering service office and this service, in turn, contacts us whenever a call comes in. The total cost includes the telephone company's installation fee, the charge for a private business line, and the charge for the answering service. The present operating expense comes to $45 a month. Such an answering service can cost as much as $125 a month, if the more sophisticated long-distance beeper service is included.

We had investigated the possibility of setting up a store-front office in the area, but found that the cheapest location available would cost $300 a month. Due to our limited finances, this was out of the question, although we realized what a public relations asset such an office would be. We were forced then to rely on the next best solution — the answering service — which necessitated our seeing patients in their homes. We realized that this would limit our contact with the public, as well as the range of services we wished to provide, such as a walk-in clinic. However, we believed it was better to establish a practice with an answering service than no practice at all.

Legalities and Policies

Each partner, as has been stated, is covered by her own malpractice insurance. The policies guiding our group practice are governed by: (1) the New York State

Nurse Practice Act, (2) the ANA's Code for Professional Nurses, and (3) the rules established by the three partners. These rules or policies which are to be regularly reviewed and updated as necessary, include:

1. All patients enrolled in our service will be covered on a 24-hour, 7-day-a-week basis.
2. All clients will be seen at any time, day or night. After 8 p.m., for safety reasons, two partners will visit all new clients.
3. Each partner will care for her own patients, but all partners will see each other's patients on an emergency basis when they are on call.
4. A complete health history will be taken on the initial visit, and each partner will be provided with a cross-file index card for every patient.
5. If a patient requires administration of prescription medications or treatments involving such medications, a written physician's order will be required on the forms provided by the practice. All medications and supplies must be provided by the patient, and no nurse will carry medication, syringes, or supplies on her person.
6. Should one of our patients be hospitalized, he will be seen by his nurse at the hospital for the purpose of maintaining continuity of care at no charge to him.
7. The fees will be $10 an hour, the amount prorated for every 15 minutes of service given. A visit may range from a minimum of 15 minutes to a maximum of two hours.
8. All fees are to be deposited in the partnership account. At the end of the month, after expenses are deducted, 25 percent of the profit will be divided equally among the partners; the remaining 75 percent will be divided on a prorated basis depending on the input of each partner.

Financial Outlay

It cost us approximately $300 to open our practice. This was covered by equal contributions by the three partners. The major expenditures were the cost of the answering service, purchase of blood pressure equipment and stethoscopes, installation of a business telephone line, newspaper advertising, and printed material. Our present operating expenses include the answering service and the monthly phone bill.

MAKING OUR SERVICE KNOWN

Now that we had our partnership, answering service, and policies, how did we go about telling people that we were available? First, we contacted the two local newspapers covering our area, and they agreed to publish news stories about our practice. We also placed ads in these papers. Second, we posted notices of our services in the local laundromats of Stuyvesant Town-Peter Cooper housing development. Third, we wrote letters to the physicians in the immediate area to inform them of the opening of our practice and the service we had to offer. We sent the same letter to the directors of nurses in hospitals and public health agencies in the area. Fourth, we notified our own professional organizations — local, state, and national — of what we were doing. And, finally, we spoke to both our professional colleagues and members of the community on an informal basis about our practice, and the services we offered.

COMMUNITY RESPONSE

The overall response of the community and other professionals has been on the whole positive. These expressions have ranged from "This is what is needed in the community," to "Can you help me?" or direct requests for services. But we have had to refer many inquiring clients to other agencies, because they lived in areas too distant from us or needed a sitter service or private duty nursing. Since we provide care for a maximum of two hours, people who wanted 8- or 24-hour nursing service were referred to other agencies. Some callers phoned for information about our service so that they would know where to call if a need arose. We have even had calls from other nurses, wanting to join our practice.

Many patients had to be referred to other agencies because Blue Cross and Blue Shield, Medicare, and Medicaid reimburse only private physicians and health agencies. Since we are not in one of these categories, we could not be paid under these plans. We in nursing need legislative input to bring about change in these laws.

Most of the clients who retained us were self-referrals (from our ads or laundry room notices) — others, through a neighbor. As yet, only one physician has referred a patient to us, although a few doctors have phoned us for more details about our services. The following are some examples of the kinds of patients we are now seeing.

Mrs. T is a middle-aged housewife with six children. She has a cardiac condition that includes occasional episodes of tachycardia with accompanying anxiety. She should be seen during these episodes in case of arrhythmia, which could require immediate hospitalization. She also needs support to allay her extreme anxiety.

Mrs. P is a 60-year-old woman in the advanced stages of cancer. She is still able to get up and about. She wishes to remain at home with her husband as long as possible. We are helping her to meet her physical and some psychological needs at home so that she can remain there as long as she is able and desires to do so.

Mrs. M is an 82-year-old widow, whose children live some distance away. Her memory is poor, and her ability to walk much farther than the corner store is limited. Her blood pressure is high, and she forgets to take her pills. We visit her daily to be sure she has taken her pills, eaten a balanced diet, and is maintaining her daily activities. Her desire is to live independently as long as possible, and her children concur in this. Through our daily visits we are trying to make this not only possible, but safe for her as well.

Miss C is a 28-year-old woman who is paralyzed from the waist down and who lives with her widowed mother and grandmother. Due to the hospitalization of her mother for back trouble, she needed someone to assist her in and out of the bath tub. We helped in this area and geared our approach to finding a means by which she could become entirely independent. We also became involved with the mother, giving support and guidance to her in adjusting to her back condition, as well as to the 80-year-old grandmother with a broken wrist, who was given support and explanation of how to exercise and care for her wrist when the cast was removed.

PROGRESS AND PHILOSOPHY

We started our practice last summer and we now have twelve patients. Responses from our clients and the community continue to be enthusiastic. Our local newspaper has published an article about our practice and the ways by which we are meeting the community's health needs. Consumers' and professionals' interest is evident; we have been asked to speak about our practice to various groups.

Independent nurse practitioner functioning, as we see it, enables realization of the entire concept of professionalism and its ramifications. We have full authority over our nursing practice and policies and assume all the responsibility for and consequences of our actions. In the words of Harry Truman, "The buck stops here." The reality of this type of practice has had a sobering and maturing effect on each of us. We are experiencing many of the things we only read about before — for example, peer review. In its pure form we each experience this type of evaluation during our weekly conferences in which we discuss our patients' care. Never has our nursing care been so carefully scrutinized.

Our relationships with other professionals has been one of collaboration, and it is very satisfying to be treated as a professional equal. We believe this attitude has been due not only to our professional manner of care, but also to the fact that we are working outside of institutional systems. Nurses have allowed the bureaucratic framework of institutions to exert a thwarting effect on their nursing care. The situation cannot be remedied by one or three nurses; instead, all nurses should act together and bring about the changes that are necessary if we are to practice as professionals within the institutional system.

In most of our cases we have achieved our goal by directly delivering nursing care to our clients. As an adjunct to our services we have acted as facilitators for our clients when there was need for another health delivery system. Our experiences as independent nurse practitioners have reaffirmed our feelings that the present system of health services is not, in fact, meeting the needs of people. New modes of delivery for health care are desperately needed, and nurses must take the leadership role in designing and ensuring utilization of new methods. Nurses are the only professional group who are prepared to deal in a holistic way with man. Therefore, they must fulfill their responsibilities to society.

EXPANDED ROLE?

Much is being said and written about what is called the expanded or extended role of nursing today. However, we believe that a private practice in nursing cannot be equated with either the extended or expanded role of nurses. Rather, we believe our practice is the fulfillment of the basic role of the nurse — providing services directly to the client. These services can comprise casefinding, health teaching, health counseling, and care that is supportive or restorative of life and well-being. To us this is the heart of nursing and the realization of the goals that Florence Nightingale established over a century ago.

IV

The Cultural Dimension
of Community Nursing

Culture has been called the "third dimension" of health care. The physical aspect of health and illness as well as the psychological dimension can easily be identified. But, in addition, all human beings behave in the context of a specific culture, which profoundly affects thoughts and feelings about health and disease. Culture influences reactions to stress; it channels attitudes toward pain. The way people feel in the face of death, the way they express grief, the way they relate to health practitioners, the way they teach children — all are affected by culture.

Culture refers to the ideas, values and behavior that are learned by members of some social group. It is a design for living. Although there are some broad cultural values shared by many who live in the United States, this society is marked by a rich diversity of subcultures. Native American groups have retained some aspects of their traditional cultures. Mexican-Americans, Irish-Americans, Italian-Americans, Afro-Americans, Puerto Ricans, Chinese-Americans and many other ethnic groups have their own subcultures. Furthermore, certain customs, values and ideas are unique to the poor, the rich, the middle class, youth, women, men and the elderly. Regional subcultures also have distinctive ways of defining the world and coping with problems. Even occupations develop their own special languages and worlds of cultural meanings. Many deviant groups such as narcotic addicts, criminals, homosexuals and skid row alcoholics have developed their own subcultures. Although most people share some features of the larger American culture, many also have learned aspects of one or more subcultures. Even nurses have their own special culture with its unique vocabulary, values, clothes and customs.

As nursing has moved outside the controlled environment of the hospital setting, the importance of these various cultural groups has become more apparent. When health professionals interact only with people of their own culture, most problems can be understood in physical and psychological terms. But when seeking to communicate across cultural boundaries, when working with people from different subcultures, it becomes important to deal with cultural influences on behavior. A missed appointment at a clinic, for example, may not mean irresponsibility or lack of interest. Instead it might be a highly rational choice in terms of some hidden cultural value such as a strong orientation to the present. A woman may avoid going to a male physician because of her cultural standards for modesty in the presence of males. A mother may fail to follow some recommendation for her child because she believes a condition is actually caused by an "evil eye." If grandmothers or other relatives have authority over the health of children, instructions to the mother alone may be to no avail. If a culture places great emphasis upon joint decisions by a group of kinsmen, urging an individual to undergo surgery may be a waste of time. Such examples only hint at the many ways culture is involved in community nursing.

One major goal of community nursing is the prevention of illness. But because prevention involves efforts to change behavior patterns, almost every attempt runs into hidden cultural barriers. Prevention is based on a strong future orientation and a certain degree of optimism about the future. This often contrasts with the present time orientation and fatalism of many subcultures. Education and teaching for high levels of health may fail because they are based on culture-bound methods of teaching. Some cultures emphasize learning by means of abstract symbols; others stress teaching by active involvement and participation. Unless the community nurse is aware of how members of different subcultures traditionally learn new things, efforts at teaching are doomed to failure.

In recent years a growing number of health professionals have become aware of the cultural dimension. In the following chapters several of these persons describe the cultures of specific groups in this society. They identify many hidden cultural barriers that confront the community nurse. They also suggest ways to deal with these barriers. Only a small number of cultural groups can be covered in Part IV but they provide examples that can be easily applied to numerous other subcultures.

18

The Cultural Context of Behavior: Spanish-Americans and Nursing Care

Madeleine Leininger

Culture is more than isolated elements of belief and custom. It is an integrated whole, a pattern of values and behavior that provide people with designs for living. The community nurse must be aware of this larger pattern that links health concerns, child-rearing practices and folk medicine to religion, politics and family structure. In this chapter, Madeleine Leininger, who is both a nurse and an anthropologist, examines the cultural context of health-related behavior in the broader context of Hispanic culture. She emphasizes the need for community nurses to become active listeners who continuously investigate the cultural patterns of those with whom they work.

In this chapter the cultural context of human behavior will be examined with respect to one particular cultural group, namely, the Spanish-Americans. An understanding of the cultural context of human behavior is important to health personnel for gaining an in-depth view of the people one is working with and to help one discover ways to tailor-make treatment and nursing care plans.[1] The cultural context approach strives for *specificity* in the consideration of patient problems and for *reducing ambiguity in nursing goals.* The approach gives full support to the discovery of cultural factors influencing or determining an individual or group health problem.

MEANING OF THE CULTURAL CONTEXT OF BEHAVIOR

The cultural context of behavior refers to the implicit and explicit behavior tendencies of a designated group of people who have lived and interacted together in a particular cultural setting according to certain values, practices, and life goals. Each cultural group in various places in the world has its own life style, its own patterns of living, and its own special way of viewing the world about it. Its special world view is the essential basis of a people's modes of acting and thinking, and its world view serves as the basic framework for their unique cultural context of behavior. The cultural context of behavior is, however, shaped and maintained by social, political, religious, economical, kinship, historical, and specific cultural factors. These factors are interdigitated and produce a certain pattern of behavior which gives "character" and distinction to a culture's mode of living. As one studies the cultural context of behavior, it is important to see how these various elements fit together to provide a comprehensive picture of

From Madeleine Leininger, *Nursing and Anthropology: Two Worlds to Blend,* pp. 111–127. Copyright © 1970, John Wiley & Sons, Inc., New York. Reprinted by permission of the publisher.

the people. The behavior of certain individuals or subgroups makes sense when perceived within the cultural context of behavior, one can predict the behavior tendencies with a fair degree of accuracy.

Anthropologists believe that one of the best ways to understand the meaning and significance of the cultural context of behavior is to become active participants in the life ways of a particular culture. Perhaps one might choose to live with a group of people for a period of time in order to gain special knowledge about the ways they interact with each other. A conscious effort must be made to know a particular group's way of living, and this effort must be directed largely towards *seeing and hearing through the eyes and ears of the people.* Empathy, interest, objectivity, and involvement are crucial means of grasping the cultural context behavior. A study of the daily, weekly, monthly, and yearly life activities of people blended with social science data about a given group can insure a good overview of the contextual aspects of human behavior. It is rewarding to put bits and pieces of cultural data together so that a larger and meaningful picture comes into existence. The whole process of determining the cultural context of behavior is analogous to putting a jigsaw puzzle together. Generally, the pieces will fit together if one is willing to struggle with the idea of a gestalt view. Since nurses may find it difficult to live with a cultural group (although it is highly recommended by this author), an alternative approach to grasping the cultural context of behavior is to be an active listener, observer, and good questioner about the people one desires to know. In addition, one can draw upon the knowledge in the literature to know "one's people." With this in mind, we turn to an exploration of the cultural context features of the Spanish-American peoples as an example of how to go about understanding the many-faceted dimensions of a cultural group.

THE CULTURAL CONTEXT OF THE SPANISH-AMERICAN

General Cultural Features

The Spanish-American people are descendants of the Spanish colonists, who date back to the eighteenth century.[2] It is generally agreed that the exact location of the Spanish colonization and cultural heritage in the United States includes the present New Mexico, Arizona, Texas, southern and central California, southern Colorado, and the east coast of Florida. Many of these Spanish-Americans share distinctive cultural features which influence their behavior in spite of their continuous contacts with other cultural groups in our society.

At the outset, it is important to clarify that the Spanish-Americans, Mexican-Americans, and Mexicans are three major subgroups of the total Spanish-speaking population. Each of these subgroups has its own cultural ways and beliefs and historical background, and so one cannot view them as identical in cultural behavior. Through time, however, there have been various kinds of interaction with a wide variety of other cultural and subcultural groups in the United States, which have shaped certain aspects of their behavior to make them similar in certain respects with one another.

The Spanish-Americans are the remaining descendants of the old Spanish colonial group who came into the middle and upper Rio Grande valleys. These people are referred to as "Hispanos," and their largest populations are concentrated in New Mexico and southern Colorado. When the Spanish colonists came to America, a low ratio of women to men existed among them, and so wives were sought among the indigenous Indian populations of the region. Intermarriage with the American Indians was a common practice until the early nineteenth century, and marriage between the Anglo-Americans and the Spanish increased. The Spanish-American of today is a genetic descendant of sixteenth- and seventeenth-century Spain, and of the new Spain with some intermarriage with the American Indians and with Anglo-Americans.

The Spanish-Americans tend to hold themselves aloof from the Mexican-Americans, since they recognize their past heritage ties while, of course, Mexican-Americans cherish their own rich background. Through the years, however, Mexican-Americans and Spanish-Americans have shown some cultural similarities because of their intermarriage practices and their ways of dealing with common social, political, and economic problems. From the Mexican-American's physical appearance, one can see a closer tie with the Indian culture of America than with the Spanish-Americans. Physical characteristics, however, are but a small aspect of the total factors influencing any culture's behavior and way of living.

Spanish-Americans became citizens of the United States by military conquest which involved no immediate necessity to modify their traditional way of life, no substantive break with their cultural traditions, and no change in residence. Today there are about 500,000 Spanish-Americans in rural and urban areas of the southwest United States.

Social and Kinship Aspects

The social life of the Spanish-American was traditionally organized (as it still is largely today) around the extended family and the church. The father is the patriarch whose authority is recognized and expected to be exercised. He is responsible for giving guidance and leadership to the family, and for making all major decisions. The role of the mother and wife is subordinate to her husband or to the father of the household. The mother's interests are primarily in bearing children, and in caring for her family, her home, and her close kinsmen. The father and husband is expected to assume material responsibility for his wife and children. His private or personal morals are his own business, but his social or group morals must be above reproach if he is to maintain his status in the family and the community. The eldest son has authority over younger siblings and has a right to influence the mother regarding family decisions. The extended and nuclear family in the rural and urban areas binds the Spanish-American family together, so that family matters always prevail over individual and nonfamily affairs.

Kinship ties extend beyond the biological ties within the family to the important institution known as *compadrasgo,* or godparents, who maintain a strong religious and social obligation toward the child. Grandparents are highly respected for their decisions and are frequently consulted for their opinions about family problems. All family and kin members are expected to show respect for one another.

The family is the chief link with the community and provides a model for relationships outside the kinship group. The family members have definite steps they follow regarding who treats illness and what specific role each person should play. The mother is first to become aware of the child or adult's illness, and then the mother seeks the father's advice. Next they seek the mother's mother for advice, and then the godparents or coparents (*compadres*). If the family remedies do not prove efficious, then the indigenous lay medical people are sought, namely, the *medicas, sobadors, curanderos,* and *albolarios.* Finally, professional or nonindigenous practitioners may be sought, particularly if the individual is seriously ill and death seems imminent. Thus the family is the group of unity and the group which deals first with a health problem. This is one of the major reasons why many physicians, nurses, and others have wondered why Spanish-American people are slow to come for professional help. Professional health personnel must realize that these people have their own health care and treatment system, including their own practitioners with whom they feel most comfortable and secure. Many Spanish-Americans still tend to seek nonindigenous help only when an illness is extremely serious or threatening to the life of a family member. There are, of course, some Spanish-Americans who are highly acculturated to Anglo-American middle and middle-upper class practices, and they seek professional help at an early time.

Religious Aspects

The Spanish-Americans are predominantly of the Roman Catholic faith. A small percent are Protestant or have another religious affiliation. Traditionally, religion was a significant factor in the people's lives, for it helped to unify and integrate their total life ways in the family and in the community. In recent years, religion has not been such a powerful force in the lives of the Spanish-American people. There is less ritualism and fewer daily religious activities; moreover, some of the major feasts and ceremonies of the Church are celebrated with less elaboration and fewer signs of external pious devotion. Nevertheless, varying degrees of religious faith continue to serve important functions and purposes for these people. It is common to hear some Spanish-Americans express regret that the ceremonial and religious activities of the Catholic Church are waning and changing. The priest continues to be recognized in many Spanish-American communities as the people's spiritual leader, and he serves as a counselor regarding temporal, religious, and community matters.

Political Aspects

Politics and political strivings are well known to the Spanish-American people, and are more apparent in some parts of their territory than others. For example, in the State of New Mexico political action has been quite noticeable in furthering the people's desires for land and general national rights. The Spanish-Americans in this state comprise more than one-half the total population of the state, and they are actively using political processes to control and protect their rights. In other states where Spanish-Americans reside, political action is not as forceful as it was in the past; however, there are today more apparent signs of overt political activity. It can be anticipated that as Spanish-Americans become more involved in national and state affairs, their traditional political methods will change along with the problems they seek to resolve. Contrary to the general public image, the Spanish-American people are not as passive and nonaggressive people as one might think them to be. When their rights, privileges and goals are at stake, they are willing to fight for them. They have been known through their culture history to rise actively and firmly to deal with matters affecting their well-being.

Political leadership emanates from the male leader of the household who learns to become a good speaker and defender of the family and community. Currently, Spanish-Americans are becoming active in Anglo-American politics in order to share in our nation's wealth, to establish democratic freedom and protection, and to obtain material, social, and political rights in our American society. New young political leaders are emerging among the Spanish-Americans, who have learned through our educational system and life experience how to obtain American rights. Reies Lopez Tijerina, for example, has been extremely active in strengthening the political movement for return of grant land to Southwest Hispanos.[3] Spanish-Americans are fighting politically for better living facilities, good schools, adequate food, and other kinds of public assistance. Political behavior as a way of influencing others to gain self and group help has changed through the years for the Spanish-American peoples, and now their behavior is becoming similar to that of many Anglo-Americans. And it is reasonable to predict that the Spanish-Americans will continue to be more open and active in national affairs than they have been in the past.

Economic Aspects

The Spanish-American way of community life has traditionally been based upon agriculture. In the past, the small irrigated farm was a prosperous and self-sufficient means of supporting a family. Today, those who have retained their lands are finding it difficult to support their large families because of rising costs related to modern technological and general farming expenses. Those who have no land live as tenants, sharecroppers, or are hired by farmers who own land. Many have joined the streams of migrant agricultural laborers who travel here and there seeking employment on sugar beet, potato, fruit, or small grain farms. As migrant farmers they find it difficult to improve their economic status, and often they go for years without any improvement in their economic status. There is, however, considerable value, among Spanish-Americans, placed on possessing their own land and raising their own crops for their family and friends. Most of the land they own is semi-arid, with limited irrigation systems. Modern irrigation and farm machinery are rarely found on their acreages. Cattle and sheep-raising supplements their livelihood. Cattle, sheep and goats are often a major source of their income, along with products from their gardens.

Industries in and near the cities have attracted many Spanish-Americans to work as unskilled and semi-skilled laborers. Only a few years ago, agriculture was the mainstay of their economy, with family wage work to supplement their agricultural production. Today, wage and salary work is the principal means of a Spanish-American's livelihood. Many families now engage in agricultural activities primarily to provide fresh food for family use and to keep "in touch" with their past cultural interests.

Only a small proportion of Spanish-Americans are wealthy. In general, their living facilities are modest and their economic status is meager (whether they live in rural or urban areas). Most Spanish-Americans have had approximately eight years or less of formal education so that it is difficult for them to compete in the industrial world with Anglo-Americans and others. Then, too, many of the Spanish-Americans speak the Spanish language and have difficulty in speaking English fluently, and this often limits what jobs are available to them. Urbanization trends continue to bring the Spanish-American people into the cities, where educational facilities are more accessible to them. There is some concern and hesitation, however, about sending Spanish-American children to these Anglo-oriented schools because parents fear the consequences of the schools' emphasis on competition, open aggression and high achievement — all values contrary to the traditional Spanish-American way of life. Then, too, they feel the children should work at home or along with their parents in their unskilled jobs in order to maintain a continuity of livelihood in the urban community.

Class differences among the Spanish-Americans do exist and range from the lower class, who are often isolated farm villagers, to a small core of upper class people who enjoy the status of their old family traditions and family wealth or who have achieved wealth in our modern society. Those who are fully acculturated to the modern American life may have today's technological conveniences and live as middle class citizens. Interestingly enough, some Spanish-Americans who have been exposed to modern ways have not given up their older life style. Doubts and suspicions exist among some Spanish-Americans about Anglo-American values and practices which they fear might change drastically or weaken their family and group life.

Health-Illness Systems

In the course of time, the Spanish-Americans have used a variety of sources for their knowledge about diseases and the treatment of illness. They have drawn upon: (1) the folk medical lore of medieval Spain; (2) the health-illness treatment practices of American Indians, especially the Mexican Indians; and (3) the Anglo folk and modern medical practices found in rural and urban areas. These sources of knowledge have been combined with their own health-illness system and adapted to other aspects of their culture.

Traditionally, the Spanish-American health-illness system was closely interwoven with faith and fatalism, and any illness could be explained; this system prepared people psychologically and culturally for life uncertainties. Their strong faith in God and their kinsmen helped to sustain them in accepting a disease and in maintaining their beliefs. Their philosophy and values of human life also helped them realize that not all of life can be fully controlled by man. To them, normal health was always subject to attack and change, just as sin and temptation always existed in the world. There was no such thing as perfect health, for health is relative to an individual and his situation. Spanish-American people realize that illness exists because perfection in health never exists completely. Being able to function adequately means wellness even though such adequacy may involve the actual malfunctioning of a body part. Good and evil are always present and are conflicting forces in man's life; so one meets and accepts illness and death, sadness and joy, good and evil.

Man is faced with the challenge of keeping his body in a state of balance or equilibrium in order to be healthy. Since the body is seen as a functioning whole, operations are viewed as dangerous to bodily wholeness. Man's body must function as a whole with the maintenance of a balance of hot and cold substances in the body. For example: (1) if your feet get wet, it is important to get your head wet, since an imbalance will lead to a sore throat; (2) one should use chili (hot food) to treat pneumonia (cold disease); (3) avoid citrus fruits (cold food) as they will cause colic; (4) drinking cold water after a hot day may cause *empacho* (indigestion). Balance must also be maintained in emotional expressions and interpersonal relationships.

Many Spanish-American people believe that they have limited control over nature. They believe that God gives health and that he sends illness to them for some reason. They recognize that some diseases are caused by accidents, the devil, witchcraft, heredity, and so on. However, they say that ultimately all diseases are caused by God. God is seen as merciful in that he gives knowledge to medical people so they can be physicians, *medicas,* or *medicos,* and can help people. An unbending faith in God and a faith in curing are essential to recovery; moreover, the cure or lack of cure is in God's hands, not in the hands of human beings. Although Spanish-Americans are knowledgeable about preventive measures and their importance, they do not necessarily think that preventive remedies are of primary relevance if an individual suddenly becomes ill, because God may have willed the illness.

A misfortune such as illness can be viewed either as a punishment from God (*castigo de Dios*) or as a cross to bear. Mental illness and mental retardation are crosses to bear for the family members. So God is primarily in charge of health, and can cause or permit illness. Pregnancy is viewed as normal, and so health personnel should not disrupt something which God controls. Accordingly, a child is in the hands of God, and it is hard to understand why immunizations are considered so important and extoiled so hard by health workers. This acceptance of and resignation to God's will provides emotional comfort and explanations of illness and health, and prepares Spanish-American people for many unexpected daily happenings and misfortunes which man faces everywhere. An assault from the unknown (*prendido*), a mysterious power influencing others, and general misfortunes can be accepted if one believes that supernatural forces control man and nature.[4]

To the Spanish-American, a healthy person is one who looks and acts healthy. A healthy adult is well proportioned, has good color, good muscles, and does a good day's work. A healthy child is plump and rosy; he eats well and is physically active. A sick person is unable to do daily routine activities and has lost strength and weight. Health is essentially a day-to-day state of being which is governed by natural and supernatural forces shaping the present. A person has to feel discomfort, otherwise he is not ill. There is limited emphasis upon causes of illness, since Spanish-American people know what probably caused the illness — either an evil force or God's will.

Diseases are classified primarily as physical or natural diseases. Some of these are similar to diseases found among Mexican-American peoples.[5] Four of the common indigenous diseases are the following:

1. *Mal ojo*, literally translated "bad eye," is a disease which is believed to afflict a person (usually a child) because someone admires or desires the child to an excessive degree. The afflicted person becomes ill with symptoms of sleepiness, general malaise, and excessive tiredness. The treatment is to find the person who has cast the "evil eye" and have him (her) caress or touch the person. Prophylactically, when a person admires a child, he should always touch the child. This gesture reduces the spell being cast on the child and protects him from illness.

2. *Empacho* is a condition in which food forms into a ball and clings to the wall of the stomach, preventing the assimilation of food. Generally, the cause of *empacho* is the poor quality of food given to an individual because of a malicious contamination of the food by a personal enemy. Stomach cramps and nervousness are common symptoms. Treatment includes a combined physical magico-religious practice in which prayers are recited while the spine is massaged gently with small doses of mercury derivative (*greta*). Other treatment modalities are also employed.

3. *Mal de susto*, or "illness from fright," is believed to be the result of an emotionally traumatic experience. The patient becomes frightened, tense, and drowsy, and experiences a loss of energy. Occasionally night sweats are noted. The treatment is directed toward relaxing the individual with herb tea (*llerba*

buena) and ritually "sweeping" the person with a branch. Again, prayers are recited during the sweeping ritual. *Susto* is caused by natural fright, such as being nearly injured. In contrast, *espanto* (fright) is caused by seeing a devil or ghost. Sometimes acculturated individuals do not distinguish between these two fright syndromes.

4. *Maleficio,* or witchcraft, is largely caused by witches or malicious friends. It is greatly feared by the people and many preventive steps are taken to avoid being bewitched. Witches are believed to obtain their power from the devil. Often those who are arousing envy and jealousy in others fear that a witch will be used to harm them. Witches can transform themselves into other persons or into animals. Their evil is worked by sympathetic image magic. Some witches force an evil wind (*mal aire*) which can produce acute pain to enter a person's body. In general, witchcraft is greatly feared by the people. They are reluctant to discuss the subject except with close kinsmen, friends, or family members.

Today many familiar diseases are recognized among the Spanish-Americans such as arthritis, asthma, cancer, colds, diarrhea, heart disease, pneumonia, tuberculosis, etc., but the people frequently recognize different causes and treatments of these diseases than those found acceptable among Anglo-American professionals. Moreover, the Spanish-American people have many remedies for disease states and known health stressors. Herbs are used frequently for ingestion, poultices, infusions, and topical cures. Massage and manipulation for illness are other therapeutic techniques frequently used, and these are referred to as *sobando* and *traqueando*.

Folk practitioners with a variety of skills are used in the treatment of their culturally defined illnesses. These practitioners are still recognized today, and are sought after for their skill in diagnosing and treating an illness. The following practitioners are found in the Spanish-American health-treatment system:[6]

1. A *sobador* is a specialist in massage, who is also known for his ability to handle fractures and bone disorders.
2. A *partera,* or midwife, is usually an older woman who has become an expert in assisting with the delivery of babies. Through the accumulated practical experience of the *parteras* with mothers and infants, she is responsible for the delivery of the infant and provides therapeutic emotional support to the mother. A *partera* has extensive knowledge of folk medicines, especially herbs and the various traditional treatments. In recent years, *parteras* are being recognized by health departments and professional personnel. They are also being exposed to professional views and practices related to maternal and child health care. The synthesis of indigenous and professional health practices should make them a special kind of health worker.
3. A *medico* is a woman or man considered as a general specialist in folk medicine. The *medico* is able to treat a wide variety of illnesses with specific local

remedies and/or with therapeutic massage. The *medico* is usually called when a sick person has not responded to general home remedies, or if the family is dissatisfied with modern professional services.

4. A *curandero* is a female and sometimes a male specialist who is equivalent to the Anglo general practitioner. Some *curanderos* are noted specialists for many kinds of diseases. They have a power to heal which they believe is a gift (*don*) from God, and so all treatments are accompanied by propiation to God or one of the saints. Often, *curanderos* have an altar in their consulting rooms. The *curandero* and patient often pray together, and the patient's payment is ritualized to show his awareness that the curer has served as God's means of helping the patient; generally, the patient leaves an offering before one of the saints. *Curanderos* claim they are inspired by God to become curers. Their training is under other practicing curers or in centers of folk curing. Treatment by a *curandero* is meaningful in the context of the patient's culture. Generally the family obtains the services of a *curandero* for their ill family member and the family is kept informed of the reasoning behind the diagnosis and the progress of the patient under treatment.

5. An *albolario* is a man, or sometimes a woman, who specializes in the treatment of victims of witchcraft. Only a few of these practitioners exist today. Sometimes a man may be known as both a *curandero* and *albolario*. They deal with witches or *brujas*.

It is of interest that when Spanish-Americans go to an Anglo-American practitioner after they have experienced no success with their home remedies, they look for a chiropractor or an osteopath because they manipulate the bones and muscles, a role similar to that of the familiar folk practitioners. In rural areas, folk medicine and folk practitioners are preferred, because of their knowledge of local medicines and the techniques of folk healing. These practitioners also take a high degree of personal interest in the patient, his family, and kinsmen, and the family can participate actively and knowingly in the treatment. Although the state and local health departments in Colorado, New Mexico, and in other states have made noticeable efforts to bring medical and general health services to Spanish-Americans, there are still rural areas which have no modern medical facilities and local folk medical treatment is used.[7] Taos County in New Mexico and Costilla County in Colorado have been places where health services and medical care programs have been established. These programs have not been too successful because they failed to accommodate cultural factors related to the health maintenance and the treatment of disease.[8] Other studies have also stressed the importance of understanding the Spanish-American culture to establish good relationships with the people and to communicate effectively with them if one hopes to have a successful health program.[9,10]

To the Spanish-American, health and illness are largely viewed as existing only in the present time, and there is little emphasis upon illness in the future. The present moment is the major concern to the people and determines how the people respond to questions about health and illness. The comment *"bueno sano"* (or well and hale) means the person is functioning well for the present.

IMPLICATIONS FOR NURSING

It is obvious that there are differences between Spanish-American and Anglo-American views of the causes, nature, and treatment of diseases; differences exist in their cultural values, beliefs, and practices. The cultural context in which health is maintained, or in which illness develops, is a broad and complex framework closely related to political, religious, social, economic, and cultural practices. For Spanish-Americans, health and illness must be assessed and treated with respect to these many factors in the patient's cultural setting. There is a particularly close relationship with the patient's illness and his religious practices and family relationships. The nurse must view wellness and illness of Spanish-Americans in connection with these variables and others, and not see illness as an isolated physical or psychological phenomenon.

In working with a Spanish-American patient and his family, the nurse will be able to understand the full nature of the patient's illness if she can speak or understand the Spanish language. Although many Spanish-Americans are becoming bilingual who live in the United States and especially in urban areas, still there are many persons who cannot speak English. These persons when ill tend to avoid contact with Anglos and to show signs of social isolation. In order to reach these people and understand their health problems, one must understand the language they speak.

Some Anglo-Americans tend to show annoyance to Hispanos who do not know how to speak English and this only aggravates and complicates the nurse reaching the patient's feelings and concerns.[11] When language annoyance occurs between Anglos and Spanish-Americans, there is often the expectation that Spanish-Americans should speak English, not that Anglo-Americans should know Spanish. This behavior implies that members of a subculture should meet the expectations of the dominant culture. As a consequence of such interpersonal encounters and attitudes, poor cooperation and feelings of resentment exist between persons from the two cultures.

Frequently one hears a comment that Spanish-Americans are "lazy," "apathetic" and "irresponsible" people. Again, labeling of a cultural group does not really help to understand the people for it does not convey an accurate picture of the people's behavior. It is a superficial label without clarification of meaning or use. Generally, the "apathetic" and so-called "irresponsible attitude" occurs as a dynamic consequence of the Spanish-American's interaction with an Anglo-American stranger. In the interactional process, the Spanish-American patient is sensitive to the behavior of the Anglo-American and often responds in an initial helpless-like manner as he feels he cannot handle the dominant and often aggressive, perceived attitude of the stranger. He then withdraws socially and appears apathetic. If one understands Spanish-American culture and the many feelings and specific attitude toward strangers, one can see that cultural labeling is superficial with the meaning of behavior being lost in labeling persons.

Gaps and distortions in communication can occur readily as a result of our use of professional expressions as well as through our many nonverbal forms of communication. Since Spanish-Americans are generally polite, deferent, and quiet in an initial encounter with strangers, they often agree with strangers in order to please them. They too may not understand the stranger's behavior and message. Since community health nurses often have contact with these Spanish-American patients in their homes, they can serve as important persons in helping them. They should be patient and allow time to listen to them and try to understand their health problems from their perspective. Most important, nurses should provide explanations which take into account the extent to which the patient and his family are acculturated and they should not assume that all Spanish-American people are equally acculturated. In general, technical and professional terms should be simply defined and clarified. Whenever possible, visual aids should be used to demonstrate health practices. A conscious effort should be made to assess ideas communicated between the patient and the nurse. Still another important communication principle is to look directly at the patient when talking to him, then to listen attentively to his comments and responses and check for the meaning of the message. In the author's recent study of several Spanish-American families, she noted that the people dislike Anglo-Americans talking to them in a hurried manner and maintaining little eye contact while talking to them, as this behavior was interpreted by them as a superficial interest in them as people.

Another way to gain cooperation and establish rapport with Spanish-American people is to use proper forms of address, e.g., saying "Mr. Martinez" rather than using his first name, "Joseph." The nurse, too, should remember to view health problems as private information and to avoid publicizing them. Maintaining an attitude of privacy is important for many reasons, but primarily because Spanish-Americans see illness as a malevolent force with secretive religious and social implications.

Health personnel must realize that it is rather useless to argue persistently with Spanish-Americans in an effort to change their traditional health practices. Instead, if a nurse strives for a warm, friendly, and understanding relationship with the family and remains consciously respectful of their traditional beliefs, she will be more likely to change some of their health practices than if she argues with them. Spanish-Americans accept suggestions and advice about new health practices once a trusting relationship has been established. Spanish-Americans like to view health workers as friends, rather than formal, indifferent, and cold strangers. If the nurse gets to know the Spanish-American family and shows signs of genuine respect and empathy for them, they will be apt to cooperate with her. One can say that the most important professional skill that Spanish-Americans look for in a nurse is her interpersonal skill and her genuine interest in them as a cultural group. This significant professional attribute is possible only when health personnel understand the dynamic cultural context of human behavior and specific cultural groups.

Hanson and Saunders have suggested that professional personnel use the "linkage" concept to help indigenous people.[12] The linkage concept refers to the conscious effort to link the traditional and current beliefs and practices of a cultural group with professional ideas that fit with the indigenous people's health-illness system. The idea of linking the health practices of two cultural groups together is a relevant one, but necessitates that one must understand the differences and similarities between the beliefs and practices of the indigenous and the professional groups. Blending indigenous beliefs and practices with our professional beliefs also requires that professional persons function as highly imaginative and knowledgeable persons about the Spanish-American culture. With the linkage approach, the therapeutic effects and their ties with other social and cultural factors are given consideration. A give-and-take attitude between the nurse and the cultural group she is working with is essential for effective work with people.

Rather than alienating them from the health plans, the professional nurse must consider the important role of the indigenous health practitioners and how they can be utilized in the care and treatment of the patient. Native practitioners are viewed as important persons in the care and treatment of Spanish-American people. They are the practitioners whom the family members call upon first when a serious illness arises, and they are valued for their ideas on ways to prevent illnesses. These practitioners should be perceived by health personnel as an integral part of the people's health-illness system and one should work closely with these people. The belief that all Spanish-Americans are persons who have some role to play in maintaining health or in helping sick persons regain their health state is an important concept to be kept in mind by professional workers. For example, a *medica* must fulfill the role of a confidant to her patients and must maintain a close personal relationship with them. *Medicas* share in the on-going joys of the family as well as in their frustrations and sorrows. They are also important psychotherapists, physical therapists as well as social therapists. To Spanish-Americans, a nurse or physician who shows an impersonal attitude, uses sophisticated language, and gives orders in a formal directive manner, does not fit well with the people's expectations of a good *medicas*. The *medicas* is the people's closest role model for conceptualizing a professional health practitioner. Excessive emotionalism, however, and too personalized behavior with Spanish-Americans may also create doubts in their minds about one's motives. A nurse who communicates genuine respect, and who offers warmth, friendliness, and overt signs of helpfulness, will be successful in interactions with Spanish-American people.

A full acknowledgment by the nurse of the Spanish-American value orientations is extremely important, and these can be briefly highlighted as follows: (1) man's nature is basically bad, and so normal health is always subject to attack; (2) man must keep his body and mind in a state of balance to get healthy; (3) man has limited control over nature and God; (4) God gives health and sends illness; (5) the present is all-important; (6) the family is the important link between the individual and the outside world; and (7) personalism and being oneself are important to man, especially in his relationship to other men. These cultural values can offer the nurse many important clues for building and maintaining a successful relationship with Spanish-American patients.

In this next section, some relevant nursing care guidelines and suggestions will be summarized. First, in planning and implementing health services for Spanish-American patients, the nurse should give full consideration to the role of the nuclear and extended family. The family is important at every phase of the curing and rehabilitation process. It is highly recommended that the nurse work toward the goal of getting family decisions about health care and treatment rather than relying upon professional pre-made decisions. In addition, individual decisions are not as effective as family group decisions unless the family is highly acculturated to middle class Anglo-American norms. Illness tends to be a social, family, and community matter rather than an illness state of one person.

Second, advice and suggestions will generally be more helpful to the patient and his family than firm directives or "physician-nurse orders." The nurse may need to offer some professional health suggestions, and she does this best by providing clear explanations and some evidence that her health practices have some positive consequences. Findings from specific research studies which are presented in a simple visual and candid manner are often helpful in helping Spanish-Americans understand professional health practices.

Third, if the nurse is working in a Spanish-American community she should involve local health leaders and indigenous health practitioners whenever she can in the health care or program plans. These health workers are generally well known and close to the Spanish-American people who take pride in seeing that local people are active participants in health activities. Health programs conducted by strangers to the community are seldom as effective as they are when the local people have an active part in the program. Of course, this is an important principle for successful work with any cultural or social group.

Fourth, ritual acts are important to Spanish-Americans. The nurse should be familiar with the positive values of ritualized health practices and ways to use rituals in helping people remain healthy. Ritual health practices can be used in the care of infants, in planning diets, and in teaching techniques for preventing the spread of contagious diseases or other illnesses. In bathing an infant, using each [time] the same techniques, equipment, and sequence of activities would help establish a ritual health practice. Ritual behavior offers security and provides guidelines for evolving specific actions to help people.

Fifth, the use of religious practices is also another point to keep in mind while working with Spanish-American people. It is particularly important to recognize Spanish-Americans' dependence on God and their theory about illness causation and cure. The role of the priest in the community should also be used in planning and implementing health programs; in general, the nurse must be aware of the important role of religion and religious practitioners in the lives of the Spanish-American people.

Sixth, the nurse must consider local, social and cultural factors producing an illness, rather than focusing upon Anglo-American views of the factors that cause illness. Every cultural group generally has different kinds of stressors affecting their health state, and we must determine what these factors are and how we can ease undue stress which causes illness. In addition, the nurse must have knowledge of the local classification of illness and how the people currently treat the illness.

And finally, if the nurse wishes to have positive experiences with the Spanish-American people, she must occasionally visit with them in their homes and community in order to see them functioning and living in their own special community. More and more nurses will be expected to know and work with Spanish-Americans in their homes and community settings in order to be of maximum help to them. Knowing the patient in *his own cultural context* means knowing the patient in a very special and privileged way.

In sum, factors contributing to an understanding of Spanish-American behavior and their health-illness system have been presented in this chapter. The cultural context approach to understanding people is a broad and comprehensive one, which makes one realize the many variables influencing behavior. The nurse can have a positive, enjoyable, and therapeutic relationship with Spanish-American people if she gives thought to the guidelines for nursing practice outlined above.

REFERENCES

1. Many of the ideas expressed in this chapter have been formulated by the author on the basis of her three years of study with Spanish-speaking families in an urban and semi-rural community in Colorado.
2. John Burma, *Spanish-Speaking Groups in the United States,* Duke University Press, London, 1954.
3. Bob Huber, "Verdict Strengthens Tijerina Movement," *The Denver Post,* Sunday, Dec. 29, 1968, p. 40.
4. Sam Schulman and Anne M. Smith, "The Concept of Health Among Spanish-Speaking Villagers of New Mexico and Colorado," *Journal of Health and Human Behavior,* Vol. 4 (1963), pp. 226—233.
5. Arthur J. Rubel, "Concepts of Disease in Mexican-American Culture," *American Anthropologist,* LXII, (October, 1960), pp. 795—814.
6. Lyle Saunders, *et al., Handbook for Public Health Nurses,* unpublished document, Santa Fe, New Mexico, June 1964.
7. Sam Schulman, "Rural Healthways in New Mexico," *Annals of the New York Academy of Science.* Vol. 84 (1960), pp. 950—958.
8. Lyle Saunders, *Cultural Difference and Medical Care,* Russell Sage Foundation, New York, 1954.
9. *Ibid.,* 377—440.

10. Robert C. Hanson and Lyle Saunders, *Nurse-Patient Communication,* The Bureau of Sociological Research, Institute of Behavioral Science, University of Colorado, Boulder and the New Mexico State Department of Public Health, Santa Fe, New Mexico, 1964.
11. Madeleine Leininger, *Field Study Observations with Spanish-Speaking Peoples in an Urban Community,* 1966—69, unpublished report, 1969.
12. Hansen and Saunders. *op. cit.,* 1964.

SUGGESTED REFERENCES

Clark, Margaret, *Health in the Mexican-American Culture: A Community Study,* Berkeley and Los Angeles: University of California Press, 1959.
Gillin, John, "Magical Fright," *Psychiatry,* Vol. 11 (1948), 387—400.
Kiev, Ari, *Magic, Faith and Healing: Studies in Primitive Psychiatry Today,* London: The Free Press of Glencoe, Collier-Macmillan Limited, 1964.
Madsen, William, *The Mexican-American of South Texas,* New York: Holt, Rinehart and Winston, 1964.
McWilliams, Carey, *North From Mexico: The Spanish Speaking People of the United States,* Philadelphia: J. B. Lippincott Company, 1948.
Suchman, Edward, "Social Patterns of Illness and Medical Care," *Journal of Health and Human Behavior,* Vol. 6 (1965), 2—16.

19

Removing Barriers to Health Care

Helene R. Robertson

Cultural differences are not always linked to racial or ethnic differences. The rich in any society develop their own special cultural traditions and ways of defining the world. So do the poor. When generation after generation of people are faced with poverty, they develop cultural attitudes and strategies for coping with this experience. Oscar Lewis, the anthropologist who first clearly identified the "culture of poverty," emphasized that it was more than poverty itself or the negative aspects of being poor. He presented a "model that describes in positive terms a subculture of Western society with its own structure and rationale, a way of life handed on from generation to generation along family lines." The culture of poverty provides people with a design for living, with ready-made sets of solutions for human problems, including those related to health and illness. Sometimes these solutions can also create barriers to improved health care. This chapter is an examination of some of these barriers and how community nurses can work with people in this culture to overcome them.

In official agencies, much of the public health nurse's effort is necessarily concentrated on the poor. Though the agency's services are available to everyone, the poor use health resources less frequently than middle-income families for a variety of reasons.

Yet the poor have the highest morbidity and mortality rates and the greatest need for preventive and curative health services. Studies in New York City give strong indication that high-risk populations are associated with poverty neighborhoods.[1] One study compares Flushing, Queens, a middle-class area that is 97 percent white, with the low-income Bedford district of Brooklyn, composed of a population one-third white and two-thirds Negro and Puerto Rican. The death rates from the ten leading diseases in the United States were higher in the Bedford district and lower in Flushing than for the city as a whole.[2]

The problem is not limited to New York; it occurs in most urban and regional areas where pockets of poverty exist. The National Health Survey reports that the prevalence of heart disease, mental and nervous conditions, and arthritis and rheumatism increases with decreasing family income.[3] The health status of the poor results from a multidimensional problem that includes inadequate and crowded living facilities; lack of education; and health services that are fragmented, uncoordinated, geographically inaccessible, and apart from those for middle-income groups.[4]

Even the term "poor" is misleading as it does not account for the variety of people included in this economic classification. The "poor" can mean the Negro, aged, uneducated, and sick. Although these groups share poverty there are cultural differences within them that contribute to behavior leading to the utilization or nonutilization of health services.

Culture can be defined as the complex of distinctive attainments, beliefs, and traditions constituting the background of a racial, religious, or social group. Within the American culture there are many subcultures which are determined by regional, racial, ethnic, religious, and national factors.

The culture of poverty, as discussed here, is that subculture within our society composed of groups caught up in the cycle of want and destitution who are third- and fourth-generation recipients of public assistance. A study of 5,000 cases receiving Aid to Dependent Children revealed that 40 percent came from families that received public assistance.[5] The poor family of today perpetuates the poor family of tomorrow and thus the cycle of poverty continues.

This culture is characterized by its members' lack of orientation to education, long-term experience of powerlessness, lack of self-esteem, sense of hopelessness regarding improvement of their socioeconomic status, and willingness to accept immediate gain rather than postpone satisfaction. They are concerned most with the present, taking their pleasures on a moment-to-moment basis, and their goals are short-termed. They have learned that it is futile to think of the future.[6]

If the needs of the indigent are to be met, health workers must understand how the culture of poverty influences the behavior of the poor, and how their own middle-class norms and values intrude and influence their value judgments and promote a negative response to health services by the poor. The poor are often stereotyped as lazy, sexually promiscuous, dirty, irresponsible, and uncaring. The person with the middle-class values of cleanliness, gratification deferment, and individual responsibility often views with contempt those with differing characteristics and those dependent on public assistance.

Although the distribution and availability of medical facilities and socioeconomic factors do influence the use of health services, personal motivation also plays an important part. For example, public health nurses repeatedly ask: "Why doesn't she keep her appointments?" She refers to the mother, who in the poverty family, is the prime mover in any effort to improve its health, as the father is frequently absent from the home.

It is indeed frustrating to the nurse who, after making several home visits and teaching the mother the importance of preventive and curative health measures for herself and her children, learns that the clinic appointment she gave was not kept. In her visits, the nurse learns about the family's environmental and economic problems and how these affect the health of the family. She fully realizes that a family in need of the basic necessities as food, shelter, and clothing does not consider health a primary need — that the mother with three or four small preschool children has difficulty in getting to a clinic. She responds by manipulating the environment by using and coordinating available community resources to promote the family's physical and emotional well-being.

When the mother complains about inadequate money for food and clothing, the nurse shows her how to budget her food allowance, and how to get the most for her money by buying cheaper cuts of meat and using protein substitutes that provide good nutritional value. At the same time, she teaches the mother good nutritional habits and principles.

When the mother complains about the children's behavior, the nurse offers advice based on accepted child-development theories on how to cope with the behavior. She may also help the mother organize her daily activities so that she can better care for her children and home, and keep appointments at the clinic. Concomitantly, she considers the cultural influences on food preferences and child-rearing practices and gears her teaching accordingly.

The nurse finds it difficult, then, to understand why this woman buys a steak or other unnecessary luxury on the day she receives her income allowance; why the home remains disorganized and unclean; and why appointments still are not kept. But in giving so much information to this mother, the nurse may have defeated her purpose if the instructions have not instilled a sense of power in the individual.

POWERLESSNESS

The feeling of powerlessness which characterizes the culture of poverty stems from poor people's dependency on organizations to meet their socioeconomic and health needs. Frequently, these agencies are impersonal, bureaucratic structures that decide how much financial assistance a family will receive for food and clothing, whether or not they will have a telephone, where they are to live, what they are to learn, and where they are to receive their health care. These decisions take away the poor person's responsibility on how he will live and create dependency which leads to hostility, apathy, hopelessness, failure to achieve, and loss of self-esteem.[7]

Given an understanding of the behavior of the poverty family and the forces that contribute to this behavior, the public health nurse should identify aspects of the patient's personality that need strengthening — areas that are within her sphere of expertise. She is not expected to effect the behavioral changes necessary to transform the patient's way of life, a way she may see as destructive and alien to the norms that our predominantly middle-class society has established as a constructive way of life. Her task is to modify the patient's attitudes toward health services that interfere with his following through on obtaining preventive or curative health care. To do this she must understand what these attitudes are.

Let us look at a typical situation — a public health nurse visiting a family who has not followed medical recommendations. The purpose of the visit is to determine why the patient has not kept clinic appointments and to assess the family's needs. The tendency therefore is to find out the mother's reasons for not appearing for the appointments and to stress the "whys" of why she should. Perhaps if the objective of the visit was changed to discovering what attitudes prevented the mother from keeping the appointments, the nurse would approach the mother or patient in a very different way.

To find the real answer, the nurse must go deeper than the surface reasons given by the mother, which may be defensive and serve as a protection in responding to one of the many authority figures she regularly encounters. These authorities tell her she must do this or that in order to receive the financial assistance she depends on; in so doing they contribute to her sense of powerlessness.

Knowing of the patient's defensiveness, the public health nurse can use her knowledge of human behavior to further understand the patient and what motivates her behavior. She will employ her most useful tool — the nurse-patient relationship. Rather than focusing on the children who need medical care or on the medical care itself, which the mother or other adult may need, she gives her attention to the person who must be reached if the recommendations are to be followed. For example, it may be the mother who is responsible for keeping appointments for her children or the patient itself, if he is the one who needs the care. The focus is kept on the person and his emotional needs, not on the disease process or ways to prevent it. This does not mean that the nurse dismisses the health needs, rather she gives them less emphasis until the patient indicates a readiness to accept instruction.

The nurse must remember that her values are not those of the patient. The patient does not have a felt need for medical care as does the public health nurse, who is health-oriented and follows the recommendations of health authorities. The nurse should direct her energies to reducing the patient's feelings of powerlessness, increasing his self-esteem, and allaying his suspicions of persons in authority. In doing so, she will be able to effect some change in the person's attitude toward health and health professionals. Nurses, particularly those in public health, stress the importance of teaching the patient. We want him to learn about his illness or how to prevent illness. Should we not stress also the importance of the patient's emotional learnings that result when the nurse-patient relationship is a positive one? It is the vehicle by which other health learning takes place.

Establishing a relationship with a person whose life is dependent on and controlled by authority figures is often difficult. The patient may perceive powerful figures as necessary but may hate them because of the power they exercise in relation to the patient's or family's needs. Past experiences may influence the patient's perception of the nurse, and she may be cast into the role of an authority figure and treated as such.

Patients learn to mask their feelings. They do not openly or directly express their anger toward people on whom they depend; instead, they often agree to any request: "Yes, I will keep the appointment." This is what the professional wants to hear. The patient does not deliberately lie: It may be a response a mother has learned to protect herself and her family. It could also be interpreted as passive aggression toward those in authority and an attempt to exercise some control over her life. Also, the mother may have learned that the social agencies that control her have not altered her situation. Why, then, follow through on an action that does not assure an improved status? Therefore, no action is attempted.

BUILDING TRUST

In the early visits to the patient the nurse should refrain from making demands on the patient and limit the instruction or information she gives to what is directly requested by the patient. Her primary goal should be to help the patient feel safe in the relationship. She encourages the patient to express what she feels. In the beginning these feelings may be complaints which are a passive approach to hostile feelings. Advice and suggestions as to how to alter these complaints should be withheld, for the patient may interpret them as criticism and as more demands to conform to middle-class norms — behavior she may be emotionally incapable of instituting — and result in deepening her feelings of powerlessness and worthlessness.

The complaints may mean that the patient is asking the nurse to appreciate and understand her problems. When the nurse responds to the complaints with true empathy, the patient feels more confidence or trust in the nurse because she perceives that the nurse understands her predicament.

Empathy involves identification with the patient, a personal though objective involvement, as expressed in the statement, "standing in the other fellow's shoes." The nurse communicates empathy when she listens and relates to the patient's complaints with understanding responses. If the nurse is preoccupied with her own problems and feelings, her responses tend to be those of an efficient information-giver, a more comfortable role for the nurse but one which may cut off communication. Each of us needs the empathy of other people, and we are reassured when we feel that someone understands us. When positive emotions develop in the patient in response to the empathy of the nurse, they may provide the major motivating force for the patient.

The nurse may then proceed to explore what the patient perceives about the medical recommendations made, what the patient knows about her own and her family's medical needs, and what her past experiences with health professionals and facilities have been. She evaluates the patient's ability to use information and gears her teaching to the patient's needs. She discusses alternatives if care is not instituted. She gives the patient a choice and lets her make the decision as to whether she wants to follow through on the recommendation or not.

For example, Wolff cites a situation in which the nurse, after several unsuccessful attempts to talk a mother into having her children skin-tested for tuberculosis, finally said: "Well, so long as you have decided so strongly against having it done, there is nothing more that I can say."[8] The mother then replied that she could take them and did. The change occurred because the nurse acknowledged the mother's right to run her own and her children's lives.

Permitting the patient to make decisions increases a mother's feeling of power and mastery over at least one aspect of her life. By crediting the mother's feelings with validity, by not suggesting that she do more than she is emotionally capable of doing, and by giving her a sense of control over her life, the nurse increases the patient's feelings of self-esteem. It is hoped that the emotional learnings which take place through the relationship will motivate the patient to follow through on the health recommendations and that there may be other personality changes as by-products of the nurse-patient relationship.

It should be remembered that the personality characteristics of the poor may differ from individual to individual and within families, as well as within cultural settings. Each person has had unique experiences derived from his cultural background and social circumstances that may influence his behavior in a more positive or negative sense. Each family must be evaluated for its existing strengths and weaknesses to guide the nurse in developing her nursing care plan. And on-going assessment of the family's ability to move toward the nurse's goals will enable her to recognize when she should withdraw or continue her efforts. She must realize that there are families in which the behavior of poverty is of such long duration that it has become a life style from which they are unable to extricate themselves.

HELPING THE NURSE

If the nurse is to realize these many objectives, the agency must provide time for her to discuss families which present problems with a nursing supervisor or a mental health consultant.

Sometimes, as in the New York City Health Department's Bureau of Public Health Nursing, all three nurses and some staff may participate in the discussion. The group setting provides the climate for sharing common problems and experiences, an atmosphere conducive to verbalizing frustrations and accomplishments, conditions aimed at supporting the nurse and strengthening her skills. The goals of these discussions are to assist the nurse in:

1. Increasing her sensitivity to the needs of poverty families by broadening her psychological frame of reference to include social systems, norms, values, and customs of families receiving public assistance.
2. Developing an awareness of society's attitudes and her attitudes toward persons receiving public assistance, and how these attitudes impede or promote the family's ability to mobilize its resources.
3. Understanding community institutions such as welfare, health, and education and their responsibility in furthering the dependency and powerlessness of the poor.
4. Defining her objectives and limitations in preparing nursing care plans for a family.

5. Expressing her feelings of hopelessness, helplessness, and powerlessness in effecting change in the family of poverty.
6. Understanding that she alone is not responsible for effecting change in the family and when to utilize the resources of others in the helping professions.
7. Recognizing when to withdraw or continue her nursing services to the family.
8. Recognizing her lack of involvement with the family and its consequences, as well as her overinvolvement and resulting lack of objectivity in formulating realistic goals.

The recent trend for consumer-controlled health services reflects a positive change in the poor person's sense of worth, self-esteem, and power over his destiny. Since these are some of the objectives of public health nursing, the profession should look to ways to encourage this trend and help to reduce illness and premature death in poverty groups and families.

REFERENCES

1. New York City, Health Department. *Annual Report, 1963–1964.* New York, The Department, 1966.
2. James, George. *Poverty is an Obstacle to Health Programs in our Cities.* Paper presented at the annual meeting of the American Public Health Association, New York City, October 9, 1964.
3. U.S. National Center for Health Statistics. *Medical Care, Health Status, and Family Income.* (Vital and Health Statistics, Series 10, No. 9) (U.S. Public Health Service Publication No. 1000-Series 10, No. 9) Washington, D.C., U.S. Government Printing Office, 1964.
4. New York State Public Health Association and Public Health Association of New York City. *State-Wide Conference on Barriers to Utilization of Health Services,* Albany, N.Y., March 13–14, 1967. New York, Public Health Association of New York City, 1967.
5. Burgess, M. E., and Price, D. D. *An American Dependency Challenge.* Chicago, Ill., American Public Welfare Association, 1963.
6. Riessman, Frank, and others, Eds. *Mental Health of the Poor.* New York, Macmillan Co., 1964.
7. *Ibid.*
8. Wolff, Ilse S. Interviewing in public health nursing. *Nurs. Outlook* 6:267–269, May 1958.

20

Cultural Understanding:
A Key to Acceptance

Rita Hoeschen Aichlmayr

Acceptance of people for what they are is a fundamental principle in all nursing activities. Acceptance is usually thought of as a nonjudgmental attitude toward individuals, accepting their physical needs, personal characteristics and emotional feelings. But in a pluralistic society, cultural acceptance is equally important. When nurses deal with people who share their cultural background, whether middle-class, European immigrant, or some other subculture, they express this cultural acceptance easily, without conscious effort. But public health nurses must constantly cross cultural boundaries within a community and interact with people from differing cultural backgrounds. Cultural acceptance means setting aside ethnocentrism — that mixture of belief and feeling that one way of life is best — and viewing the practices and values of another culture from a nonjudgmental framework. It means the nurse must express a positive feeling, not merely for individuals, but for their culture with its different traditions and values. In this chapter, a specific case of working with native Americans clearly demonstrates both the need for cultural acceptance and the means of achieving it.

If public health nurses are to be effective in working with the increasing number of community action groups springing up throughout the country, they must develop an understanding of the different cultures, customs, and values of the people comprising these various groups.

But to gain understanding of a group's mores creates a double challenge to the nurse. First, she must find a way into the community group and gain acceptance by the members; and second, she must continually analyze her role behavior and her activities in relation to the group's membership and values.

Often, we characterize people from minority and ethnic groups, or lower economic levels, as culturally deprived. In reality, it is not deprivation but cultural pluralism that exists — the culture of the nurse and the culture of the community group, each with its own values and pride. To gain acceptance and establish a working relationship with a community group that has values other than her own, the nurse must not only recognize and understand these differences but must reinforce by her behavior the group members' cultural pride and values.

Accomplishing this task is a long slow process that if hurried may result in the group's rejection of the nurse or the nurse's rejection of the people. To resolve this dilemma several groups of senior baccalaureate students and I worked with an Indian group on a reservation in northern Washington state during five academic quarters.

Our project began when six students, in the community health nursing course, observed an interdisciplinary health and welfare meeting, whose purpose was to explore the health needs of the Indian people and the health resources available to them. The students felt that the dignity of the Indian had been affronted when the guest speaker, a government official, spoke to the Indians in a condescending manner, and they were angry when he unwittingly failed to acknowledge either the Indians' contributions or their expressed health needs. The students returned to the health district where they were assigned for their community health field practice and pleaded that something be done to achieve better understanding of Indians and their culture. They wanted to meet with them, themselves.

After a discussion with the health district administrator, we approached the director of the Office of Economic Opportunity responsible for the Community Action Programs as the most logical contact, since he worked closely and well with the Indian people and employed several of them as community aides. He was reluctant to allow students to meet with Indian groups who, he felt, would not accept them on the reservation.

Previously, white people had come to the reservation with prescribed programs, and some through verbal and nonverbal communication had expressed negative attitudes toward the Indians. As a result, the Indian people refused to cooperate and accept the programs, and the white people rejected the Indians, stating that the Indians were "unappreciative" and "unreachable." The director believed that our presence would only widen the gap between the red and white communities.

We had earlier learned of the white community's attitude. Professionals as well as other white people asked us: "Why do you want to meet with the Indians?" "They are all lazy." "You can't do anything with them." The blame for failure to reach an understanding was always laid to the Indians.

Finally, we convinced the director to set up a meeting for us with the Indian community aides. At the meeting, we explained our wish to meet with the Indian people and provide health assistance in any way that they desired. Silence followed. We then restated our request that we wanted to know the Indian people, but that they would have to decide what they wanted of us. With this, the Indian aides began discussing among themselves the high infant mortality rate and incidence of communicable disease, and the inaccessibility or nonexistence of medical facilities for their people. The director was as surprised as we were to learn of these concerns. We all agreed that the place to start was with the Indian women and a meeting was arranged. The community aides agreed to inform the women and to provide transportation to this meeting which would explore their felt needs and convey to them our interest in them and their culture.

We were excited as we drove to our first meeting with the Indians, but fearful that we would be rejected or that we would say something wrong. Once there, our apprehensions grew when the Indians responded to many of our statements and questions with long periods of silence that we could not understand. Again, we explained that we had come to the Indian reservation without plans, and that we were interested in helping in any possible way.

This statement precipitated many negative feelings. One Indian woman expressed it this way: "We are tired of having people come to the reservation with their prescribed programs and telling us what our needs are and how we should live." She cited some white groups from large cities who came to tell the Indians that they should bathe every day, without consideration to the availability of bathing facilities, or quantities of water that would have to be carried and heated to bathe all the family members every day. Others told of classes given in interior decorating and design, when families could not afford wallpaper, paints, or other costly materials.

We listened intently and in awe, and began to understand how the Indians felt. Then they expressed their immediate concerns and needs. Priority was given to first-aid classes, especially classes in artificial respiration, because of the number and kinds of accidents on the reservation. The people earn their living by fishing in Puget Sound; they received no government subsidies. When fishing or drowning accidents occur, immediate medical attention is called for; however, the nearest medical facility is 12 miles and the Indian health hospital over 35 miles away.

At the following meetings, we focused on mouth-to-mouth resuscitation, back-pressure arm-lift artificial respiration, and first-aid measures including splinting, bandaging, and control of bleeding. An informal lecture-discussion method was used to present the material; two students amused the children while their mothers participated in the sessions.

One morning, before the third meeting, we received a call from an Indian aide *ordering* us to go immediately to the reservation. We arrived fearful that we had done something wrong only to find that the Indian women had prepared a pot-luck lunch for us. This gesture marked our acceptance by the group, as Indians eat only with social equals. Months later, we learned that our acceptance began when the Indian women saw that we were not there to prescribe a program to them. By providing baby-sitting services, we had recognized the women's need for help with child care and showed our concern for their children.

As the quarter ended, the Indian women were sorry to see us go and asked that the sessions continue. Although we were eager to comply and would have students enrolled during the summer, the Indian women lacked the time. They participated in the Office of Economic Opportunity's summer programs which included Head Start, social enrichment, and a tutorial program for children having difficulty in school. However, we felt that we had to keep the program idea alive because of their interest and our promise to return. If we failed to fulfill our promise, we could easily be perceived by the Indians as white people who don't keep their word or have a sincere interest in the concerns of the Indian people. Therefore, we used the summer months to learn about the reservation and the Indian's values.

ESTABLISHING RAPPORT

During the next weeks, we made frequent visits to the reservation and established rapport with the Indians through casual conversations about their salmon fishing and their way of life. Lacking a written record, the Indians told us their history of how five diverse, but neighboring, tribes left their long houses in the 1860's following a treaty agreement with the government and moved to the new and foreign land designated as their reservation. Distrust of the white man grew when many moons passed and the Indians did not receive the housing, equipment, or provisions promised them in the treaty. During this period of relocation and on through the next generation, many Indians died of starvation, exposure to the cold, and communicable diseases that were rampant among them.

The Indians' lot has not improved very much in the past hundred years. Indians have the lowest income, most unemployment, least education, poorest housing and health of any ethnic group in the state.[1] A recent survey showed 67 percent of Indian families with annual incomes of less than $3,000; 17 percent less than $1,000.[2] Included in the latter are those families who fish for salmon from May through September and earn as little as $600 a year.

Although families may engage in seasonal farm work, a 40 percent unemployment rate persists. Lacking formal and technical education, they cannot acquire industrial jobs in nearby towns. The eighth grade is the median education level and the high school dropout rate is estimated at 80 percent. On some reservations, this rate reaches a staggering 100 percent.

Unsanitary and inadequate housing, inadequate nutrition, and a high incidence of communicable disease result in an infant mortality two and one-half times the national average and a life expectancy of forty-four years as estimated by the Bureau of Indian Affairs.[3] Despite these devastating economic, social, and health conditions, an Indian will not complain of his poverty; rather, he will present to the world his highest values — courage and pride. The Indian people are proud of their culture and heritage, and will not bemoan their difficulties. Rather, they will express concern for someone less fortunate.

During our summer visits, we were introduced to a white woman without any acknowledgment of who she was or why we were being introduced. We then learned that she was part Indian — one of the most highly respected people on the reservation, and an important link between the white and red man's culture. We talked with her as she quilted and interpreted Indian's thinking and values.

Weeks later, we learned that we had been introduced Indian fashion. To add comfort and ease of conversation, white man's etiquette requires that a proper introduction consist of a resumé of the person or his interests. In contrast, the Indian wishes to remain anonymous. To indicate his status, achievements, or interests would be considered boastful and embarrassing. Consequently, an Indian will introduce you to someone he likes and trusts without giving any identifying information about his friend. In turn, you must be warm, friendly, and convey acceptance of this new friend. If you fail to do so, you have lost two

friends — the new and old. But, if you are successful and convey a genuine interest in the new friend, then both of them will be friendly and open with you.´ In
the future, you will be expected to introduce this new friend by name and by
order of age if he is with someone. The oldest is introduced first; not to do so
would cause resentment.

EXPLAINING VALUES

The respected white lady was invaluable in helping us analyze our role behavior
in relation to the total group. We had felt uncomfortable during silences at the
meetings. She explained that the Indian people were not uncomfortable: they
value patience and the ability to wait for others to speak. Patience is also related
to their concept of time. If a meeting was planned two to three weeks in advance,
few Indians would come to it, and, if it were set for 11:30 in the morning, they
might arrive 30 to 40 minutes late. But, if they were told one day in advance to
come around lunch time, they would usually arrive at 11:30 a.m.

We learned at first hand their time values. Sudden illness delayed attendance
at one meeting for two hours. We were expected to wait. To have left would
have been considered impatient. How different from the white man's compulsive
concept of time. How easy for us to interpret the Indian as lazy, irresponsible,
or rude!

Sometimes our professional words and values create cultural conflicts. Indian
people value sincerity, honesty, and absolute trustworthiness. When working
with the Indian people, one must always keep his word if he is to be trusted.

Sometimes the nurse's professional vocabulary creates a conflict. For example,
a public health nurse may state that she is visiting to "help them" and then gives
the name of an agency to call or a place to visit where the patient or family may
receive service. This cannot be seen as help, when the recipient does not possess
a telephone or a car for transportation. If we are really helping, why not bring
the concrete service to the Indian or take him to the source of help? We see then
that a nurse's professional value of "making people independent" interferes with
actually helping the Indian people.

Through our baby-sitting service, we learned of the closeness Indians feel to
their children, who are a source of pride and joy to their parents and the group.
We found a relationship could always be established when we turned first to their
children. Elementary school classes are held on the reservation, and the children
love to learn about and are taught to be proud of their heritage. However, when
the teenagers attend the city high schools, they feel like outsiders with their poor
clothes, divergent reactions, and noncompetitive values. They are exposed to
subtle or harsh prejudices that teach that it is a liability to be an Indian which
creates severe obstacles to the teenager's completion of school. We listened with
compassion as an Indian lady told us of incidents of prejudice displayed toward
their highly valued children and Indian culture.

Indians also place high value on generosity. They share everything: food, cars, clothing, and income. Their unsurpassed generosity provided us with a key in approaching them: we met them on a compassionate level as though they were doing us a favor by letting us help them. Because of their generosity and strong sense of responsibility toward their families and tribe, the Indians are very perceptive of the needs of others and orientated to the total group — the tribe. Being from the white culture where needs are frankly voiced, we had to increase our astuteness and perceptiveness if we were to ascertain the Indian's health needs.

The Indian concern for others was noted when a supply of clothes was offered to them. Those present took only what they needed for themselves and for anyone not present. If nothing is needed, nothing is taken. Compared to white middle-class values, those of the Indian become quite striking: sharing versus saving; cooperation versus competition; anonymity versus individuality.

The Indian's value for anonymity created our greatest problem. In the fall quarter, after our six months' acquaintance with them, silences continued when a specific question was directed toward an Indian woman. Sometimes the question would be answered by a friend sitting next to her. Finally, we realized that, by asking a direct question, we were forcing the Indian woman to violate her value of anonymity. They would not speak of themselves, but would express the feelings and thoughts of their friends. This was opposed to our professional orientation to speak directly to the person and not to gossip about those present. When we learned the art of "professional gossip" our long periods of silence ceased and we learned more about the Indians' feelings and concerns and gained further rapport.

EVALUATING CLASSES

During the fall quarter, the Indian women helped us to evaluate the effectiveness of our teaching. Previously all classes had been held in an informal lecture-discussion method. Class topics at this time included birth control, splinting, treatment of burns, and artificial respiration. During our class on artificial respiration, the women practiced back-pressure, arm-lift respiration on one of the nurses. As each took her turn, they began laughing and teasing the victim. Then they practiced 5-man carry lifts and teased the victim that they would drop her. As the Indian women left, they all commented that this was the best class; hence, it was apparent that the Indian women learned best when the situation was less formal, and they were actively involved.

Prior to the winter quarter, we held a meeting with the director of the Office of Educational Opportunity and the community aides to discuss future health meetings. To our surprise, the Indian people began teasing us in our initial greeting and during the meeting. We, in turn, teased, laughed, and joked with them. Then, the Indian women suggested that we begin meeting in their homes rather than in the tribal hall. We were perplexed by this behavior, and approached the respected white woman. We related the tenor of the past meeting and she stated, "Now you are really accepted. They do not tease anyone that they do not accept."

Next, we were casually introduced to an Indian woman, who we later discovered was one of the tribal leaders. We felt our original double problem was being resolved when she told us, "Many people come out to the reservation, but they soon leave. They never know what they do wrong and we never tell them. But, you, we tell." And, indeed, they do. From that day on, we were told what words we could use, where we could visit, and how we should act. One woman said, "From now on, you must never use that word. You cause resentment in the tribe when you call things by their wrong name."

The students in the winter quarter had the advantage of all that we had learned during the past nine months. From the very beginning, they were accepted; silences were replaced by gaiety, teasing, and laughter at all the meetings in the Indian homes. For this group, the Indians requested classes in child care, prevention and treatment of colds, and care of children with seizures.

We had been working with the Indian people for 15 months, when a cut in federal funds eliminated all but one community aide, who had to assume responsibility for all the community aide duties. Her compounded duties prevented the meetings from continuing. But, our social and professional contacts with the Indian people have not ceased. We are called upon for professional advice, and invited to tribal meetings and social gatherings. In turn, the Indian people visit our homes and when the possibility or the request arises for health classes, they will continue again.

Looking back, we have not found any set of rules that leads to success when working with people of differing cultures. Displaying patience, compassion, acceptance of each other's differences, and respect for each person are basic prerequisites to gaining acceptance. Beyond these fundamental values, an analysis of one's own role behavior within the context of the other person's culture is worthwhile, as well as gaining an understanding of the culturally ordained concepts upon which the other's behavior is based.

REFERENCES

1. *Seattle Times,* June 30, 1968, p. 92.
2. Interview with director of Office of Economic Opportunity.
3. U.S. Congress House. *American Indian: Message from the President of the United States Transmitting Message Relating to Problems of American Indians, Mar. 6, 1968.* (90th Congress, 2d Session, 1968. House of Representative Document 272) Washington, D.C., U.S. Government Printing Office, 1968.

21

Health Care of the Chinese in America

Teresa Campbell
Betty Chang

Many health professionals fall back on two ways for dealing with people from other cultures. The first uses stereotypes for understanding others. The second strategy employs psychological insights to interpret behavior. A person from another culture may thus be seen as unmotivated, hostile, belligerent, unwilling to cooperate or even irresponsible. But both these approaches — stereotypes and psychological analysis — only build further barriers to cross-cultural understanding. It is important to replace stereotypes with informed knowledge about cultural differences, and to shift from treating problems as purely psychological or individual ones. Many of the difficulties confronted in community nursing stem from profound cultural differences. In this chapter how the Chinese subculture in American cities influences health care and interactions with health professionals is shown. This subculture, like many others in our society, has ways to deal with illness, a unique system of folk medicine. Such traditional ways of dealing with illness affect the practice of nursing.

Chinese people in America prefer to work in restaurants, laundries, and sewing shops; they have a low rate of juvenile delinquency; they always take care of their own; they are "inscrutable." These stereotypes are about as far as most non-Asians go in thinking about the Chinese who live in this country. Their superficial ideas result from limited personal contact and from a paucity of literature on this group.

The stereotypes are rooted, in fact, in the history of the Chinese people's adjustment to an alien society. During the settlement in America, as an example, the Chinese handled racial hostility by developing businesses and seeking employment where there was little competition from the white population. Today, many new immigrants, although better educated than their predecessors, are limited by language and continue to seek menial jobs in the restaurants, laundries, and sewing shops of Chinatown. This does not mean, however, that such occupations are part of their "culture."

Similarly, the fact that for many years the Chinese enclaves in American cities were populated by men fostered the myth of a low juvenile delinquency rate. (The Exclusion Act of 1924 prevented the entry of Chinese women into this country.) However, the arrival of Chinese wives starting in 1943 and new immigrants starting in 1965 changed the composition of Chinese families and increased the number of Chinese youths in the United States. Today, the delinquency among the young in Chinese communities is a serious problem.

In China before the revolution, the lineage and clan, as well as numerous specialized associations, were the means for fulfilling the social needs of the individual in the village. When Chinese first entered this country over 100 years ago, they established the same type of formal groups they had known at home — the family name associations, tongs, and benevolent associations — to meet their social welfare needs. However, their increasing social and health problems now demonstrate that without help the Chinese can no longer "take care of their own." Among their health problems are a high incidence of visual problems, immunization deficiencies, and dental caries; in San Francisco the tuberculosis rate among Chinese is three to four times that of the city as a whole.[1] In addition, the environmental conditions in San Francisco are particularly poor, with a very high population density — often whole families living in two rooms and sharing a community toilet facility and kitchen with other families.

The legend of "inscrutability" may derive from different orientations to body language. An observer of one nationality, for instance, may see things in body language that are completely missed by someone of a different nationality.[2]

Because of this and other differences in cultural orientation, health professionals would ideally belong to the same ethnic group as the population they serve. If this is not feasible, a knowledge of customs and culture will help any health worker serve more effectively. Certainly a knowledge of Chinese folk medicine and health practices, attitudes, and beliefs as they are manifested by the Chinese in America is very important.

The number of Chinese people in this country is relatively small — a little over 435,000, according to the 1970 census. Most of them live in the urban central city, mainly in the western states, although the largest Chinese-American community (over 69,000) is in New York City. San Francisco runs a close second.

Population statistics, however, should be of little concern to the nurse caring for a Chinese-American patient or family; no matter how few members of this ethnic group she sees, she needs the health-related information.

THREE MAIN GROUPS

The Chinese people in this country fall into three main groups: (1) individuals who were born in China and immigrated from rural villages 40 to 50 years ago — they are the strongest believers in Chinese folk medicine and continue to influence the health practices of their immediate families; (2) new immigrants who have arrived over the past 20 years from a number of Asian countries and Hong Kong; and (3) first- and second-generation American-born Chinese. Members of this last group, while oriented to Western medicine, bow to the pressures of their elders in practices of folk medicine. One young pregnant Chinese woman who was a registered nurse, for instance, routinely followed her obstetrician's orders, but at the same time, under pressure from her mother and mother-in-law ate special foods and herbs to insure the birth of a healthy baby.

Chinese folk medicine evolved from an Eastern philosophy which holds that the elemental forces controlling the universe pervade all aspects of human endeavor. The universe is thought of as a vast entity, each organism in it conceived as an open system that interacts and is affected by others in the universe. The energy for regulating the universe is composed of two opposing forces, the Yin and the Yang.

YIN AND YANG

The Yin represents the female, negative force: darkness, cold, and emptiness. The Yang represents the male and positive force, producing light, warmth, and fullness. All things or beings in the universe consist of a Yin and a Yang, and if peace and harmony in society and health in the mind and body are to be maintained, the two energy forces must be in perfect balance. An imbalance is thought to cause catastrophe and illness.

The Yin and Yang energy forces are embodied in the autonomic nervous system as elsewhere in the body. Thus, the sympathetic system responds to stress by mobilizing the body for defensive action, much as the Yang is said to protect the body from outside infiltrations. An excess of Yang causes fever, dehydration, irritability, and tenseness.

In contrast, the parasympathetic system is generally concerned with restoring and conserving body energy and controlling the digestive processes, and Yin is thought to store the vital strength of life. A person with too much Yin catches cold easily, is nervous, apprehensive, and predisposed to gastric disorders. Further, various parts of the body correspond to principles of Yin and Yang. For example, the body surface is Yang; inside is Yin. Some organs are Yang; others are Yin.

When a Chinese person is ill, he may go to a Western doctor or to a practitioner of Chinese medicine. Or he may see both. The Chinese specialist will be an acupuncturist, an herb pharmacist, or an herbalist, whose treatments often overlap and duplicate each other.

The herbalist diagnoses by interrogating, observing color, tongue, and perspiration, listening to sounds of the body and taking the pulse. He will then formulate a prescription of herbs that either he will fill directly or that can be filled by the herb pharmacist. A patient may also go directly to the herb pharmacist, tell him his symptoms or what he wants, and receive a prescription.

An acupuncturist will use basically the same procedure as the herbalist for making a diagnosis. He then treats the patient by inserting fine needles into a number of the 365 body points where channels or ducts called meridians extend internally. Acupuncture is gaining in popularity in San Francisco and was recently included as acceptable treatment by Teamster Local 856 for medical insurance coverage.

CHINESE VS. WESTERN MEDICINE

Some persons believe that Western medicine is for Westerners and Chinese medicine is for Chinese. Others think that Western medicine is best for some diseases, like tuberculosis, but that Chinese medicine is more effective for skin diseases and blood disorders. Still others believe that a combination of both provides the best treatment. Therefore, the professional health worker should encourage a Chinese patient to let his Western doctor know what medication he is receiving from his herbalist. Herb prescriptions may contain the same chemical ingredients as Western medicine and might result in an overdose or adverse reaction in the patient. For instance, Ma Huang, or Chinese ephedra, a major source of ephedrine, is an herb used in the treatment of pulmonary disease. Ginseng, one of the most commonly used herbs, is viewed in Chinese folk medicine as a panacea. However, it is classified by many Western physicians as a tonic-stimulant and its use is contraindicated in hypertension.[3]

Chinese patients frequently switch doctors and herbalists and may see two or three during the same period. This shopping around for doctors is an attempt to find the most promising cure. It is important for the health professional to know what medication the patient is receiving from each doctor, and the patient must give this information to his doctors. But a Chinese patient is often reluctant to tell his doctor directly that he is seeing another one for fear that the doctor will "lose face."

The professional in such a situation can obtain the patient's permission to let him tell the doctor, and it is important to have the permission. Irreversible distrust developed in one family toward a community health worker who, without the family's knowledge, told the doctor that his patient was seeing another doctor as well.

One conflict between Chinese folk medicine and Western medical practice is medication. Increasingly, Chinese people are recognizing the value of Western drugs, but they continue to use herbs for certain ailments as they see fit. And the health worker cannot always justify one type of medicine over the other. A diabetic woman, for instance, refused to continue taking her oral hypoglycemic agent and, instead, started taking a medicine prescribed by an herbalist. On later home visits, the health worker found that the patient's urine tested negative on the Clinitest, her arthritic pain had diminished, and she seemed to be progressing without any apparent problems related to her diabetes.

SOME DIFFERENCES

An important difference between Western medicine and Chinese folk medicine is the administration of medication. When a patient receives one dose of a prescription from an herbalist for instance, he is told to return if he doesn't feel better — one dose of any correct medication should cure him. And so the patient has difficulty comprehending why Western doctors give so many pills to be taken over a long period. The health professional working with a Chinese patient must help him understand that there is a difference between Western medicine and Chinese medicine. Concrete illustrations help. If the patient's blood pressure has stabilized, for instance, the health worker can explain how the medicine he is taking has helped.

Another difference is the form of the medication. A Chinese person boils the herbs he has received from the herb pharmacist in the amount of water and for the time prescribed to get the right concentration of broth. Liquid medications cleanse the intestines, stimulate the circulation, and restore the balance between Yin and Yang. Why is Western medicine dispensed in pills or capsules and with few directions?

The health professional again must explain that Western medicine is different from Chinese medicine — that it comes in different forms and must be taken over a longer time. He can also explain that just as herb broth comes in child and adult doses, so, too, does Western medicine. If one pill is for the treatment of a child, then two pills may be necessary to treat an adult.

CHECKING THE MEDICATIONS

Some Chinese keep all the medicine they have received and take it at their own discretion at various times for numerous ailments. They also tend to borrow and loan medications at will. The health worker visiting in the home should ask to see all the medications the patient has and learn which ones he is taking. Although he can try to persuade the patient to dispose of all old medications or let the professional destroy them, he is usually not successful. As an alternative, he should have the patient take the medications to the doctor.

It is clear from these examples that extensive health teaching and supervision is necessary to help Chinese believers of folk medicine understand the correct use of Western medicine.

FOOD AND DISEASE

Food is thought to play a part in the cause and treatment of diseases. In Chinese philosophy, *chi* (literally, "air," "breath," or "wind") is an energy present in all living organisms. Food, when metabolized, is transformed into *chi* and becomes either a cold Yin energy force or a hot Yang energy force. Illnesses caused by Yin excesses are treated by hot foods; those caused by Yang excesses are treated by cold foods.

This theory is demonstrated in the following instances. Cancer is viewed as a cold disease. When a Chinese child in a large San Francisco hospital was diagnosed as having leukemia, the mother immediately asked the Chinese student nurse whether it resulted from improper eating — possibly too many cold foods in the diet. In another situation, a Chinese patient suffering from an ear infection, a hot disease, refused scrambled eggs, a hot food, because a hot illness needs to be treated with cold foods such as wintermelon. The common ginger root is believed to be a hot food and is used to strengthen the heart (Yang organ) and to prevent and treat nausea and dyspepsia (Yin excess disorders).

The knowledge of hot and cold foods is passed down in the family by tradition and practice. At present, there is no complete listing of hot and cold foods. A health professional in an institution might encourage family members to bring in Chinese dishes which support the Yin and Yang beliefs if the foods are not contraindicated.

FOOD HABITS AND NUTRITION

Like those in any other ethnic group, Chinese have definite food preferences based on cultural eating patterns. A health professional needs to be alert to food patterns so that a therapeutic diet compatible with the patient's beliefs and preferences can be selected. Some older Chinese, for instance, believe that drinking ice water shocks the system and is harmful to health. Also, because of a history of inadequate sanitation in China, Chinese have habitually boiled their drinking water.

As a result, many Chinese prefer to drink hot water, which is often brought to the hospital in a Thermos by their families. If there is no family to bring a Thermos to a patient, the professional might inquire if the patient would like hot drinking water.

Similar unsanitary conditions have made raw vegetables generally unacceptable to Chinese from overseas, where organic fertilizer was used. Uncooked vegetables caused illnesses, and, as a result, eating them has not been a regular part of the dietary pattern.

Then, too, milk and milk products have been scarce in the Far Eastern countries, and people's taste for them may not have developed. Thus, they tend to dislike foods containing milk or milk products — particularly in dishes like cheese and creamed foods where the milk or cream flavors is not disguised. In diets that call for a higher intake of calcium, health professionals can suggest modifications or substitutes: custards are usually well-liked, and milk with Ovaltine, or simply warm milk with sugar added. Green leafy vegetables also contribute a large part of the total calcium in the diet.

Another example is rare beef, which may not be acceptable, since in most Chinese foods beef is cooked until the blood is no longer apparent. The health professional can list for the dietitian all the various food likes and dislikes of the patient, so that meals can be as appetizing as possible.

It is common knowledge that the preparation of Chinese food requires soy sauce. Its high sodium content makes it a problem in restricted-sodium diets, for experience has shown that it is useless to instruct the patient to eliminate soy sauce. Greater success has been attained by having the patient measure and limit the amount of soy sauce for cooking. He should also avoid dried, salted, or preserved foods. The San Francisco Heart Association has diet instructions and sample menus printed in Chinese and English for Chinese patients on restricted-sodium diets.

FOOD SUBSTITUTIONS

Although health professionals are knowledgeable about the "basic four" in nutrition, they need to know about using food substitutions for a Chinese diet. One such is the versatile tofu, a soybean curd made by precipitating protein of soybean milk by the use of calcium or magnesium salts. Tofu is a commonly used food in the Chinese diet that is a good source of protein, relatively high in iron, and if made with calcium salts can contribute a considerable amount of calcium, which is often deficient in the Chinese diet. A 2-inch cube portion of tofu can substitute for a protein equivalency of two to three ounces of hamburger, or two eggs.

Half a cup of rice or *mein* (Chinese noodles) can be substituted for one slice of bread or a serving of potatoes. In a diabetic diet, Oriental foods can take the place of Western foods, which may not be familiar to the patient. Emphasis should be placed on approximate portions of meats and starches rather than exact measurements. There are relatively few concentrated sweets in the Chinese diet, so eliminating them is not a problem for most Chinese persons with diabetes.

CARE DURING PREGNANCY

Folk medicine practices during the childbearing periods are assiduously enforced in many Chinese families. Practices vary from family to family. For instance, some Chinese women avoid excessive use of soy sauce during pregnancy so that the baby will not be too dark. Shellfish during the first trimester may be shunned in the belief that the baby will thus be prevented from developing allergies later in life. Some young women refuse to take iron supplements because they think that the iron will harden the bones and make delivery difficult. During the seventh and eighth months of pregnancy, ginseng is sometimes taken as a general tonic to strengthen the expectant mother.

The health professional supervising the care of a Chinese family may acknowledge that these are indeed the family's practices and help by suggesting some scientifically based health measures that are not in conflict with folk medicine beliefs. Eating foods from the family's usual diet that are high in calcium and iron can be stressed.

Major conflict with Western medicine occurs during the postpartum period when the health professionals' recommendations are incompatible with principles of Yin and Yang. The traditional postpartum convalescence consists of a one-month period during which the new mother's dietary and health practices are directed toward decreasing the Yin energy forces or cold air in the body. The pores are believed to remain open for 30 days postpartum, during which time cold air can enter the body.

As a result, a new Chinese mother is forbidden to go outdoors or to take a shower or tub bath. The health professional can demonstrate an understanding of the Chinese mother's beliefs and support her in continuing with sponge baths, emphasizing pericare, breast care, and other activities contributing to her total comfort and well-being.

The classical Chinese postpartum diet is high in hot foods. Most fruits and vegetables, considered cold, are avoided. Basic mainstay of a postpartum and lactating diet generally consists of rice and eggs and a chicken soup containing pig knuckles, vinegar ginger, rice wine, and sometimes peanuts. Because the vinegar in the soup helps to transfer tricalcium phosphate from the bone of pig knuckles into solution, the traditional soup may supply some of the calcium essential in the diets of postpartum and lactating women. The alcohol in the rice wine may stimulate bleeding, and its addition should be postponed for at least two weeks postpartum.

The health professional can be supportive to the new mother who eats this soup but should encourage her to supplement her diet with other foods that are culturally acceptable as well as nutritious, such as eggs, meat, or liver.

IN THE HOSPITAL

Members of the Chinese community are most reluctant to be admitted to hospitals. They feel: (1) hospitals are unclean and individuals die there; (2) there will be no one to translate for them; (3) surgery, considered very mutilating, may occur; (4) a patient's spirit may get lost and be unable to find its way home; and (5) Chinese food will not be served. Ideally, Chinese patients would be admitted to hospitals staffed by Chinese-speaking professionals, but this is seldom possible. Bilingual family members, however, can be encouraged to remain with the non-English-speaking patient.

The importance of having an interpreter at hand was made clear when one young Chinese woman who attempted suicide was admitted to the emergency room of a large hospital. The non-Asian doctors examined her and sutured her lacerated wrists, but because of the language barrier, they did not discover until later that she had also swallowed poison.

When a Chinese person is admitted to a hospital, his family usually leaves some valuable jewelry on him for status, and some jade for good luck. To avoid loss, family members should be encouraged to take all jewelry with them.

Elderly Chinese patients may have large amounts of money hidden in the linings of their clothing. The nurse should see that some member of the family removes most clothing until the day the patient is to be discharged. If a patient dies in the hospital, the family may then be reluctant to accept his clothing, for it is considered to contain evil spirits. Or the family may return later and request all or part of the deceased person's clothing. The health professional should therefore itemize the clothing of the deceased and keep it in a safe place.

UNDERSTANDING EACH OTHER

Health professionals frequently label the practitioners of Chinese folk medicine ignorant and superstitious. In turn, the practitioners of Chinese folk medicine frequently reject Western medicine because it is alien to their basic philosophy and beliefs. Better understanding of Chinese folk medicine by health professionals will contribute to the acceptance of health care by a portion of our community which is still for the most part not reached.

REFERENCES

1. Chinatown U.S.A. 1970. *Calif. Health* 2:27—28. Feb. 1970.
2. Fast, Julius. *Body Language.* New York, Pocket Books, 1971, p. 157. (Originally published by M. Evans and Co., 1970.)
3. Zacharoff, Lucian. A new look at ginseng. *San Francisco Examiner Chronicle* Feb. 13, 1972, p. 5.

22

Maternity Nursing and Navaho Culture

Flora L. Bailey

The Navaho Indians of the Southwest are the largest native American group in the United States. Many Navahos remain on the reservation while others have moved into towns and cities. In addition to presenting insights into Navaho culture, this chapter shows how health care professionals must go beyond mere understanding and appreciation. Is it possible to change the system of medical care to be more compatible with the variety of subcultures in this society? Flora Bailey makes such specific suggestions as allowing women to deliver babies in the traditional kneeling position, providing certain foods important to Navaho women and carrying out traditional customs regarding newborn infants. In a pluralistic society it is necessary to work toward a health care system that allows cultural differences to flourish.

Some interesting and valuable suggestions on the implementation of health education and medical procedures among the Navahos have been made by Alexander and Dorothea Leighton.[2] Since I agree with them that a sympathetic approach to this important problem is necessary, I should like to offer a number of additional suggestions based on my investigation of the beliefs and practices of the Navaho Indians pertaining to the reproductive cycle.[3] This material was gathered from three areas in New Mexico, namely, the Ramah, Pinedale, and Chaco Canyon regions. Sixty-six informants, both men and women, furnished the data. The investigation was made with a view to laying the background for a better understanding of Navaho attitudes toward health and particularly toward the problems of childbirth. Hospitals which serve the Navahos, both government and private, have made efforts to inculcate certain health principles into the minds of those whom they contact but the extent to which they have been successful is undetermined. Recent figures estimate that perhaps 25 percent of the women seek medical assistance during childbirth.

In analyzing the data, a considerable degree of homogeneity of belief was found to exist, with certain deviations of opinion surrounding the central pattern. Definite patterns of thought, however, could be distinguished throughout all the material. For example, Navaho beliefs and practices pertaining to the reproductive cycle are dependent upon mythological and religious sanctions. Pregnancy restrictions and behavior patterns for facilitating delivery are based on the premise that *like produces like,* or that an effect resembles its cause, and various forms of sympathetic magic are indulged in so that nature will be forced into the path

From "Suggested Techniques for Inducing Navaho Women to Accept Hospitalization During Childbirth and for Implementing Health Education,"[1] *American Journal of Public Health,* Vol. 38, No. 10, pp. 1418–1423, 1948. Reprinted by permission of the publisher and the author.

which is desired. It was also discovered that there is a strong emotional response in relation to hospitalization and medical aid. Although many informants did not refer to hospitals, others expressed a violent feeling either for or against these institutions and even mentioned individual doctors by name, discussing them with strong feeling.

Because certain Navaho practices are sanctioned by mythology and reinforced by ritual, they offer great resistance to change unless such changes can be made to fit the pattern of Navaho logic rather than that used by administrators of educational and medical programs. It is suggested, therefore, that medical workers and health educators accept without adverse comment the pregnancy restrictions and rules of conduct which are traditional with the Navaho. Then, using a pattern of logic which parallels that expressed in Navaho thought, they could present new restrictions and rituals based on modern medical knowledge which would assist the woman to achieve the desired result, namely, the safe and easy delivery of a healthy child.

Specific recommendations, based on these conclusions, have been proposed and will be presented here in conjunction with the native practices which can be used to reinforce or redirect the pattern.

It is of primary importance to gain the support and confidence of influential members in each family group if a program of health education is to be successfully implemented. Group decisions in matters of health are a common practice when a healing ceremonial is involved. There is considerable carry-over, it is safe to venture, in decisions regarding hospitalization. There is little doubt that many women would welcome medical advice and assistance during pregnancy and childbirth if they had the support of older members in the family and heard favorable reports from those of their friends who had experienced hospital care.

One *singer* reported, "For a while, after one woman around here had gone to the hospital and come back with the news that they gave her something to put her to sleep and she had no pain with the baby, many women thought it was better to go to the hospital than to stay home." If, as a result of one woman's confidence and satisfaction, "many" women wish to make use of medical assistance, it should be a matter of principle for each woman receiving help to be sent away feeling secure and happy so that her enthusiasm would create support and confidence among her neighbors.

In explaining why women hesitate to make use of medical facilities the statement was made, "Women know what to do at home, and they don't know about hospitals, so they don't go to hospitals." This, according to Dr. Clyde Kluckhohn's analysis of Navaho thought patterns,[4] is a basic reaction closely linked with others by which they win security. Regarding unfamiliar human beings as threats the women withdraw and do nothing when confronted with a new and potentially dangerous situation. Facing such a situation, with which she feels unable to cope, the woman solves her problem by refusing to have anything to do with doctors. The medical staff, by anticipating this reaction, could prepare the way for a more constructive solution of her problem through field clinics, individual conferences, and educational procedures designed to reassure the patient through an explanation of hospital routine.

Even a white patient, entering a hospital for the first time, is confused and apprehensive if the routine has not been explained. How much greater must this apprehension be for a woman who enters an alien world where the language is strange, where nothing fulfills her expectations of how things should be done, and where she is liable to "ghost infection" (as the Navahos term the disease) if she comes in contact with articles previously used by those who have died there.

After orientation and reassurance have been given her, the staff of the hospital, or the visiting field worker, should continue to seek ways of reinforcing the woman's emotional security and peace of mind. The fear and anxiety of pregnant women in connection with hospitalization could doubtless be reduced by encouraging early admittance, thereby lowering the mortality rate. Reports show that the majority of maternal deaths in the hospital are caused by a retained placenta since the women are so afraid to face an unknown situation that they arrive at the hospital only in time to die there. One young woman remarked, "If a baby doesn't come for two or three days they get scared and go to the hospital." This tendency to seek hospitalization only in an emergency, or if death is imminent, is not unusual. As a result, one hears such bitter reports as that which came from an older woman who had lost two daughters in childbirth at the hospital after each had successfully delivered other children at home. Obviously, in her opinion, there was only one deduction — the white doctors had killed her daughters!

Any effort made by health educators, therefore, to persuade women to seek hospitalization at the proper time would be valuable in that rumors of death due to the fault of the hospital would be minimized, and the fear which serves as an emotional block for some women could thereby be counteracted.

One anxiety, however, which might be exploited in persuading women to accept aid is the extreme fear of contact with the birth discharge. It is linked with the even greater fear of contact with menstrual blood. One man reported, "This blood is not as bad as menstrual blood but it will break the back or the breast." The "breaking" thus referred to is *arthritis deformans,* for it is believed that deformation will result from contact with the birth discharge. Other ill effects were detailed by a young woman as follows: "If a ghost-bird, or a blue-bird, or a coyote eats it, the woman won't get well for a long time; she stops having babies; it gives the woman more pain; it kills the mother; the baby won't have any sense; it will cripple animals; and witches will get it." In the face of such formidable dangers which follow the improper disposal of the birth discharge, medical authorities might offer to relieve the woman of this responsibility, assuring her that if she comes to the hospital the nurses would take care of the disposal, thereby avoiding the possibility of exposing any of her family to contact with the blood and the resulting infection.

In dealing with patients during pregnancy, as well as after their admission to the hospital, it is important to phrase medical suggestions in terms of Navaho logic. For example: Navaho methods of keeping the fetus small, to insure an easy delivery, include hard work, exercise, and not sleeping in the daytime, as well as the magical application of certain medicines which work on the *like produces like* formula such as sucking honey from the pentstemon (called hummingbird's food) or eating a hummingbird's egg, shell and all, because this bird is so tiny. If the medical worker suggests other methods such as moderate exercise, the use of vitamins, or an increased calcium intake, he might explain them by using the Navaho phraseology, "It will make the baby strong, even though he remains small, so he will be born easily." It might also be pointed out that exercise keeps a person lean and in good condition, therefore it would, as they say, "keep the baby small."

There are certain parallels between Navaho and white medical practice which might be capitalized on by the hospital staff to expedite the delivery in a manner satisfactory to all concerned. Since the woman is accustomed to the native pattern of male assistants in the hogan, the presence of a male physician should be acceptable to her, and the Navaho practice of manipulating the abdominal walls in order to secure a favorable presentation could be related to any similar manipulation which might be undertaken by the doctor. Both these patterns have mythological sanction, for Washington Matthews notes that abdominal manipulation to secure a favorable presentation was used by the two male gods, Talking God and Water Sprinkler, when they assisted at the delivery of Changing Woman and White Shell Woman.[5]

Native forms of modesty should be respected for a Navaho woman expresses her modesty in a slightly different manner from a white woman. That is, she does not consider exposure of the breasts an immodest act but places great emphasis on being adequately covered from waist to ankle. In their ceremonials women strip to one or two skirts and are very skillful in participating in events, even in the ceremonial bath, without exposing the lower part of the body. It is not strange, therefore, that hospital procedures involving a short bedgown and exposure during nursing care should be disliked. Manual examination should be undertaken with as little exposure as possible. However, since women are accustomed to a *singer* pressing and manipulating the body for ceremonial purposes, the doctor might minimize his problem by relating his examination to some such act with which she is familiar.

If internal version is indicated there is precedent in native practice for this also. Cactus salve is rubbed on the hands to make them slippery and the midwife then reaches into the orifice, using her hands as forceps, to deliver the child. However, one woman said, "It is a bad thing to reach in for the baby. I saw it done and it killed the woman." It should be explained to the patient, therefore, that under sterile conditions such emergency measures involve less danger than she anticipates in the hogan.

Navaho medical practices include the application of medicines externally and drinking of draughts during the period of pregnancy as well as at the onset of labor. Thus, any medicine which needs to be administered could be given with the explanation that it will, as the Navahos say, "help bring the baby easier," or "bring the placenta right away," or "stop the pain and clean out the blood." These are the results toward which their native medications are oriented and will, therefore, have meaning for them. No more than the exact amount, however, should be left where the patient has access to it, unless drinking a large quantity will make no difference, for the usual dose of native medicine is prescribed as "drink lots of it, drink one or two cups of that medicine."

If there is need for the use of diathermy, X-ray, or similar treatments these might be related to the healing properties of the sun prominent in Navaho ceremonial lore.

Since women are used to hot applications (made by heating the branches of juniper and packing them around the body) a parallel will be easily grasped, if heat needs to be applied, by using the Navaho cliché, "it will stop the pain."

If lacerations occur it is customary to use lotions, salves, or dusting powders. Steam baths, produced with water and herbs called Life Medicine, are also recommended. If similar treatments, ordered in the hospital, are tactfully introduced, objections might be avoided. Surgery, however, is not a native practice and this would have to be presented as a special technique used by white doctors.

A few days after delivery the woman takes a bath in certain herbs, including those called Life Medicine, to counteract the danger from contact with the birth discharge. It would be easy for a nurse to mention that the daily bath water contained a kind of Life Medicine possessing purifying qualities, thereby easing the patient's mind.

If a woman does not have sufficient milk to nurse her child she may resort to artificial means of increasing lactation. This follows the familiar pattern of *like causes like* since liquids (particularly soups) are taken internally, and milkweed plants are applied to the breasts. On the basis of Navaho logic, therefore, the staff could introduce milk into the diet or, if desirable, force liquids. Certain other practices which have mythological sanction and therefore deep emotional significance for the parturient might be permitted, or even suggested, by the medical staff. If the doctor, for example, would advise the woman to have a Blessingway ceremonial sung for her, prior to entering the hospital, it would fall into a pattern which is familiar to her and make her feel that there was sympathetic cooperation between the white doctor and the native *singer*.

The kneeling position, which the woman by tradition assumes for her delivery, has mythological sanction and is more in keeping with her sense of modesty than the modern obstetrical position. If the hospital could adapt its methods to allow delivery in the native position it might reduce emotional tension and prove valuable psychologically. Perhaps the dragrope, which in the legend was either a rainbow or a sunbeam, could be adapted for the woman's support, and certainly such small rituals as placing pollen ceremonially on the objects to be used, or applying pregnancy charms to her body, could do no harm. Corn pollen, sprinkled on a living horned toad at the moment it is born and then gathered, is always carried by a pregnant woman for use in this emergency. They say, "Take live pollen from the horned toad's babies and when the pains begin the woman takes a pinch and drops it inside her blouse because when the little toads are first dropped they can run away fast. They are strong." Mythologically the horned toad is protected against danger. For a nurse to suggest that the woman make use of such ritual assistance might easily serve to strengthen her feeling of security so that the subsequent ordeal would be eased.

Since the ritual act of *untying* plays an important part in native precautions at birth, if the woman were allowed to unbind her hair and remove her jewelry, and in cases of unusual emotional tension if the nurses would also make some gesture toward untying or unbinding their own persons, this would reinforce her morale.

The Navahos say, "No one should be around who gave any trouble to his mother at birth." Perhaps the hospital assistants could let it be known that they themselves had been born with great dispatch and little trouble. Anything that can be related to the *like causes like* formula would serve to bring reassurance.

That Navaho women find the smell of blood objectionable is evidenced by the fact that they use pungent herbs as an inhalant with the explanation that this will prevent fainting from smelling the blood. This may be partly psychological, related to the fear of contact with the birth discharge, but it would be easy to present the woman with a small bunch of sagebrush or a twig of wet juniper and might help her through a trying time. Familiar odors are known to be powerful stimulants to the emotions and would be gratefully welcomed in an atmosphere of strong, unfamiliar, and doubtless unpleasant odors.

One of the reasons women dislike hospitalization is that the food is unfamiliar and sometimes, to them, unpalatable. The food which the post-parturient expects to receive immediately after delivery is a ceremonial food sanctioned by mythology. It is a special type of blue cornmeal mush without the juniper ashes usually added to cornmeal breads. Any woman who has eaten mush ceremonially must eat it following childbirth. Where Navaho women assist in the hospital kitchens it should be possible to serve this specialty and thereby add to the patient's mental and physical comfort.

Since the woman is used to having the newborn baby close to her side it might be advantageous to let the infant remain near its mother in the hospital rather than to exile it to the nursery. This practice is not without precedent in certain modern hospitals where the philosophy of purely objective routine and seclusion for the infant has been replaced by one advocating closer physical contacts.

Molding or pressing the body of the newborn baby is believed to produce strength and beauty. This manipulation is based on mythology, being related to the pressing in the "Girl's Puberty Rite." Women who have had children born in hospitals say that the children did not develop normally due to lack of this ritual. One young mother said, "You press his forehead and nose, and body to make him beautiful. My oldest girl was born in the hospital and they didn't do that to her, and her nose is little and her forehead sticks out." Certainly it would do no harm to suggest this ritual pressing and would satisfy a need.

Legend tells us, "It is thought the sun fed the infant on pollen, for there was no one to nurse it." This statement gives the sanction for the first food given to the child. Allowing the mother to offer a pinch of corn pollen to her baby would do him no harm and might do the mother considerable good. It might be practical, also, if the mother has enough milk, to allow her to nurse the child whenever it cries. This would follow a familiar native pattern yet would not be out of line with [acceptable] practices in child care.

If the mother remains in the hospital until after the navel of the infant has healed it is important that the cord be given her to take home rather than discarded. The strong emotional tone in which the magical properties of the cord are discussed would indicate that cooperation in its proper ritual disposal would be appreciated.

When the mother and child are discharged from the hospital it is to be hoped that confidence will have been established between the medical adviser and the Navaho patient. Toward that end the preceding recommendations have been offered with the hope that they may point out specific ways of adjusting one culture to another and of lessening the tensions which are inevitable from such contacts.

REFERENCES

1. This paper was presented before the Section on Anthropology of the American Association for the Advancement of Science at the One Hundred and Fourteenth Meeting in Chicago, Ill., December 26, 1947.
2. Leighton, Alexander H., and Leighton, Dorothea C. *The Navaho Door.* Cambridge, Mass.: Harvard University Press, 1944.
3. The writer is indebted to Dr. Clyde Kluckhohn of Harvard University and Dr. Leland C. Wyman of Boston University for their encouragement and advice in the conduct of this study.
4. Kluckhohn, Clyde, and Leighton, Dorothea. *The Navaho.* Cambridge, Mass.: Harvard University Press, 1946.
5. Matthews, Washington. "Navaho Legends," *Memoirs.* American Folklore Society, 5, 1897, p. 231.

23

The Stigma of Obesity

Beatrice J. Kalisch

It is easy to see that culture is important for people who live with a specific religious or ethnic subculture. But cultural patterns affect everyone and play some role in most health problems. This article examines the cultural influence on a problem that seems to be personal or psychological — obesity. Food is culturally defined in every society including what is good to eat, how much one should eat and how often to eat. Standards of beauty, body build and weight are all culturally learned. Beatrice Kalisch examines obesity and how the health professional might deal with it from a cultural perspective. The author shows how such cultural stigmas as being "fat" influence those with overweight problems. By recognizing the cultural as well as the psychological factors involved, the health professional is in a better position to work effectively with obese individuals.

Society stigmatizes people with any characteristic it considers undesirable. The characteristic may be labeled a handicap, shortcoming, failing, disgrace, weakness, or, in the words of a leading authority on the theory of stigma, a "spoiled identity."[1] While the degree of undesirability may vary extensively, the common factor in such characteristics is lack of full social acceptance. The afflicted person is deprived of his right to be evaluated according to his unique personality.

In our society, the obese are invariably subjected to stigmatizing attitudes. Obesity has most commonly been considered completely physical or psychological, or both in origin; however, it must also be viewed as a social phenomenon. The ways that various cultures and even subgroups within the same culture define it in terms of beauty and ugliness gives weight to this. One has only to look at Renaissance art to discover that plumper body types were favored at that time. In some cultures where food is scarce, a high status is accorded to those who weigh more because this indicates financial success.

Social class has also a potent influence on weight in our society. A study of the residents of a central area in New York City showed that extreme overweight was seven times more frequent among women of the lower socioeconomic class than those of a higher class. In men, the same relationship existed, but to a lesser degree.[2]

The fact that obesity is a social phenomenon within our culture is seen also in dieting patterns. Wyden notes that even though only 11 percent of the total United States population falls in the upper- or upper-middle classes, these classes contain 24 percent of all dieters.[3]

Women diet more than men and teen-agers more than adults.[4,5] That obesity is a greater social disadvantage for a woman than a man in our society may account for this difference between the sexes. The obese woman finds it more difficult to move up the social ladder, relate to others, and obtain a suitable marriage partner than does the obese man. Moreover, the self-concept of American women is connected with physical desirability. The appearance of men is important, but financial status, educational achievement, and occupation affect his value more.

Another cultural influence is that the shape of men's clothing conceals body form and thus can hide bulges, while women's clothing is designed to reveal the configuration of the body. Adolescents diet more than adults probably because physical appearance is of great importance at that period of life and teen-agers tend to regard any type of deviation from the peer group norm as negative.

WHY WE STIGMATIZE

What causes a person to stigmatize another? It stems from our self-concept. Upon seeing a distortion, we feel threatened, probably because it reminds us of our own unearned good luck and our vulnerability. Stigmatizing attitudes increase our feelings of well-being, safety, and superiority. In other words, this mechanism allows us to dissociate or deny our common condition of vulnerability with the afflicted. Those with strong egos have less need to reject than those with weak ones.

DEGREE OF STIGMA

Studies have been directed to finding out how serious is the stigma attached to obesity in the United States. Richardson and his associates investigated how 650 boys and girls 10 and 11 years of age, reacted to the physical disabilities of other children.

The children were shown six black-and-white line drawings of a child with no physical handicap, a child with crutches and a brace on one leg, a child sitting in a wheelchair with a blanket covering both legs, a child with one hand missing, a child with a disfigurement on one side of the mouth, and an obese child. The results showed that, almost unanimously, the normal child was the most preferred and the obese child the least desirable.[6]

Using this same ordering task of the six drawings, Maddox and others conducted a study with various adult groups, including persons they defined as most likely to be indifferent to the societal preference for leanness (elderly persons, Negro men, low-income persons). These groups, too, considered the picture of the obese child to be the least desirable and likable.[7]

Obese applicants to colleges were found to be less likely to be accepted than the nonobese, even though there was no measurable difference in academic achievement, social class, and motivation.[8]

Physicians have also been found to have negative attitudes toward the obese whom they described to be more "weak-willed," "ugly," and "awkward" than other patients.[9]

REASONS GIVEN FOR STIGMATIZING THE OBESE

One justification frequently given for the negative connotation fatness carries in our society is that success depends to a great degree on physical attractiveness. Another reason given is that excess weight is detrimental to health, and health is a valued measure of status and security. A relationship between thinness and length of life has been reported frequently with reports indicating the obese are more prone to diabetes mellitus, cardiovascular, digestive and renal diseases.

Some interpretations of these relationships have recently been criticized for oversimplification. Formerly the weight-height tables used by the insurance companies disregarded the influence of body type and composition. Later they added modifications for frame size, without precise definitions of frames. Using the standards of height, age, and sex, today overweight refers to heaviness while obesity refers to excessive amounts of body fat. It is possible to be overweight and not overfat and vice versa. Body type determines how much of excessive weight may be due to muscles, bones, fluids, and fats.

The Build and Blood Pressure Study, 1959 by the Society of Actuaries has largely influenced the belief that excess weight is associated with poor health.[10] The findings, which revealed a consistent gradient advance in mortality with increasing degrees of overweight, have propagated the notion that all degrees of excess weight constitute a risk to longevity and health. A 1966 reevaluation of the 1959 study demonstrated that there was no significant excess in actual over expected mortality until the level of extreme obesity was reached. At this point, the mortality ratio rose in a very steep progression.[11] The source book on Obesity and Health states that "The association of body fat and mortality below the level of frank obesity is not clear."[12]

Obesity is regarded as more than a beauty and health issue in our society, however. Many look upon excessive weight gain as immortal. Historically, the Protestant ethic emphasized impulse control and thus, in this case, abstinence from overeating. And gluttony, of course, is one of the seven deadly sins. Fatness is not necessarily due to eating large amounts of food. Many Americans may be obese due to the sedentary lives they live. Yet, people associate the handicap with gluttony and self-indulgence.[13] Under controlled, hospitalized conditions some persons find it most difficult to lose weight and numerous physiologic factors affect the process.[14]

However, society continues to place the blame on the individual. Maddox found that, while the obese were held responsible for their own condition, people with other handicaps were not so blamed.[15] And Goffman points out that whenever the stigmatized are believed to be the cause of their condition, the irrational, prejudicial attitudes are exaggerated.[1]

RESULTS OF STIGMATIZING ATTITUDES

An obese person finds his condition a constant barrier to attaining the privileges, opportunities, and status accorded to others. Physical and bodily discomfort that stems from obesity seems to be of less significance to him than the suffering imposed by the socially derogatory attitudes held by those around him. Fat people are ridiculed, despised, and often avoided.

When an obese person seeks medical care, his personal tragedy may equal or exceed that of patients with more socially accepted physical diseases. The suffering and frustration associated with the obesity, however, may go beyond that of other physical ailments.

For an overweight person, hospitalization often mandates exposure of his overweight condition. On admission the routine weigh-in may humiliate him; he realizes the results will become part of his chart for the hospital staff to see. A hospital gown may not fit and, even if it does, gives little protection from exposure. His body is exposed for treatments, bathing, and other procedures, and his food intake is monitored. Even though the nurse may not be critical of him, he may feel that she is.

As Goffman points out, the worst result of stigmatizing attitudes is that the afflicted come to accept the negative evaluations of the society.[1]

In a study of high-school girls, for example, such personality traits as withdrawal, passivity, expectation of rejection, and extraordinary concern with self-image were found to characterize the obese.[16] The obese, then, tend to live up to the expectations that others have of them, accepting a tremendous amount of blame for their predicament – a typical, unfortunate example of the self-fulfilling prophecy.

An examination of physicians' attitudes revealed that they thought that obesity was either incurable or only slightly amenable to help.[17]

One cannot help but wonder if the reported low success rate in the treatment of these individuals is related to the expectations of failure by physicians, nurses, and other helpers.

COMBATING THE STIGMA

Before a nurse can build a relationship with an obese patient which will help him strengthen his self-concept she must first examine her own feelings about obesity. She may well hold many of the unwarranted prejudices of the general public and might find it helpful to separate myths from reality.

Most stigmatizing attitudes stem from erroneous assumptions, and when rational understanding is achieved the stigma is eradicated. However, achievement is not easy because it must be preceded by the difficult and painful process of becoming self-aware.

Unconditional acceptance of the person is the key to helping the obese. Cahnman concludes from his study of obese adolescents that acceptance of the individual must come *before* the weight reduction.[18] To mention weight control to a person before a relationship based on genuine acceptance is developed, is one way to doom the efforts to failure. Because of the shame and guilt many obese persons experience, it may be difficult for them to talk about their true feelings and concerns.

Often, persons who have succeeded in reducing their weight to the normal range are unable to eradicate the self-hate and inadequacy they felt when they were overweight. Because we humans strive for self-consistency, if a formerly fat person does not revise his self-concept, he will most likely be unable to retain the weight loss. The nurse can help the patient adjust to his new identity, to help him retain his weight loss.

A typical response when normal individuals interact with the stigmatized is to pretend that the stigmatizing condition such as obesity does not exist. The person is aware that he is not genuinely accepted. In such a relationship, if a nurse advises or lectures the patient, he may build defenses to ward off anxiety. A common coping mechanism is denial. This defense interferes with his losing weight or adjusting in other positive ways.

Beyond assisting the patient to work through his problems by accepting him, the nurse can help him deal with the negative societal reactions. He should be helped to become aware of, and resistant to, stigmatizing attitudes rather than returned "cold" to the community. An understanding of why people react in the way they do will help the overweight person to cope with pressures he will undoubtedly face.

Goffman demonstrates that because the stigmatized are cut off from society, they associate with a group of persons, known as the "own" group who share the stigma.[1] With these persons, the obese can gain "instruction in tricks of the trade" as well as acceptance. This may account for the epidemic spread of the "Weight Watchers" and other reducing clubs. It may be appropriate for the nurse to encourage certain patients to join clubs of this type so that they will have a subgroup to relate to and thus gain moral support.

It is important to start with the assumption that people don't want to hurt others. In hospital or other institutional settings, group sessions in which the staff can talk out their feelings and concerns about the obese would likely be helpful. A change in attitudes, however, is not likely to occur overnight. If any staff member continues to stigmatize obese patients, or for that matter any patient, the nursing leader must make the situations unrewarding for him either by reprimanding or dismissing him. This should be an established policy rather than an occasional informal action.

Helping the people abandon stereotypes and helping the stigmatized reconstitute their self-images are two sides of the same rehabilitative coin. All too often, however, the nurse neglects her responsibility for education of the public.

In the expanding role of the nurse, it seems imperative that she assume responsibility, along with other health professionals, for such programs.

Health education is still a largely unstudied field and outcomes of programs may be unexpected. For example, in York and Reading, Pennsylvania, a one-year campaign to decrease the negative, stigmatizing attitudes toward epilepsy was instituted. But instead of eradicating the stigma, the campaign tended to polarize attitudes and many were found to be more prejudiced after the campaign than before.[19] Thus care must be taken in setting up and carrying out such a program. It is a fairly well-established fact, however, that dwelling on the differentness of the stigmatized is an error. The most successful programs have emphasized how the handicapped person is like normal individuals.

Effective nursing of the overweight patient requires that both the nurse and patient focus on an obesity destigmatization process. Above all the patient should be appropriately involved in an assessment of his strength and limitations in relation to his condition so that he does not feel manipulated and misunderstood. With acceptance from others as he is, the individual is then more likely to be able to deal realistically with his feelings and excessive weight. A corollary is to work with other health personnel and the public to develop accepting and empathic attitudes toward the obese.

REFERENCES

1. Goffman, Erving. *Stigma; Notes on the Management of Spoiled Identity.* Englewood Cliffs, N.J., Prentice-Hall, 1963.
2. Moore, M. E., and others. Obesity, social class, and mental illness. *J.A.M.A.* 181:962–966, Sept. 15, 1962.
3. Wyden, Peter. *The Overweight Society.* New York, William C. Morrow and Co., 1965, p. 8.
4. Dwyer, J. T., and Mayer, J. Potential dieters; who are they? *J. Am. Diet. Assoc.* 56: 510–514, June 1970.
5. _____, and others. Body image in adolescents; attitudes toward weight and perception of appearance. *J. Nutr. Educ.* 1:14–19, Fall 1969.
6. Richardson, S. N., and others. Cultural uniformity and reaction to physical disability. *Am. Socio. Rev.* 26:241–247, Apr. 1961.
7. Maddox, G. L., and others. Overweight as social deviance and disability. *J. Health Soc. Behav.* 9:287–298, Dec. 1968.
8. Canning, H., and Mayer, J. Obesity – its possible effect on college acceptance. *N. Engl. J. Med.* 275:1172–1174, Nov. 24, 1966.
9. Maddox, G. L., and Liederman, V. Overweight as a social disability with medical implications. *J. Med. Educ.* 44:214–220, Mar. 1969.
10. The Society of Actuaries. *Build and Blood Pressure Study. Volume 1.* Chicago, The Society, 1959.
11. Seltzer, C. C. Some re-evaluations of the build and blood pressure study, 1959, as related to ponderal index, somatotype, and mortality. *N. Engl. J. Med.* 274:254–259, Feb. 3, 1966.
12. U.S. Public Health Service, Division of Chronic Diseases. *Obesity and Health.* (Publication No. 1485) Washington, D.C., U.S. Government Printing Office, 1966, p. 6.
13. Dwyer, J. T., and others. Social psychology of dieting. *J. Health Soc. Behav.* 11:269–287, Dec. 1970.

14. Gordon, E. S., and others. New concept in the treatment of obesity. *J.A.M.A.* 186:50–60, Oct. 5, 1963.
15. Maddox, and others, *op. cit.,* pp. 296–297.
16. Monello, L. F., and Mayer, J. Obese adolescent girls, an unrecognized "minority" group? *Am. J. Clin. Nutr.* 13:35–39, July 1963.
17. Maddox, G. L., and others. Overweight as a problem of medical management in a public outpatient clinic. *Am. J. Med. Sci.* 252:394–403, Oct. 1966.
18. Cahnman, W. L. Stigma of obesity. *Sociol. Q.* 9:283–299, Summer 1968.
19. Leonard Wood Memorial. *Combating Stigma Resulting from Deformity and Disease.* New York, The Memorial, 1969.

V

The Nursing Process

The nursing process provides a guideline for all community nursing activity. Sometimes called the "problem-solving process" or the "deliberative process," it is a series of steps that, when taken, lead toward the goal of effective nursing action.

Simply stated, the steps or phases of the nursing process include assessment, planning, implementation and evaluation. Each phase requires thoughtful deliberation on the part of the nurse. In the assessment phase the nurse is gathering and analyzing data. From this information inferences are drawn and diagnoses are made. During the planning phase possible actions are considered and then the best one is selected. This plan of action is carried out in the implementation phase. Finally the results are evaluated. On the basis of this evaluation new data is gathered and the process starts over again.

The term "nursing process" is preferable to "the problem-solving process" because the latter suggests exclusive concern with problems. Community nursing also emphasizes health and normality so that dealing with problems is only one part of the community nurse's activity. The nurse is encouraged to use the process in all nursing actions. For example, to help a young couple understand normal child development, the nurse will need to use each step of the nursing process. First, data must be gathered and analyzed. What does this couple already know about child development? What stage of development is their child in now? What are the parents' chief interests? Perhaps they would like to know how to provide an enriched, stimulating environment for the child. Second, the nurse will select the best approach to presenting the needed information. She may choose to suggest to the couple that they read and discuss selected articles on child development together. Next, the plan is carried out. Finally, the nurse must consider the effectiveness of this action. What did the couple learn? Were they satisfied with the material presented and the method used? What further information would they now like?

It takes conscious effort by the nurse to develop skillful use of the nursing process. Part V includes several ways to improve the community nurse's use of the process.

24

The Relevant "Who"
of Problem Solving

Muriel Standeven

The process of solving health problems is a joint venture between the community nurse and the patient or family. Each step of the process requires input from those involved to achieve accurate problem definition and effective problem resolution. Yet a serious error is often made, this author contends, by not considering all the persons relevant to the problem. Individuals are not isolated entities; they are members of groups, socially and culturally. In the problem-solving process the community nurse must consider and include all those persons whose relationship has an important bearing on the problem.

Problem solving is usually more effective when those who are involved in the problem or affected by the solution have a say in bringing about the solution. However, the commonly described method for problem solving indicates the action to be taken but leaves out who should be involved at each step. Indication of the relevant "who" for each step of the problem-solving method can serve to remind the problem solver that there are, perhaps, out-of-view others who should be included. This in turn can contribute to obtaining a more complete history of the problem situation, a clearer definition of the problem, selection of a solution that is agreeable to all who will be affected by the solution, more complete implementation, and result in better problem solving.

Through the use of a problem-solving method, nurses seek to assist patients and their families with their health needs and problems. Many times health problems are resolved but often the nurse along with her patient are in such haste to solve the problem they frequently commit an error of omission which results in ineffective problem resolution. The nurse works only with those people involved in the problem — those who are in her immediate view; she overlooks the out-of-her-view relevant others who are also a part of the problem situation.

The traditional problem-solving method contributes to this omission. Generally it is outlined as (1) gather the data, (2) identify the problem, (3) consider possible solutions, (4) select the best solution, (5) carry out the plan, and (6) evaluate the results. The method clearly describes the action to be taken but who is involved at each step is left up to the problem solver. It would seem that if how well each step is performed determines how effectively the problem is solved, including or overlooking the relevant "who" in each step would also influence the effectiveness of the solution.

From *Nursing Forum*, Vol. 10, No. 2, 1971, pp. 166–175. Reprinted with permission from Nursing Publications, Inc., 194-B Kinderkamack Road, Park Ridge, New Jersey 07656.

IDENTIFYING THE RELEVANT "WHO"?

Essentially everyone participates in one or more groups in the course of his every-day living — family, extended family, groups at work or school, and friends and interest groups. Each group constitutes a social system and is, simultaneously, a unit or part of a larger social system. A person is a unit of the various social systems to which he belongs, and performs to some degree the expected behaviors of the positions he holds in them. The expected behaviors or roles contribute to the continuity and smooth functioning of the system.

Social systems, according to Warren, have a proclivity for equilibrium and a built-in resistance to change:

A social system is a structural organization of the interaction of units which endures through time. It has both external and internal aspects relating the system to its environment and its units to each other. It can be distinguished from its surrounding environment, performing a function called boundary maintenance. It tends to maintain an equilibrium in the sense that it adapts to changes from outside the system in such a way as to minimize the impact of the change on the organizational structure and to regularize the subsequent relationships.[1]

Solutions to most problems require some change of behavior for the involved persons. Change in the behavior of one person in a social system influences the behavior of others in it, requiring some degree of change in their behavior. Over-coming the resistance to change becomes a critical issue in the solution of prob-lems. Watson has recommended the following principles that indicate the impor-tance of involving the relevant "who" in bringing about any change. Resistance will be less:

1. If participants have joined in diagnostic efforts leading them to agree on what the basic problem is and to feel its importance.
2. If the project is adopted by consensual group decision.
3. If proponents are able to empathize with opponents, to recognize valid objections, and to take steps to relieve unnecessary fears.
4. If it is recognized that innovations are likely to be misunderstood and misinterpreted, and if provision is made for feedback of perceptions of the project and for further clari-fication as needed.
5. If participants experience acceptance, support, trust, and confidence in their relations with one another.[2]

The relevant "who," then, are members of the involved social systems who are affected in some way by the problem.

BACKGROUND OF THE PROPOSED PROBLEM-SOLVING METHOD

Holland, Tiedke and Miller propose a theoretical model for community health action which when combined with the current, commonly used problem-solving method produces a model that enables the problem solver to know who should be included and what should be done in each step of the problem-solving proce Though they discuss each phase of their model in terms of community health action, for the purposes of this article each phase will be discussed as it pertains to the problem-solving process. There are five analytical components to the Holland, Tiedke, and Miller process: (1) convergence of interest, (2) establishment of an initiating set, (3) legitimation and sponsorship, (4) establishment of an execution set, and (5) fulfillment of a charter.[3] The first four components relate to "who" needs to be involved, the fifth relates to action only. The following is, in essence, their explanation of each component.

Convergence of Interest

For action to take place, there must be some convergence of interest of those actors in the social system who have appropriate sentiments, beliefs, and/or rationally calculated purposes with reference to a problem. The motivation behind their interest in the problem does not matter at this point. The important thing is that there is convergence of interest.

Establishment of an Initiating Set

The initiating set evolves from the group with converging interests. The internal organization of the set must be such that all those with the right to initiate and those with the obligation to respond are included in it. Those in the initiating set must develop common group goals — goals which may arise out of individual motives but are the goals of the group. These become its charter and formalize the relationships of the initiating set.

The members of the set must believe the charter (goals) can be fulfilled and see the availability and accessibility of the means to fulfill it. They must also develop within the set acceptable justification of the need and their right to initiate the action specified by the charter. This may occur before or after agreement on goals, but must occur to promote internal security of the set and as a basis on which to approach others involved in the problem or its solution.

Legitimation and Sponsorship

By this is meant the acceptance of the right of the initiating set to initiate action and the approval of the goals it established by those who have a say in the matter and by those who control the resources necessary for the action. If these persons are not members of the initiating set, their legitimation and sponsorship must be obtained by the initiating set before action is taken if the goals are to be realized.

Establishment of an Execution Set

The execution set is the group that will carry out the action to fulfill the charter. It may or may not include all of or more than those included in the initiating set. It may include people who are interested in the charter but who, unlike the initiating set, have neither the right to initiate nor the obligation to respond. The members of the execution set must accept the goals of the charter and have access to the resources necessary to take action.

Fulfillment of the Charter

Fulfillment of the charter is described as the action taken by the execution set toward achieving the goals of the charter and not the degree of success in achieving the goals.

THE COMBINED MODEL

The following is an outline of the problem-solving method indicating both *who* needs to be involved and *what* needs to be done.

1. The convergence of those who have an appropriate interest in reference to a problem.
   a. Gather data
   b. Begin to identify problem areas
   c. Identify those who should be a part of the initiating set
2. The development of the initiating set (those who have the right to initiate and those with the obligation to respond).
   a. Gather further data
   b. Identify and define the problem
   c. Develop group goals
   d. Consider possible solutions
   e. Select the best solution
   f. Hold the belief that the goals can be fulfilled
   g. See the availability and accessability of the means to reach the goals
   h. Develop within the set acceptable justification of the need and right to initiate action
3. The acceptance and approval of the right of the initiating set to take action toward fulfillment of the goals by those who have a say in the matter or who control the resources.
4. The establishment of the execution set (all or part of the initiating set and others who have an interest in and accept the goals).
   a. Carry out the plan
   b. Evaluate the results

The following illustrates the application of the combined model to a hypothetical situation in community health nursing.

The *convergence of interest* occurs when Mrs. Manders, a community health nurse, makes an after-school home visit to the Davis home in response to a hospital referral of 13-year-old Tommy Davis, newly diagnosed as a diabetic. Tommy and his mother agree to discuss the situation with her. Mrs. Davis, Mrs. Manders, Tommy, and Dr. Brown, the referring physician, have an interest in Tommy and his condition, but the motivations behind their interests could be quite different at this point. Some initial data gathering and beginning identification of the problem areas takes place as the mother, boy, and nurse talk together. Those others who are involved in the problem areas, who have a "right to initiate or the obligation to respond," now need to be identified and included in the discussions thus *developing the initiating set.*

Because of problems such as reactions to the diagnosis, understanding the disease condition, how to explain it to others; what insulin does, how to administer it, the possible side effects of too much or too little; the food to be eaten, how to prepare it, what to eat at school; how the disease will affect Tommy's total growth, current activities, and adult life; and the feelings and fears associated with each aspect of the disease, the initiating set could involve Tommy, his father, his mother, Janie, his 10-year-old sister, other members of the extended family, his physician, the school nurse, his teachers, his closest friends, and possibly others. These people are the members of the social systems in Tommy's life. Failure to include any one who has the need and the right to be involved could result in less effective problem solving. This is the time for the nurse who is involved as a health teacher and coordinator to consider those who though invisible to her are the relevant "who" who should be included in the gathering of further data, defining problem areas, developing group goals, determining best solutions and making plans, identifying resources, and developing justification of the group's need and right to initiate action.

In this hypothetical illustration, acceptance and approval to initiate action takes place when the goals and plans, or the appropriate parts of each are accepted and approved by Tommy's physician, the school principal, and parents of the close friends who would participate in some of the plans. Tommy's father is frequently away from home, therefore he is a contributing but not an active member of the initiating set. But as an involved member of the family who also controls some of the resources needed to carry out the plan his acceptance and approval of the plan are specifically obtained.

The acceptance and approval of the right of the initiating set to take action toward the fulfillment of the goals by those who have a say in the matter or who control the needed resources is a step in the problem-solving process which the nurse commonly neglects or only partially recognizes. That is because in her planning she overlooks those relevant "who" who are invisible to her. The community health nurse frequently sees only the mother of a family, so falls into the practice of planning and implementing her nursing actions in terms of only the mother. The father, and the children who are old enough to participate in solving problems that include them, are overlooked. A community health nurse seldom forgets to include the patient's physician at the appropriate times, although he is invisible to her, because she is accustomed to working with physicians. However, she frequently forgets the relevant "who" of other involved community systems — the school, the welfare and penal systems.

Establishment of the execution set evolves along with the development of the plan of action. What needs to be done arises out of the identified goals, and who will do what may be based on who needs to learn to do it, who can best do it, whose responsibility it is to do it, or who needs something to do. Those in the set have to be in agreement with the goals and plans and have access to the resources necessary to carry out their part of the plan. For instance, Mrs. Manders could teach Tommy and Mrs. Davis to give the insulin; Janie could draw a chart for her brother to keep a record of urine tests and insulin dosages; the whole family and Tommy's closest friends could study the signs and symptoms of insulin reaction and what to do in the event it happened. Mrs. Davis could study food exchange lists and prepare sample menus for the nurse to review, Tommy and his friends could make up a list of snacks he could eat after school or at parties; Dr. Brown, Mrs. Manders, Mr. and Mrs. Davis, and Tommy could discuss the effect of diabetes on Tommy's future life; Mr. and Mrs. Davis and Tommy could have a conference with the school nurse, Tommy's home room teacher, and his three other teachers to discuss any limitations in activity and what to do in an emergency. The school nurse could discuss Tommy's diet with the lunchroom supervisor and assist in arranging for appropriate food intake. Each one carries out his part of the plan with some degree of success and, ideally, everyone who has participated will be involved in evaluating the results of his own efforts; those responsible for over-all planning will evaluate over-all results.

This particular example describes a medical situation. The problem-solving method can as easily be applied to a health promotion problem: a child-raising problem, e.g., discipline, language development or sibling rivalry; or a home-making problem that affects health, e.g., improving the nutrition of the family, or planning for recreation for the family; or problems in ward or office management.

REFERENCES

1. Warren, Roland, *The Community in America*, Chicago: Rand McNally and Co., 1963.
2. Watson, Goodwin, "Resistance to Change," *The Planning of Change*, (Edited by Warren G. Bennis, Kenneth D. Benne, and Robert Chin), New York: Holt, Rinehart and Winston, Inc., 1961, pp. 488–497.
3. Holland, John B., Miller, Paul A., and Tiedke, Kenneth E., "A Theoretical Model for Health Action," *Rural Sociology*, 22: June 1957, pp. 149–155.

25

The Process of Contracting
in Community Nursing

Margaret R. Sloan
Barbara Thune Schommer

Patient and family self-determination has become an increasingly important concept for community nursing. Assisting patients realistically to discover and develop their own strengths is a means of promoting self-actualization as well as positive health practices. An effective means whereby the community nurse can accomplish this is the use of contracts. In this chapter the authors present a helpful description of the steps involved in the contracting process.

A contract is a valuable tool that the community nurse can use to involve the patient and family in their own health care. As an example, witness a particular nurse, patient and family deeply involved in discussing what each will do to achieve the mutually set goal of weight loss. The patient agrees to follow a weight reduction diet, the family agrees to learn how to prepare foods according to the diet and the nurse agrees to discuss nutrition with them. After four weeks they hope to accomplish their goal of the patient losing eight pounds.

Many community nurses are unfamiliar with this tool. Others either reject the use of contract entirely or fail to use it effectively in their nursing practice. The effective use of contract is dependent on understanding (1) the difference between the contract in a legal agreement and the contract in community nursing; (2) the philosophy underlying the use of contract; and (3) the operational definition of the process of contracting.

In this chapter we shall examine each of these areas and present a model of the contracting process. Our model represents an operational definition of contracting and includes eight activities that are necessary elements in the negotiations between patient, family and nurse. The activities are goal-oriented within a mutually agreed time period.

Although we believe the contract can be used effectively with many families, it is not a tool that can be used indiscriminately. In certain situations only a modified use of contract is appropriate. We shall describe situations where the nurse needs to take a more affirmative approach or action rather than negotiate a contract with the patient.

LEGAL CONTRACT AND THE COMMUNITY NURSING CONTRACT

The legal and business form of contract has been in use for many years and is a familiar concept. We contract to buy an automobile or a home. A contract describes the terms of agreement in marriage, employment or union negotiations.

This chapter was written especially for this book and has never been published before.

In each case the contract is a written binding agreement between two parties. It is an obligation created and determined by the two parties in which each is pledged to carry out his promise. The signed, notarized agreement is recognized by law.

Only in recent years has the contract been adapted from the business and legal field to the human services professions as a tool for developing helping relationships. This has occurred primarily in the fields of mental health, counseling, education, social work and community nursing. The community nursing contract is similar in most aspects to the business and legal contract with a major difference being that the community nursing contract is usually less formal. It is not usually legal and binding on the two parties although some aspects of the contract may be legal, like the fee.

The lack of acceptance and use of the contract as a tool for community nursing practice is frequently related to the legal aspects of the term itself. Failure to fulfill a business contract may lead to legal action. Nurses who attach this legal connotation to "contract" may have difficulty accepting "contract" in helping relationships.

In community nursing a contract may be defined as any working agreement, continuously renegotiable, between nurse, patient and family (see Fig. 1). Community nurses have a beginning contract when they agree to make home visits to families who have agreed to such visits. Some nurses may prefer to call this

---

Contract for Service

1. Goals:

2. Length of contract:

3. Client responsibilities:

4. Nursing responsibilities:

5. Home health aide responsibilities:

6. Fee determination:

    Signatures:_____ Client

                  _____ Community nurse

                  _____ Home health aide

Figure 1. Contract for Service utilized by Anoka County Comprehensive Health Department, Public Health Nursing, 1973 (this is not a legal document).

process the development of mutual objectives and responsibilities rather than contract. The agreement may be formal or informal, written or verbal, simple or detailed, signed or unsigned by patient and nurse.

PHILOSOPHY UNDERLYING USE OF CONTRACT

Patients' involvement in their own health care has become an increasingly important concept in nursing. A contract is one means for developing and ensuring patient involvement. Contracting is based on the belief that all men have the potential for growth and the right of self-determination, although their choice may be different from ours. The helping person who involves the patient in health decisions is demonstrating his belief in the dignity and worth of man.

This philosophy of patient involvement encourages the individual to act for himself and to maintain his autonomy. Relying on the patient and family for decision making concerning their goals for health affirms their ability to solve their own health problems and their right to accept or reject nursing services. It affirms that the patient's health is his decision and his responsibility.[1]

Carl Rogers eloquently describes the act of involving the patient as a partner in his health care. He speaks to one of the most basic, important elements in a helping relationship, that of seeing the patient as a person of unconditional self-worth.[2] By encouraging patient responsibility for helping to set goals, to plan and participate in regaining health, nurses are able to communicate respect for individuals as cognitive human beings and for their decisions. We all need to know that someone is interested in us, accepts us as we are and cares about us before we are able to reveal ourselves to others and move constructively forward.

An important element in community nurse acceptance and use of contract is the willingness to accept this philosophy as well as to view the patient and family as having responsibility for making decisions about their health. Mutual involvement by patient and nurse in a meaningful contract will include the building of trust between them as a result of unconditional caring and acceptance of mutual responsibilities.

THE PROCESS OF CONTRACTING

The effective use of contract is dependent on implementing the operationally defined activities indicated in the model (see Fig. 2). The flow of activities is accomplished through mutual agreement and may overlap. A contract is most effective when family as well as the patient is involved in its development.

To help clarify these activities we include an example of contract use with Linda and her two children, Billy, age 5, and Katie, age 6. Linda's husband was not a part of the original contract. Linda was referred to community nursing by the outpatient pediatric clinic at City Hospital. She had complained to the clinic nurse that she could not stand the constant bickering between Billy and

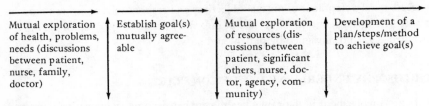

| Mutual exploration of health, problems, needs (discussions between patient, nurse, family, doctor) | Establish goal(s) mutually agreeable | Mutual exploration of resources (discussions between patient, significant others, nurse, doctor, agency, community) | Development of a plan/steps/method to achieve goal(s) |

Figure 2. An Operational Definition of the Contracting Process in Community Nursing. (According to Burd and Marshall, "An operational definition provides statements of all observed behaviors that are associated with the concept in the order in which such behaviors emerge in the observed."[3]) Figure is adapted from "The Process of Contracting in the Helping Relationship," by John K. Sauer.[4]
Key: → Flow of activities; ↕ Mutuality of contracting

Katie, and had tried everything she knew to alleviate it. She agreed to community nurse visits, and a referral was sent.

Identification of Problem — Mutual Establishment of Goals

The community nurse will begin the process by assessing the problems or needs of family or patient. The added dimension of contract involves the mutual identification of the need by both nurse and patient. The patient is encouraged to articulate his need to a helping person who will listen and collaborate with him by following through this problem with the other activities of the contracting process. The patient's perception and statement of his problem is given much value in determining nursing care, and he becomes a partner in planning his care from the very beginning.

Along with identifying needs, the partnership will attempt to set reasonable mutual goals which will lead to a solution. Both partners must discuss together such questions as the following: What can we do together to solve the problem? From what side do we want to attack this need? What kinds of things are realistic for us to work on at this time? Again, these are mutually set goals, articulated as much as possible by the patient.

In our example, Linda and Pat, the community nurse, have been talking for a while, and they are now identifying Linda's needs and setting reasonable goals for themselves.

Linda: I'm having trouble with my kids, they fight with each other, they don't mind me, and I'm always getting mad at them.
Pat: Would you like to try working together on these troubles?
Linda: Yes, I could use some help.
Pat: O.K. Let's see. . . . Let's talk about what it is that we really want to change here.
Linda: Well, I want to get less mad at the kids, and I want them to stop fighting.

Linda and Pat may discuss the alternatives for a while and decide that they cannot change the children's behavior just yet, but will attempt to help Linda change her behavior first. They will work on changing the children's behavior as a later

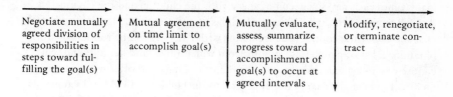

Negotiate mutually agreed division of responsibilities in steps toward fulfilling the goal(s)	Mutual agreement on time limit to accomplish goal(s)	Mutually evaluate, assess, summarize progress toward accomplishment of goal(s) to occur at agreed intervals	Modify, renegotiate, or terminate contract

goal. There is much dialogue at this point as they attempt to arrive at workable, realistic goals.

Mutual Exploration of Resources

After the goals are set, the nurse and patient must mutually explore the resources that are open to them for meeting their goals. What are the special qualities each offers the relationship? What is each partner willing to offer? This exploration allows each partner a chance to become more familiar with the other person, and to gauge the depth of his commitment to and understanding of the problem and the goals they have chosen. Another aspect of this step involves each partner indicating what he expects from the other person. This helps to clear any misunderstandings based on unstated assumptions. For instance Linda relates the following to Pat: "I can offer to be open and honest in telling you my feelings about the kid's fighting, I will keep our appointments, and I will listen to your suggestions. I will expect you to offer suggestions, listen to my side of the story, and keep our appointments."

Develop a Plan

After the patient and nurse have set their goals and have examined the resources each will offer, they can begin to mutually develop a plan or method for meeting their goals. Questions they may ask include: What kinds of things can we do right now to meet our goal? How much time shall we give ourselves? Where shall we start? Is one of our goals or a part of a goal more important than the others?

In the example, Linda and Pat decide that to meet their goal of changing Linda's behavior, they will talk about the times Linda gets angry when she is with the children, they will meet weekly for one-hour sessions, they will talk about ways to involve Linda's husband in their sessions, and they will begin looking for a parenting group for Linda and her husband to attend.

Division of Responsibilities

The patient and nurse next will determine which activities each one will be responsible for completing. Both nurse and patient will be responsible for certain specified things, and by mutually agreeing upon these, both know what each other will be doing. Each has an idea of what to expect from the other during visits as well as for the next visit.

In the example, the partnership agreement is that Linda will keep a list of how many times each day she becomes angry with the children and the circumstances that led to the anger, talk about her feelings of anger with Pat and talk to her husband about the contract she is making with Pat. Pat will be responsible for obtaining a list of parent[ing] groups from which Linda and her husband will choose one to attend, reviewing the list kept by Linda and offering suggestions on how Linda might change her approach to the children. Linda and Pat are also responsible for discussing any negative and positive feelings resulting from each other's comments and/or actions.

Set Time Limits

Now the patient and nurse are ready to set time limits on their contract. These time limits act as a built-in check on their progress. Without time limits, the contract and the care may continue for long periods of time, with no concern given to looking at whether or not the goals had been met. Without time limits, patients and nurses often fail to review the care, with the result often heard, "We just aren't getting anywhere with that family." By setting time limits in contract both partners know when they will be reviewing their work to determine whether they have met their goals. If more work is needed, they may renegotiate for another time limit or choose another more realistic goal. In whatever manner this is accomplished, the mutual setting of time limits is an important part of the contracting process.

Linda and Pat agree to weekly visits for a period of four weeks to carry out their goal. At the end of four weeks, Linda and Pat each summarized their contributions to the progress of Linda's goal to change her behavior.

Evaluation

An important activity in the contract is mutual evaluation of the contract and the care. Were the goals met? If not, do they need to be revised to be more workable? Is there a new problem or need that must be met? Does the contract need to be renegotiated? Are we finished with the problems, and should visits be terminated?

At the end of four weeks, Linda and her husband requested joint sessions with Pat. The three of them renegotiated the contract to focus on family relationships rather than just on Linda's anger. One of their new goals was that Linda and Jim wanted to learn to cope with anger from each other. Another goal was to spend more time with their children.

Renegotiation

The actual contract may be as informal or formal as the partners agree upon. Some find an informal contract that is verbally agreed on to be the most expedient, as the partners feel freer to renegotiate the activities of the contract at any point along the way. Others find a written contract very effective. The goals and responsibilities are down in black and white, and perhaps less easily forgotten, yet renegotiation is just as possible. The important consideration in the contracting process is not what form to use, but rather that mutual involvement in goal setting, implementation, and evaluation has taken place.

MODIFICATIONS IN USE OF CONTRACT

In certain situations a patient may not be able to immediately contract with the community nurse for health care, and the nurse may modify the contract in working with that patient. The nurse should use creativity in modifying the process so that a contract is made with a patient at this level of understanding. A modification of the process may be equally as effective as the outlined steps because the patient's individual situation was taken into account. The authors are concerned that strict application of the contracting tool is not appropriate for every situation.

The stage in the health-illness cycle of a person must be taken into account when deciding to use a contract. Acute situations, whether physical, psychological or emotional, requiring immediate professional attention are not appropriate for the time and discussion of the contracting process. For instance, a person recovering from a heart attack is a much better candidate for a contract than one who is experiencing a heart attack. However, as the person becomes less acutely ill, the nurse may begin to involve him in care by contracting with him for problems or needs which he identifies, and thus begin contracting at a level understood by the patient. The nurse will need to be aware of and be working on other problems associated with the acute nature of the patient's illness, which he may not readily identify. By contracting at the same time with the patient for a problem he wants solved, the nurse is able to involve him and help him to begin establishing trust.

The opposite is also true — a patient and nurse may have contracted for a particular problem and the patient becomes acutely ill. The nurse will attend to his acute needs, while attempting to maintain some connection with their contract.

The presence of physical impairments may hinder appropriate contract use. Included here would be gross hearing loss, brain damage or injury to the point that the patient does not understand the meaning of contract. The community nurse may find an alternative in contracting with a family member in addition to providing care for the patient.

One area in which contract modification takes place is in postpartum home visits. Young mothers are not always able to define what they wish to accomplish with a nurse, and may hesitate to allow visits. The nurse may begin by contracting for a certain number of visits to teach baby care. At a later time when the mother has established greater trust, she may wish to contract at a deeper level in other areas where she wants assistance.

BENEFICIAL EFFECTS OF CONTRACTING

Appropriate and informed use of the contract results in beneficial effects for both parties participating in the agreement. For patients and families contracting results in increased self-esteem, recognition of personal and family strengths, maintenance of independence and experience in solving problems successfully. The family experiences increased self-esteem as a result of being treated with dignity and respect. With a contract the nurse shows confidence that the patient and family are persons who have good reasons for what they do.

The contracting relationship is basically and fundamentally honest. Nothing is hidden. No solution or plan of treatment is imposed on the family. They have had a part in all the decisions made. If only the nurse identifies the problems, other areas of concern to families that may be far more important may be closed off.

Helping the patient to identify and recognize his strengths for carrying out his part of the contract helps him to solve his own problems. Patient and family gain strength and energy from having the nurse recognize what they can do for themselves. The nurse utilizes the knowledge that patients and families tend to behave responsibly if they are expected to behave responsibly. Families gain strength from honest identification of the ways in which they have the ability to help themselves.

Utilizing the contracting relationship is a means to help patients to achieve physical and emotional independence from the beginning of the helping relationship. Making the patient and family dependent on the nurse postpones their ability to gain personal security. It adds another problem to be solved because independence from the helping person must ultimately be achieved. What the nurse does for the family always must be tested with the question, Do I leave the family better able to fulfill their own needs?

With the nurse's assistance the patient and family carry out their responsibilities in the contract. Success in fulfilling their agreements in the contracts results in successful solution of their problems. From this experience the family gains skill and confidence for solving their future problems.

In contracting the nurse is kept from having unrealistic expectations of self or the family. The nurse participates in those aspects of the contract seen as useful by the family. Energy is not expended uselessly. Nurses experience less frustration from participating in more meaningful and realistic family goals. Greater satisfaction is experienced from seeing the family develop increasing ability to solve their own problems.

REFERENCES

1. Blair, Karyl. "It's the Patient's Problem and Decision." *Nursing Outlook*, 19:588–589, September 1971.

2. Rogers, Carl R. "A Counseling Approach to Human Problems," *American Journal of Nursing*, Vol. 56, No. 8 (August 1956), pp. 994–997.
3. Burd, Shirley, and Marshall, Margaret. *Some Clinical Approaches to Psychiatric Nursing*. New York: Macmillan, 1963, p. 359.
4. Sauer, John. "The Process of Contracting in the Helping Relationship," *Minnesota Welfare*, Summer 1973.

ADDITIONAL REFERENCES

Downey, Dorothy. "Contract for Health Care: Significance, Uses and Method of Achieving a Health Care Contract" (unpublished manuscript, University of Minnesota, School of Public Health, 1969).
Davis, Robert C., and Woodcock, Edwin. "The Nursing Contract: An Alternative in Care," *Journal of Psychiatric Nursing and Mental Health Services*, Vol. 9, May–June 1971, pp. 26–27.
Rogers, Carl R. *Freedom to Learn*. Columbus, Ohio: Charles E. Merrill Publishing Company, 1969.

26

Crisis Intervention — The Pebble in the Pool

Janice Marland Hitchcock

The community nurse frequently faces a patient or family in crisis. Does crisis intervention require special skills and knowledge? In this chapter the author shows how using the problem-solving process coupled with simple techniques and attitudes pertinent to crisis intervention can equip the nurse to offer effective crisis intervention.

Although nurses have always spent much of their time dealing with crises, an opportunity to view intervention in an organized way has emerged only in the past few decades.

Caplan defines crisis as "psychological disequilibrium in a person who confronts a hazardous circumstance that for him constitutes an important problem which he can for the time being neither escape nor solve with his customary problem-solving resources. During the upset, the individual works out a novel way of handling the problem through new sources of strength in himself and in his environment."[1] During the period of upset many different abortive attempts at solution are made.

An individual in crisis feels himself involved in a totally subjective experience. He is caught in a state of great emotional upset, and he is open to intervention. Like the pebble thrown into a pool, a minimal response by a helping person at this time can have a widening impact. Frequently, what a person in crisis needs most is someone who will truly listen.

The umbrella over all crisis intervention is the problem-solving process. This process is composed of logical steps, each dependent on the one preceding. We often use this process unconsciously, but we probably can be more effective if we understand the steps and consider them more directly.

The first step is *assessment* of the person (or family or community or agency) and the factors influencing his disequilibrium. The data emerge as the person tells about his difficulty. Questions should be asked to elicit past coping mechanisms and other available resources. How has he handled a similar situation before? Whom can he talk to at home? What community contacts has he, such as church, school, or work? How well is he managing his daily activities at present?

After these basic facts have been assessed, the next step is to *plan specific therapeutic intervention.* Does he need psychiatric referral? If the nurse has a good relationship with the patient and consultants available and if the patient seems to have community resources and seems able to ask for help, it is usually

[1]Caplan, Gerald. *Principles of Preventive Psychiatry.* New York, Basic Books, 1964, p. 53.

better for the patient if his nurse continues to work with him rather than suggesting that he go elsewhere.

Are medications advisable? This decision calls for introspection by the staff nurse to be sure that it is the patient's and not the nurse's or the doctor's crisis that is being alleviated by drugs. For instance, when a patient learns he has a fatal disease, do we consider medicating him because he can't tolerate his intense feelings about his illness or because we can't deal with the many facets of his grief?

Intervention may take the form of continued discussion to elicit feelings and to shift attitudes so that the patient can begin to see alternatives to his plight. Environmental manipulation may be required to find food, housing, or a job. The client may need a specific direction, such as, "When you feel like crying, do what you feel rather than force yourself to be active or stoic."

The final aspect of intervention is *evaluation and anticipatory planning.* Is there a difference? Is action being taken to help resolve the crisis? What has the patient planned for the future and what has he learned that can prevent other crises? Does he wish help in dealing with other issues this crisis has uncovered? If so, what plans can he make for continued counseling? When these points have been resolved, the crisis is over and equilibrium has been restored.

To illustrate the process, I will describe a client whom I saw in a crisis clinic for one session of approximately two hours.

Jim was a 20-year-old whose presenting crisis was a dilemma about his impending marriage to Joan, who was 17. He had called off their wedding the night before he saw me, but was now torn between guilt over that decision and panic at the thought of marriage when he knew he wasn't ready to take on that responsibility.

As we talked about his conflict, Jim began to see that part of his guilt stemmed from his conviction that Joan would return to her old friends whom he considered a bad influence on her. His need to rescue her seemed a greater motivation for the marriage than his love for her. Joan and her mother, Jim said, had put pressure on them to get married, although they had met only the previous summer and had seen little of each other during the winter when he was at school.

Jim believed he had open communication and a good relationship with both his parents. They were not happy about the engagement, thinking that both of them were too young and unprepared for such a major step. However, his parents had indicated that they would respect his decision and not interfere.

As he told his story and I assessed the situation, several points seemed relevant:

1. He was an intelligent young man who seemed willing to use his several sources of support (parents, aunt, and uncle).
2. The primary crisis seemed to be a maturational one which had been brought to a head by the imminent marriage. He was forced into making decisions

about what he wanted to do with his life and had to decide whether to take on the responsibilities of marriage now or postpone it, with the possibility that he might lose Joan.
3. He was describing events, but not expressing feelings about them.

With this assessment in mind, I planned the following intervention:

1. Attempt to elicit feelings caused by this conflict, that is, *anger* at being forced into a position (as he saw it) by Joan and her mother, but with no understanding by Joan about his feelings in the matter; *relief* at getting out of the situation; *guilt,* precipitated by his relief and anger and also related to letting down Joan and allowing her to return to her rough friends; *anxiety* at the prospect of going through with the plans; *helplessness* and *hopelessness* about taking definitive action.
2. Help him sort out his feelings once they were verbalized and help him consider the available alternatives and the possible consequences of each one.
3. Help him think through each alternative to a decision and then consider with him his plans for carrying out his decision.

I could not be sure that such a plan would fall into place and I was open to altering my goals, if necessary, as new data were presented. I did have a hunch that he would be able to work out the conflicts with guidance from me because he had been able to present his problem in a way that showed he had been grappling realistically with many of the issues. He had thought of some possible relevant action but his ambivalence at the moment did not allow him to take action. If some of this ambivalence could be resolved, then, I believed he would be able to make a constructive move.

In the conference, I mentioned that he had said a great deal about the events that had occurred and about his concern for Joan's feelings and reactions to his behavior, but really he said little about his own feelings. He admitted that he was not clear about what he felt, didn't know whether he loved her or not, was feeling guilty about the possibility that he might be leading her on, and was scared that the marriage wouldn't work.

Then Jim brought out more information that helped to substantiate my hunch that this situation was part of a larger maturational life crisis. He had not dated girls much except in the past three years. When he had met Joan the previous summer, it was on the rebound from breaking up with Judy, a girl he'd gone with for two years. After the break-up, he'd come to San Francisco for the summer, begun dating Judy's cousin, and met Joan, a friend of this cousin.

He said that he was still very unsure about what he wanted to do with his own life, let alone how he could manage a wife and possibly children. He was beginning to see more clearly that his own feelings for Joan were influenced by many things besides his possible love for her and that a marriage at this time would be on shaky ground. However, his own guilt about letting her down if he didn't marry her was interfering with his ability to evaluate her behavior.

Joan apparently was saying that the marriage must occur now or not at all and she was threatening to go back to an old boyfriend if Jim didn't do things her way. Her concerns seemed to be much more with the image of marriage than with its interpersonal aspects. I reminded Jim at several points that there seemed to be rather poor communication between them. Gradually, he began to recognize the truth of that and was able to give additional examples that illustrated their faulty communication.

During further discussion, I reflected back his own statements, supported his gradual awareness that Joan was not accepting her responsibilities to him, encouraged his exploration of alternatives with a reminder that any decision he made would cause some pain, and helped him consider the consequences of his actions. He now recognized that he had hoped for a painless alternative.

Jim decided he would leave San Francisco, go home where he would have family support and friends to talk to, and where he also knew of the mental health center. When he left, he looked more relaxed and said he felt relieved and able to follow through with his decision.

This example illustrates two additional points about crisis. First, the intervenor must assume there has been a loss of some kind. (Jim was concerned with the loss of his fiancée and the unresolved loss of his previous girlfriend.) Secondly, crisis intervention is directed toward removing or ameliorating a symptom so that the person can function and nature can continue the healing process.

Jim had not worked out all his feelings about becoming a man, but the resolution of the immediate problem freed him to move in that direction on his own, using the new ideas he had begun to think about during our session.

In my work with Jim, I used certain specific techniques that are pertinent to crisis intervention.

1. I believed Jim had the capacity to work out his problem and offered him support for his strengths rather than his weaknesses.
2. I helped him verbalize his feelings of hostility, guilt, and so on. Often a person needs help to put a label on his feelings in order to focus on what he's experiencing.
3. I sometimes intervened on a hunch rather than waiting to collect more information. One must move in rapidly, but with an openness to change as more data are provided. I had to set my priorities quickly in terms of what I saw the crisis to be and then move on my assumptions.
4. Although I was assessing the situation internally, my responses were on an affective level. I used short, clear sentences reflecting back Jim's own words, and did not give long, involved, intellectualized explanations. A person experiencing high anxiety cannot respond to complex verbal intervention.

5. I directly interpreted what I thought was going on. If an interpretation is offered with feeling and concern, it acts as a mirror for the patient of what he is experiencing and saying. No harm is done provided there is no insistence that he go along with the interpretation. If he is not ready to deal with the information, he will deny its relevance.
6. I allowed Jim to express his feelings and his view of the situation without questioning whether it was factually true or not. The important point was that the experience was valid for Jim and I was dealing with his *felt* need.

If one encourages appropriate expression of feeling, one must also provide appropriate controls for the patient's impulses and find new ways to channel them. The first step is to imply that feelings exist and help make their existence acceptable. One might say, "You sounded angry just now. From what you have just told me, I'd say you had good reason for having these feelings." Then, offer a reason for their denial: "It isn't nice to feel angry toward someone we feel needs our acceptance. Most of us would feel bad about the anger." Be critical of unrealistic, omnipotent ideas: "You must be God if you think you have that kind of influence over someone else." It is well to encourage the expression of guilt about feeling angry along with the feeling of anger itself or the patient may be left grappling with unvoiced guilt feelings in addition to his anger.

In the initial stages of crisis, one must often allow quite a bit of dependence. For a while the patient's autonomy is sacrificed. He is tired from trying to solve a problem and failing. He needs answers *now* and support to make his own decisions gradually. He may need your telephone number so he can call you between the times you see him, or some comparable interim support. A public health liaison nurse between hospital and home often fills his need. Frequently, a situational change is mandatory, such as helping him to find housing, food, or a job, before other issues can be dealt with. Often this change is enough to free a patient to manage his own affairs.

It is important to anticipate a patient's doubts, concerns, and worries in order to respond in advance whenever possible. Preoperative teaching is a good example of this advance intervention. One keeps in mind the patient's high anxiety level and low learning capability and anticipates his need for repetitive explanation at a later date. Arrange to see the patient according to his needs rather than your own.

In crisis intervention, it is imperative to share one's thoughts with the patient. It is important, but extremely difficult, to say to a patient, "I find myself getting bored as I listen to you right now. Perhaps we're getting away from what is really on your mind. Let's explore further what's happening." In general, nurses are oriented to keeping their thoughts to themselves, but in crisis intervention, one must be right in there with the patient.

Natural responses to crises have often been educated out of us: "Don't sit at the bedside." "Be objective!" "Why are you still visiting that patient? She'll become dependent on you." Empathic responses, so vital for effective crisis intervention, require us to be in charge of our own feelings, not to negate them.

Much of the effectiveness of crisis intervention lies in the humanity of the intervenor and his positive attitude toward the strengths of the person in crisis. Actual words are of relatively little significance. Crisis therapy is not depth therapy, but dealing supportively with here-and-now issues. This takes skill and a fund of knowledge, but not an extensive theoretical and experiential background in psychiatry or psychiatric nursing. Any nurse with warm feelings toward patients, ability to express her belief in another human, and sufficient interest to learn the simple steps can offer effective crisis intervention.

BIBLIOGRAPHY

1. Aguilera, D. C., and others. *Crisis Intervention: Theory and Methodology.* St. Louis, C. V. Mosby Co., 1970.
2. Lindemann, E. Symptomatology and management of acute grief. *Am. J. Psychiatry* 101:141–148, Sept. 1944.
3. Parad, H. J., ed. *Crisis Intervention.* New York, Family Service Association of America, 1965.

27

Problem-Oriented Medical Records — Not Just Another Way to Chart

Pamela L. Schell
Alla T. Campbell

Paperwork is often described as the least desirable aspect of the community nurse's responsibilities. To many it has seemed like a waste of both time and talent. A better system for nursing-care planning and recording has been needed. Problem-oriented medical records can be a solution. It offers a systematic method for identifying and analyzing data as well as planning for and evaluating nursing intervention. Ultimately it can help to develop the nurse's potential for critical judgment and decision making while contributing to improved patient care. This chapter presents a detailed description of the use of the problem-oriented medical record system.

The problem-oriented medical record (POMR) can revolutionize health care practice, the education of health practitioners, and the evaluation of health services. Properly used, this record system has tremendous implications for nursing as well as for medicine and other health care disciplines. Although one cannot be knowledgeable about all of the changes being proposed in the health care field, everyone working within it — particularly those who are shaping the future of health care in this country — should have some understanding of the concept of the problem-oriented medical record.

It was less than a year ago that we became aware of this system of medical record keeping developed by Dr. Lawrence Weed.[1] The system was being introduced into a nearby medical center, and Dr. Weed was invited to describe his system to the staff. We attended his lecture and decided to examine this new concept more closely.

Since 1968, frequent references to the Weed system have appeared in medical journals, but only recently have two articles about it appeared in the nursing literature.[2,3] However, both those articles stressed only certain aspects of the system — improved charting, better communication among members of the patient care team, and improved patient care. While these are important goals of the POMR system, there is much more to this revolutionary health care concept.

PHILOSOPHY OF EDUCATION

In order to fully comprehend the implications of this system — particularly for the education of health care personnel — it is necessary to understand Dr.

Weed's philosophy of education, which he described in the lecture that we attended:

... One of the premises [in education] has to do with memory ... that there is a core of knowledge that people should know, that you should give it to them, that you should test them on it, that this will be useful in the practice of medicine, [that] it's absolutely necessary, [that] you can then take their grades and equate them with how good they are [as practitioners] and with what they might do in the future. *My* premise is that there should not be a core of knowledge, that you should never have a memory-dependent system, and that you should teach a core of *behavior* so that the person becomes thorough, reliable, analytically sound, and efficient.

We have been conditioned to accept people who *know* a large number of facts as *educated* people, implying that memorizing facts is the process of education. The rapidly expanding scope and variety of facts that are part of medicine today, however, make a memory-dependent system of education incongruous. Since our educational system perpetuates the illusion that our answers must come from memory if we are to function effectively, the time has come for educators in the health care disciplines to face up to reality. Total performance includes not only cognitive ability, of which memory is a small part; it also includes affective or attitudinal ability and manipulative or psychomotor ability.[4] Since a student can learn rather easily to extract facts from the literature, the educator's task should be to teach students how to deal with the facts in a thorough, reliable, analytically sound, and efficient manner.[5]

The POMR is a means whereby this philosophy of education can lead to the achievement of specific, attainable goals. Through the development and proper management of the medical record, the performance of those providing patient care is exposed to critical assessment, just as scientific investigations are open to the evaluation of other scientists. An on-going detailed scrutiny of records can also serve to promote professional growth and development. But, before discussing the many other implications that the POMR has for nursing, let us examine the system itself.

POMR COMPONENTS

What are the components of the POMR system? Basically, there are four main elements: a data base, a problem list, an assessment and plan for each problem, and progress notes for selected problems. (These and the following explanations and samples are based on Weed's problem-oriented medical record system.)

Data Base

The same type of baseline information obtained in the admission work-up — initial history, physical exam, and laboratory tests — and recorded in traditional medical records is included in the data base for the POMR. With the POMR, however, the information is standardized, which means that those concerned with the delivery of health care to a given population have defined the content of the data base prior to instituting the use of the POMR system. The specific information to be included is that which these practitioners believe to be necessary if they are to provide efficient, economical, comprehensive health care to the given population.

To assure uniformity and standardization of the data base, this information must be obtained from every patient who receives service. Properly developed, the system refines clearly what data must be collected in a consistent manner for each patient. The following example of a data base was developed for a population of cardiovascular patients in a medical center and, with use, it has been revised. Refining and updating the content of the data base increase its appropriateness to the population and are continuous responsibilities of those providing health care.

Chief Complaint. A brief statement (if possible, in patient's own words) concerning his reasons for coming to clinic or hospital.

Patient Profile. A brief narrative about the patient and his way of life that includes name, age, sex, race, occupation, hometown or area, referring physician, domestic matters (age, number, and health of dependents; marital history; source and extent of income; living conditions), level of education and ability to read or write, religion, and how he spends an average day.

Psychological State. General statement regarding patient's present adjustment, including significant related factors.

Past History. Includes hospitalizations and dates, operations and dates, past illnesses and/or serious injuries and dates, medications for past conditions, smoking, drinking, and allergies.

Family History. Ages and causes of death of parents, grandparents, siblings, and children; history of congenital heart disease, diabetes, tuberculosis, rheumatic fever, high blood pressure, heart attacks, strokes, renal disease, cancer, mental illness; and age and health of living family members not previously mentioned.

Present Illness. Brief narrative regarding present health problems, each discussed individually. Includes onset of the problem, progression, signs and symptoms, treatment (any attempts by patient to solve problem), and patient's understanding of the problem and its treatment.

Current Medications. Those prescribed and taken as directed, prescribed and not taken as directed (explanation), self-administered, patient's knowledge of drug actions (if not recorded previously), administration and dosage, side effects, ability to obtain drugs, and any other significant factors affecting current medication regimen.

Diet History. Typical food consumption in a 24-hour period, whether a prescribed diet and its type, and patient's understanding of diet and any problems with it.

Present Activity Level and Limitations. Stable, improved, or decreased tolerance in relation to last clinic visit, brief statement regarding how patient sees his present activity level in relation to past pattern of activity (active vs. sedentary life), and future activity goals (leisure time, occupation, etc.).

Present Physical State. If patient has experienced any of the following or if any are noted by examiner, describe: angina (kind, pattern, changes), dyspnea, paroxysmal nocturnal dyspnea, orthopnea, cough; palpitations and/or tachycardia; dizziness and/or headache; visual disturbances; problems with hearing or speech; problems with orientation; syncope or blackout spells; numbness, tingling, claudication; nervousness, sweating, dry skin; pallor or cyanosis; fatigue or weakness; signs or symptoms of bleeding (nosebleed, hemoptysis, etc.); abdominal pain, nausea, vomiting; nocturia; edema; fever; pain other than previously mentioned; miscellaneous.

Physical Exam. Skin (hair, nails, skin turgor, color, temperature, etc.); neck (veins, carotids); lungs (rales, respirations, etc.); heart (rate, rhythm, gallops, murmurs); abdomen (liver); extremities (edema, peripheral pulses, color, temperature); neurological evaluation; BP/TPR, height, weight; obvious physical defects not previously noted.

Laboratory Data. Blood work, urine, x-ray, electrocardiogram, etc.

Problem List

Patient problems are identified from the data base. The more adequate and appropriate the data base, the more comprehensive the identification of problems. Problems are numbered, titled, and listed on a sheet at the front of the chart. This problem list is similar to a "table of contents" for the entire record. *All* the patient's known problems are listed — physiological, psychological, and socioeconomic.

A problem title is not entered as a specific diagnosis unless it can be unquestionably confirmed by the data. Therefore, each problem is titled according to the level of sophistication that is appropriate for it. Titles are changed as more information becomes available; for example, "jaundice," "blurred vision," and "poor memory" are acceptable problem titles. "Jaundice" may later become "serum hepatitis" or "carcinoma of the pancreas," when data confirm these diagnoses. Expressions such as "rule out," "probable," and "impression" are either diagnostic hunches or plans and should not be included in the problem list.

The problem list is updated by any member of the patient care team as more information is obtained, new problems are identified, or active problems become inactive. The team member (patient, physician, nurse, dietitian, and so forth) should communicate new information and make appropriate changes on the problem list or see that they are made. Maintaining a comprehensive, accurate problem list is a continuing responsibility of the patient care team, and the patient must be allowed to share in this responsibility. Many health practitioners review the problem list with the patient. It is the patient's record, and a complete problem list is an integral part of his care.

Problem Assessment and Plan Formulation

Each problem is individually described and evaluated, and an initial plan is formulated for each one. These and all subsequent data (orders, plans, progress notes, etc.) are recorded in the body of the record under the numbered and titled problem to which they are specifically related. The majority of these entries follow a specific format (SOAP is the acronym) as indicated below:

Subjective data (S) — the problem from the patient's point of view, how he feels, any changes he has noticed.
Objective data (O) — physical and laboratory findings, other pertinent observations or developments regarding the problem.
Assessment (A) — has the status of the problem changed? By what criteria?
Plan (P) — diagnostic plan, therapeutic plan, and plan for patient education.

Recording data in this manner encourages the development and use of sound logic in problem analysis and plan formulation.

Progress Notes and Related Data

Notations made by members of the health team other than the primary physician are not recorded as separate parts of the record; nurses notes, physical therapy notes, consultation or other notations are recorded as progress notes and entered in a continuing sequence. The series of progress notes regarding specific patient problems and the format (SOAP) requiring explicit recording of data are two means by which the POMR becomes a tool for improving communication among members of the patient care team.

For complex problems, flow sheets may be kept in addition to progress notes. The flow sheet is used to record specific parameters in a tabular or graphic manner. The example on page [241] was devised for a clinic patient with multiple problems, including aortic stenosis, hypertension, obesity, nervousness and anxiety, and impotence. Monitoring various parameters is necessary for the proper management of complex problems. The patient care team devises a flow sheet to facilitate comprehending and interpreting changing, interrelated variables. The sheet helps the team follow the progress of such problems and may be the only progress notes in the record for certain rapidly moving problems.

ADVANTAGES OF THE SYSTEM

Properly developed, the POMR provides a logical, explicit description of all the patient's problems, the current treatment for each problem, and the plans of the health care team in relation to each problem. Reviewing such a record is an efficient means of evaluating the team's performance and providing the team

Flow Sheet

Date	6-18-71	9-17-71	12/17/71
T-P-R	99^{2}-70-16	98^{4}-66-16	98^{-}64-18
B/P Standing	160/90	162/88	188/128
B/P Lying	168/90	170/90	190/120
Headache &/or Blurred Vision	"Sev. Times a Week"	"Several times a week"	"2-3 x/week"
Edema	None	None	None
Anxiety	Mod-Severe	Moderate	Moderate
Sexual Function	Impotence x 2-3 wks	Continued Impotence	"Normal-Satisfactory"
Daily Activity Pattern	Stable	Stable	Stable
Weight	201 ½	204	196 ½
Electrocardiogram	Unchanged-Stable	Stable	Stable
Lab Data	WNL Except ↓ K+ (3.2)	WNL	WNL
Diet Since Last Clinic Visit	Low NA 1800 Cal.	Low Na 1800 Cal — ↑ Banana c̄ OJ intake	Low NA 1800 CAL
Medications Since Last Clinic Visit	Digoxin 0.25mg QD Diuril 500 mg qam Aldomet 250mg Tid	Digoxin 0.25mg q.d. Diuril 500mg q.am. Hydralazine 10mg q.i.d. Librium 10mg. tid	Digoxin 0.25mg QD Diuril 500 mg QAM Librium 10 mg TID *Prescribed but not taken by PT: Aldomet 250 mg TID

with immediate, meaningful feedback on the quality of patient care. Such a record audit thus becomes both an educational experience for health care personnel and an essential instrument for quality control of health care services.

However, a record system that may expose practitioners to criticism presents some elements of threat. Bjorn and Cross, who have used the POMR in their private practice for some time, report:

Most of us are not conditioned to welcome criticism, and we tend therefore to equate being corrected with being accused of stupidity or inferiority. Medical audits of the type described here, based on structured records, must become an integral part of medical practice if standards of quality are to be assured.... Although we agree that it is more ego-threatening to be audited for performance than for knowledge, periodic audits of our practice have been exciting and intellectually rewarding exercises.[6]

With the POMR, every time someone is audited, someone is educated; and every time someone becomes educated, someone receives better care — what Dr. Weed calls "the multiplier effect." Education of health care personnel and quality control of health services are concomitant and result in improved patient care. Because of the system's potential for change and improvement in health care, POMR has implications for current issues that nursing faces.

IMPACT ON NURSING EDUCATION

The report of the National Commission for the Study of Nursing and Nursing Education (NCSNNE) pointed to the need for developing a health core curriculum, which the commissioners defined as "a central body of basic knowledge, understanding, and skill that should be commonly known to all recognized health practitioners."[7] This definition suggests what might be called "the old premise" in education. Using Dr. Weed's theory that a core of behavior rather than a core of knowledge should be taught, the definition might be: *a central body of behavior — all recognized health practitioners should be thorough, reliable, analytically sound, and efficient. The primary and common goal of all educational programs should be the development of our most basic resource — the individual's capacity to learn and think on his own.* Within this new frame of reference, the content and development of a health core curriculum would be viewed in a very different light.

Education is relevant when it teaches students a core of behavior which is applicable for a lifetime, rather than a set of facts that become outdated a few years after graduation. If we teach a core of behavior and use the POMR as a tool for monitoring that behavior, the student learns from real data. With this philosophy, there would then be no question about the relevancy of "training" in educational programs.[8] However, there is question about any educational program that spends (wastes?) a great deal of time emphasizing the learning of facts.

The kind of learning that the POMR approach provides is applicable not only to basic nursing education, but also to continuing education. In fact, it is the essence of continuous learning. Nurses have seldom consistently had the challenge that the POMR can provide in their work-a-day world. Through daily practice in its use, nurses could experience the intellectual stimulation derived from sharpening their ability to define and assess patient problems explicitly and to plan, implement, and evaluate their patient care — not in isolation — but in coordination with the efforts of the interdisciplinary team. In addition, use of this new educational philosophy and concept of record keeping would alter the goals, content, and development of continuing education programs in nursing.

OTHER NURSING IMPLICATIONS

Other areas of nursing concern would benefit from use of the POMR. Chief among these would be research. The need for increased research in both the practice of nursing and the education of nurses has been recognized as one of the basic priorities for optimum change. The NCSNNE report contained many recommendations as to the kinds of research to be undertaken. However, good records are a prerequisite to scientific research and to clinical investigation for improving nursing practice and measuring the benefits of this practice for the client. Because the POMR, unlike traditional medical records, presents a logical and more explicit set of data, its use would make possible more *accurate* clinical research. Nursing then would be able to answer with greater authority the question: how can nurses be utilized more effectively, efficiently, and economically?

Another important question in nursing today involves licensure and related issues such as accountability, peer review, professional certification, and continued competency. Nurses are beginning to face the problem that a one-time licensing examination does not assure competency to practice for a lifetime. The POMR provides a tool for on-going, meaningful audit, enabling nursing practice to be evaluated on the basis of readily available and definite criteria. Thus, the record would assist in the determination of professional accountability and continued competency in performance.

The evolution of professional roles in nursing, medicine, and other health professions has been recently receiving much attention. The expanding role of the nurse in areas long assumed to be the sole domain of the physician has prompted extensive discussion about the critical need for joint action among the professions in planning and articulating congruent roles. Expanded roles for nurses will require major adjustments in the orientation and practice of both nursing and medicine.[9] The problem-oriented system of record keeping and patient management could provide that common approach for nursing and medicine, as well as for other health professions. This mutual orientation would enhance collaborative efforts to define and develop congruent roles.

In addition, utilization of the POMR, with its improved documentation of clinical information and activities, would increase the accuracy of the cost-benefit analyses and similar economic studies recommended in relation to extended nursing practice.[10]

CONCLUSIONS

The systematic method of recording utilized in problem-oriented record keeping illustrates the manner in which the system preserves recorded data in a standardized, explicit form.   Familiarity with and use of this system are important to all members of the health care team and have implications for better, more comprehensive health care, as well as for improved methods of educating health care practitioners and evaluating the quality of patient care.

REFERENCES

1. Weed, L. L. *Medical Records, Medical Education, and Patient Care.* Cleveland, Press of Case Western Reserve University, 1970.
2. Bloom, Judith T., and others. Problem-oriented charting. *Am. J. Nurs.* 71:2144–2148, Nov. 1971.
3. Field, Frances W. Communication between community nurse and physician. *Nurs. Outlook* 19:722–725, Nov. 1971.
4. McDonald, F. J. *Educational Psychology.* 2d ed. Belmont, Calif., Wadsworth Publishing Co., 1965, p. 391.
5. Weed, L. L. Medical records that guide and teach. Parts 1 and 2. *N. Eng. J. Med.* 278:593–600; 652–657, Mar. 14, 21, 1968.
6. Bjorn, J. C., and Cross, H. D. *Problem-Oriented Private Practice of Medicine: System for Comprehensive Health Care.* Chicago, Modern Hospital Press, McGraw-Hill Publications Co., 1970, p. 67.
7. National Commission for the Study of Nursing and Nursing Education. Summary report and recommendations.
8. *Ibid.,* p. 282.
9. Extending the scope of nursing practice. *Nurs. Outlook* 20:48, Jan. 1972.
10. *Ibid.*

28

Adapting the POMR to Community Child Health Care

Marilyn L. Bonkowsky

The problem-oriented medical record (POMR) is not an end in itself but a tool that can increase the effectiveness of community nursing practice. Its adaptation for use in one community nursing setting is described in this chapter. In addition, the author discusses the advantages that it provided the agency.

The roles of nurses in health care are expanding in all directions. Nurse practitioners, clinical specialists, and community and clinic nurse specialists are being accepted and welcomed on health care teams because of their contribution. However, the effectiveness of a team approach to comprehensive patient care necessitates an accurate, efficient patient care record. And many nurses still tend to rely on verbal communications or lengthy narrative notes for transmitting patient information. The time has come to revise the organization of nursing records.

One group of nurses, determined to change their record system and improve communications among themselves, other nurses, and team members, were employed in a federally funded project. The overall goal of the project was to provide comprehensive health services to children up to the age of nineteen, living in a defined geographic area of the District of Columbia near the Children's Hospital. Primary care was delivered through three satellite clinics, each staffed by a team of health professionals — medical, dental, nursing, psychiatric, psychologic, and community health workers. The teams aimed at reaching children in the catchment area who were not receiving medical attention.

Each member had his own responsibilities, but worked with other team members in evaluating patient needs and planning and administering therapy. The facilities and resources of Children's Hospital were used by the team for referral and consultation when necessary, but responsibility for the overall care of children remained with the team.

The nursing staff at these satellite clinics included registered nurses, licensed practical nurses, and nursing assistants. During clinic sessions, they were responsible for assisting physicians, giving treatments, counseling parents, and assessing children's growth and development. Registered, and some practical, nurses also extended their services into the community — making home visits, helping with local school health problems and health education, and providing guidance for youth groups concerned with a variety of health and social issues, such as drugs, sex, and venereal disease. They made nursing assessments, diagnoses, and judgments and instituted nursing care plans based on these evaluations.

BETTER CHARTING NEEDED

Charting these nursing activities, however, was haphazard and random and under-taken largely to satisfy the requirements of the nursing department and those of the program. The nurses relied on verbal communication to transmit information to each other; their nursing notes, written in a lengthy, poorly organized style, were often ignored by other health workers. For example, one could not tell from patients' records whether nursing observations were different from those of other health workers, or whether patients were being given consistent advice. What was needed was a better method of charting.

Since some of the nurses were familiar with the problem-oriented medical record system,[1] they suggested that it be tried. The group agreed, but realized that they could not change the record system of the entire program. Therefore, they decided to adapt the problem-oriented approach to the record requirements of the program, and began to familiarize themselves with the use of the POMR system.

Weed has stressed that comprehensive medical action comprises four basic parts: (1) accumulation of a data base, (2) development of a problem list, (3) plans for management of problems, and (4) plans for follow-up. Logically, the first step should be to determine what kind of information is to be included in the data base. According to Weed, the items included in this base may vary from one type of practice to another; however, the content must be defined explicitly.[2] Unfortunately, there was little agreement among the nurses as to what informa-tion should be included. However, they soon realized — at the first audit of their records — the need for a more clearly defined data base and some inclusive yet concise way of recording the initial assessment of the patient.

From this experience, they decided on what information they would obtain on first meeting a patient. Then they organized it under six headings: physical status, growth and development, nutritional data, behavioral assessment, environ-mental assessment, and socioeconomic data. Further information was added to the data base on subsequent visits as it was required. A sample record of nursing assessment and follow-up notes written primarily by the nurse caring for the patient and family is shown on pages [247–248].

Next, a problem list [see page 249] was formulated for each patient, based on the nurse's assessment and other information available about the patient. This list included all recognized problems of the patient — medical, nursing, social, psychological, and so forth. An effort was made to include the entire clinic staff in formulating and reviewing the problem list and keeping it up to date — that is, revising the list as problems were resolved and new problems identified.

PROBLEM LIST AND NOTES

The problem list was attached to the inside cover of each patient's record, where it was easy to consult. Each problem was given a title and number and the list

Nursing Assignment and Progress Notes

1-27-71   Nursing Initial Assessment
Referral from C. Hospital for follow-up of pt. admitted at age 8 days. Diagnosis "MI and resulting CHF." Discharged yesterday.
Socio-economic — Mother is 18 yr. old. Father in school in Kentucky, will graduate in June and return to area as electrician. Baby and mother live with MGM and several other family members.
Environment — House clean and in good condition. Baby sleeps in own crib in same room with mother.
Nutrition — Baby takes 4oz SMA formula q3h. Nothing else at present.
Behavior — Sleeps most of day, awake most of night. Alert and active when awake.
Growth & Dev. — Appears normal on gross observation. DDST deferred.
Physical Status — See below.

Problem #1 ROUTINE HEALTH SUPERVISION
Physical Status
Subjective: Mother reports rash over J's face, appearing after bringing him home. She has been using Vaseline on his skin and hair.
Objective: Fine raised red rash over entire face and neck.
Assessment: Probably dermatitis due to Vaseline.
Plan: *Rx* — Discontinue Vaseline to skin and hair. Wash with mild soap and water, dry well, put nothing on skin.
Pt. Ed. — Explained to mother natural qualities of baby's skin, how Vaseline clogs the pores and how skin is easily irritated by lotions, etc.
Follow-up — Mother to contact me if no improvement in 2-3 days.

Problem #2 CONGESTIVE HEART FAILURE
Subj: Mother states she is much less anxious about J than when she first brought him home.
Obj: J resting quietly, appears in no distress. PR=140, reg, good quality. RR=38, reg.
Plan: *Pt. Ed.* — Reviewed cause and effect of illness, medications and importance of mother's observations of color, respiratory distress, coughing. Encouraged her to call Dr. or nurse immediately if any question or problem. Discussed diet and importance of not adding anything until ordered by Dr. Mother seemed to understand and has a healthy concern for J.
Follow-up — Will visit weekly for support and supervision.

2-19-71   New Problem Problem #3 HYPOPLASTIC LEFT HEART SYNDROME
Obj: Cardiac cath done 2-17 at hospital showed severe cardiac anomalies: mitral and aortic stenosis, patent ductus, small left ventricle.
Assess: Doctors are considering surgery; they feel prognosis very poor with or without surgery. Problem #2 is doubtless due to these anomalies.
Plan: *Pt. Ed.* — Discussed findings with mother after they were explained by Dr. She understands physical abnormalities and how these affect baby. Seems to be coping well.
Follow-up — Will visit in 4 days, available anytime to talk.

Nursing Assignment and Progress Notes (continued from p. 247)

2-22-71   Phone call to J's mother by Nutritionist
          Problem #1 ROUTINE HEALTH SUPERVISION – Nutrition
          Diet: SMA formula 1-1½ cans concentrate per 24 hrs. Taking 4-5 oz.
                 every 3-4 hrs. Rice cereal given 3 times a day.
          Diet appears to be adequate and appropriate.
          Advised: Continue formula. May use barley or oatmeal cereal. No wheat
                    or HiProtean cereal. Start apple juice. No orange juice yet.

3-10-71   Problem #1 ROUTINE HEALTH SUPERVISION
          Behavior
             Subj: J sleeps most of day and has fewer periods of activity. Watches
                    mother, laughs spontaneously, reaches for objects.
             Obj: Sleeping at time of visit.
             Assess: Development normal for age. Need lot of rest. Mother
                    reassured by my visits.
                    Follow-up – Will visit weekly. Clinic apt. 4-1,

          New Problem Problem #5 DIAPER RASH
             Subj: Mother reports diaper rash. Has been using Vaseline on area.
             Obj: Diaper area red and excoriated.
             Plan: *Rx* – Leave open to air as much as possible. Keep diaper area
                    clean and dry. Use light for 20 min. qid.
                    Pt. Ed. – Instructed in use of 40w light bulb, distance, etc.
                    Follow-up – Mother to take J to clinic if no improvement in 2 days.
                    I will visit next week.

3-17-71   Problem #5 DIAPER RASH – Resolved

---

thus served as an index to the areas of concern for that patient. Since the primary
goal for all children served by the project staff was preventive health services,
problem number one was always "Well Child Supervision" or "Routine Health
Supervision." This rubric included continual follow-up in the six areas that comprised the data base.

Nursing follow-up notes, headed by the problem title and number, were
written following the format suggested by Weed – subjective data, objective data,
assessment-discussion, and plan (SOAP). These notes were written in sequence
by date of entry and identified by problem title and number. All nurses having
contact with a patient were encouraged to contribute to the record, using the
appropriate problem title or listing a new problem if indicated.

When a minor problem developed in one of the areas included in "Routine
Health Supervision" which was easily handled through counseling and resolved
quickly, it did not become a separately listed problem (for example, see Progress
Notes, 1-27-71, rash on face, in illustration). If however, the situation appeared
severe or was not resolved easily, it then was noted on the problem list and was
followed separately from routine health supervision [see Problem List, Problem
#5, diaper rash, on page 249]. Whether or not to list a problem separately

Problem List

1	1-27-71	Routine Health Supervision	
2	1-27-71	Congestive Heart Failure	
3	2-19-71	Hypoplastic Left Heart Syndrome	
4	3-4-71	Anemia	
5	3-10-71	Diaper Rash	3-17-71
6	3-17-71	Conjunctivitis	

required discretion by the nurse — a judgment that was part of the evaluation of her performance during the record audit by team members.

Both illustrations — the Progress Notes and Problem List — were taken from one patient's record to demonstrate how the problem list was formulated and revised for this patient. The patient was referred to the nursing staff initially with a diagnosis of an "MI with resulting CHF." Upon cardiac catheterization, he was found to have a hypoplastic left heart. This was listed as a new problem, and Problem #2 was revised accordingly. If and when a problem is resolved, the date of resolution is listed, as in the 3-17-71 notation on diaper rash in the Progress Notes.

CHART AUDIT

The final step in the recording process is chart audit. Three months after the nursing staff began using the problem-oriented approach to record-keeping, a peer review of records was organized. Each nurse evaluated ten records of another nurse for basic content and asked herself: Are the health-related problems clearly identified and are they all listed? Is there a plan of care directly related to each of these problems? Can the current status of the patient be easily understood?

Everyone involved in the audit found it a profitable experience — both the nurse doing the audit, as well as the one being audited. Each nurse realized how much important information she had assumed the reader would know, but had not been stated. To increase the value of the audit experience, the nurses invited a physician familiar with the philosophy and use of the problem-oriented record system to join them at a post-audit session. He discussed the use of the system in general, pointed out the importance of nursing initiative in record-keeping, audited a few charts, and discussed the use of flow sheets. The physician's views proved not only helpful, but were reassuring; the group felt that their efforts were resulting in better communication and patient care. In fact, the sessions occasioned a lively exchange of questions and ideas about the patients and their problems and ways to improve their care.

Other members of the health care team were quick to recognize the usefulness of the problem-oriented medical record and followed the nurse's lead. An example is the nutritionist's note in the Progress Notes dated 2-22-71, in which she titled her note appropriately and organized her comments in a format equivalent to "objective, assessment and plan." Other staff members — social workers and physicians — sometimes copied the format in their notes as well.

OTHER ADVANTAGES

When problem-oriented charting was first used, the nurses found it required more time, thought, and effort on their part. Previously many of them had not followed a defined protocol in patient evaluation and had not organized their thinking or their nursing notes in a systematic way. However, within weeks of using the new system, they became adept at sorting out complicated problems of some patients and at devising and completing care and follow-up plans for each of them. As a result, they felt they had improved their overall comprehension of the patients, and their work became more stimulating and rewarding to them.

With the POMR system, specific patient problems were evident to the nurses. This directed their attention and study and in turn led to further inquiry and consultation with experts in appropriate fields. The nurses' own professional knowledge was enhanced and their learning was firmly grounded in the reality of the patients' conditions. Some nurses were stimulated to devise explicit nursing care plans and instructions for patient and parent education for such areas as hemoglobinopathies — particularly SC disease (an inherited disorder similar to sickle cell anemia), lead intoxication, and care of pregnant adolescents.

Auditing records also contributed to further improvements in charting which helped assure more thorough and thoughtful patient management. This peer-review "feedback loop" was felt to be essential to the success of the project.

Finally, problem-oriented records eased the ever-present staffing problem. It became less difficult to fill in for another nurse temporarily or to assume an entire caseload because the current active problems of the patients and plans for each problem were easily discerned from the record. A look at the problem list made it easy to grasp the salient features about an unfamiliar patient. Similarly, the progress notes enabled the nurse to learn quickly the specific plans for each active problem and the instructions the family had been given.

Other nursing efforts to institute problem-oriented charting as reported in the literature have also been of value. Field described how problem-oriented communication was proving useful to community nurses in rural areas and to the physicians who referred patients to them.[3] In the hospital setting, however, the traditional unnecessary division between physician and nurse progress notes vitiates some of the value of this method of recordkeeping. Bloom reports a movement in hospitals toward the goal of using a single problem-oriented record for patients, with contributions by all members of the health care team.[4] But anachronistic hospital rules present obstacles for attaining this goal. When nurses' notes are incorporated directly into a single set of progress notes, they are of real value in patient care. Also, nurses will spend less time writing for the pointless purpose of having a note on each patient's chart for their shift.

A LOOK TO THE FUTURE

Thus, the problem-oriented record, kept with pen and paper, appears to represent an advance in the system of patient care. Probably of greater significance in the long run will be the use of computers to assist in record-keeping; the problem-oriented format will serve as a basis for the system. Weed and his co-workers report that this goal has been achieved in a hospital ward.[5] Of course, computer storage and retrieval of medical information seem remote to most of us, but the incredible accomplishments of technology have surprised us too often for us not to realize that computerized records may be closer than we think. At any rate, improved records are sorely needed, and the promise of eventual computer-assisted storage and retrieval makes the problem-oriented record doubly important.

Is it not time for nursing schools and continuing nursing education courses to teach problem-oriented charting? Should not audit of nurse records be part of the training and evaluation of the student nurse and of the practicing nurse? I would answer "yes" to both questions. From the experience described above, I believe that nurses can learn, use, and teach the problem-oriented approach to recordkeeping quite easily and to real advantage for themselves and their patients.

REFERENCES

1. Weed, L. L. *Medical Records, Medical Education, and Patient Care.* Cleveland, Press of Case Western Reserve University, 1970, p. 6.
2. *Ibid.,* pp. 16–19.
3. Field, F. W. Communication between community nurse and physician. *Nurs. Outlook* 19:722–825, Nov. 1971.
4. Bloom, Judith, and others. Problem-oriented charting. *Am. J. Nurs.* 71:2144–2148, Nov. 1971.
5. Schultz, J. R., and others. An initial operational problem-oriented medical record system — for storage, manipulation and retrieval of medical data. *U.S. Armed Forces Inst. Pathol. Conf. Proc.* 38:239–264, 1971.

29

A Search for Assessment Criteria

Marlene G. Mayers

An important but sometimes neglected step in the nursing process is evaluation, measuring the effectiveness of care given to each patient and family. What criteria does the community nurse use in assessing this effectiveness? Based on a study that she conducted, Marlene Mayers offers some insights into criteria that can be used by community nurses in assessing their own nursing care.

How can community health nurses assess the effect of their care upon patients when so few systematic methods of evaluating this care are available?[1-3] Even the few that do exist are not consistently used, because they are considered too time-consuming or fail to provide the kinds of information agencies consider important. The need is for criteria — clear, understandable, and in acceptable terms — that will reflect the effects of nursing care on patients. For these reasons, I decided to study the nursing assessment process as the first step in eventually identifying concrete, meaningful indicators of achievement that can be measured in terms of patients' progress and growth.

My decision grew out of my own experience and what I learned from conversations with other nurses in public health nursing. The nurses felt frustrated and they resisted specifying outcomes of their services. They rationalized their resistance by explaining that the desired outcomes for each family or patient were so individual and special, and so dependent upon a wide variety of factors relating to each family, that it was difficult, even unwise, to attempt to make generalizations. This attitude, so common among community health nurse practitioners, apparently leads them to assume that if certain accepted nursing strategies such as teaching, counseling, referring, and home visiting are effectively implemented, then positive outcomes for patients will follow.

Such reasoning left me unsatisfied. I believed it was possible to develop an evaluation tool or guide composed of generally accepted concrete criteria against which patient progress or the relative success or failure of nursing intervention could be measured. But where to begin?

After considering various alternatives, I decided to observe the visits of community health nurses and discover, through interviews with them, what criteria they used in actual family situations. I assumed that as practicing nurses they would be expert on the criteria they actually did use in practice. Furthermore, the factors they identified as important in assessment and evaluation would provide clues to what these nurses believed was relevant and pertinent. By use of this method, I thought, my eventual tool would not be too idealized or remote from actual practice to be useful to nurses.

In apparent support of this method, Vickers has stated: "There are, I suggest, three contributions that public health can thus make to the setting of its own goals. It can evaluate health by the criteria that we currently use. It can criticize these criteria and thus help to deepen and refine them. And it can explore the processes of decision by which public health policy is defined and implemented."[4]

Using Vickers' guidelines, I set up the first phase of a 3-phase study to discover the criteria that public health nurses use when they assess a patient's status at a given point in time. (Subsequent phases of the study will be devoted to obtaining relevant criteria from patients and a panel of experts. This information will make it possible to evaluate and perhaps supplement the criteria elicited from the nurses. The resulting criteria will then be refined and standardized through extensive field testing.)

METHOD AND SAMPLE

The participant observation method of field research was used to gather the data.[5] I chose at random 16 community health nurses to observe and interview about visits they made to a total of 37 families. This direct contact with the nurses and their patients during the home visits enabled me to gather real life data about the process of nursing decision making and the criteria upon which it was based. However, I was aware that my presence as an observer-participant might modify and influence this nursing process.

I accompanied the selected nurses in their normally planned home visits, and they knew that I would discuss each situation with them afterwards. However, they were assured that my purpose was not to evaluate their performance but rather to discover the dynamics of nursing practice as they themselves perceived it — to discover what *was*, not to judge.

The sample of nurses and patients was considered complete when (1) by the standards of participation-observation methodology, no new additional data were discovered — that is, when similar instances kept recurring; (2) the patients within the sample represented a wide range of cultures, ethnic groups, and problems; and (3) the nurses who were observed and interviewed reflected a wide range of age, educational, and experiential backgrounds.

PATIENT ASSESSMENT CRITERIA

After each visit, the nurse was asked whether she believed the patient was doing well or poorly, and what there was in the patient or his situation that led her to her conclusion. After brief reflection, the nurse would then list those behavioral or situational clues that were the specific criteria upon which she based her decision. Some examples of nurses' responses to these queries are:

He's in trouble because of his physical signs and symptoms — diaphoresis, shortness of breath, pain on breathing, and pallor. I also think he is so tired and full of wine that he is unable to make decisions for himself.

The positive things I noticed about her are that she is coherent — able to make decisions. She seemed to be stubborn or opinionated. It's a good thing; she has individuality. I also felt that she wasn't telling me everything. I mean she had the mental ability to think — even to decide what to tell and what not to tell.

These statements of specific patient-centered criteria were recorded, thoroughly analyzed for similarity of content and meaning, and then placed in general categories — that is, they were clustered in groups of similar content. These major groupings became the basic core of nurse-elicited criteria for use in the tentative assessment-evaluation tool.

The criteria that the nurses used in assessing a patient's status, in the order they were most frequently mentioned, were as follows:

1. *Ability to act independently* — a patient's statements regarding successful or unsuccessful management of past or present problems, specific behavior indicating a satisfactory level or ability in the management of present health problems, and evidence of keeping or not keeping medical appointments and of following the doctor's orders.

2. *Physical condition* — a patient's general appearance, presence or absence of pathophysiological signs and symptoms, and level of growth and development.

3. *Congruent feelings or affect* — the patient's general mood; whether or not he expresses congruent affect, behavior, and conversation; his physical posturing; and other clues to serious problems.

4. *Interpersonal ability* — evidence of interdependence within the family, the patient's management of the interpersonal situation with the nurse, his socialization pattern, evidences of trust (with the nurse and others), and the nurse's sense of comfort or discomfort in the interpersonal situation with him.

5. *Verbal ability* — the patient's ability to talk about himself and his concerns, and his ability to become specific and to be reflective about his successes and failures.

6. *Ability to meet role expectations* — the patient's observed ability to meet his role expectations (job, parenting, wage-earning), and his stated and implied feelings regarding his own accomplishments.

7. *Congruent life style* — observable signs that the patient's life style was consistent with his culture, and evidence of critical factors that might upset this life style, such as impending eviction from his home.

8. *Appropriateness of future plans* — the patient's intentions in terms of future health and other plans.

9. *Intellectual ability* — the patient's vocabulary, apparent general intelligence, coherence, and ability to solve problems and make decisions.

These criteria that the nurses used in making judgments about their patients tended to reflect a holistic view of patient assessment — that is, they were not based on a narrow diagnostic approach. With minor modifications, these criteria appear to be generally applicable to any client setting, or to any diagnostic category or program area. Also, they may well be what practicing nurses believe to be the most significant and critical characteristics or phenomena relevant to a patient or his situation and important to note and appraise when evaluating their patient's status.

SOME SURPRISE FINDINGS

Although the study was principally designed to identify the criteria by which nurses assess patients, perhaps the most significant development was the discovery of four other factors closely correlated with nurse-perceived coping abilities of patients: ease or difficulty of entrée, open or closed environment, ability or inability to focus, and a positive or negative mood-response pattern. Interestingly, these factors were not explicitly mentioned by the nurses but became evident as I reviewed the data and contrasted the situational phenomena in families whom the nurses perceived as "coping" with those they called "non-coping." A brief description of each of these factors follows.

1. *The ease or difficulty with which a patient allows entrée to his home.* Easy entrée is described as a relatively quick response by the occupant to the knock or the ring of the doorbell, a cordial smile, an invitation into the home without significant hesitation, and a courteous and pleasant invitation to be seated or to be comfortable. Difficult entrée is described as a delayed response to the knock or ring without explanation, hesitancy to admit visitors or to invite them to be seated, and the presence of physical or mechanical barriers, such as many complicated doors and locks. Two of the field notes reflect easy and difficult entrée in the following words:

Mrs. G answered the door promptly. She seemed very glad to see the nurse. She seated us in her small living-dining room. She served tea. . . .

The patient was very slow in answering the door. She hesitated with the door partially closed for a few seconds and then wordlessly opened it. She sat rigidly on the edge of a straight-backed chair. She did not invite us to sit, but we did when she did.

2. *Evidence of an open or closed environment.* A patient's environment is described as open if there are signs of books, papers, room decoration and color, records, television, functional furniture, cushions, food or food preparation materials, new possessions, or evidence of care, such as covered or repaired furniture, and so forth. A closed environment is cluttered, dusty, dirty, without decorations, stark, cold, has broken furniture, is chaotic or dark. The terms

open and closed were used because they aptly reflect the visual impact of the contrasting environments. Examples of both environmental systems are described in these field notes:

There's no sign of life in the place. It's stark and dark. There are no books, magazines, or newspapers, and the kitchen shows no evidence of being used. The whole apartment looks like before someone moves in — stark and dead.

The E's live in a three-room apartment that is nicely furnished and pleasant. The baby has a lovely new crib, many toys, a walker, etc. The living room is strewn with books and papers that Mrs. E is studying....

3. *The ability of a patient to focus his attention and conversation.* This characteristic relates to a patient's ability to follow a line of thought, to stay on the subject, and to respond in a congruent or relevant manner. Persons who are unable to focus attention change the subject frequently and are easily distracted. They tend to circle back to the same few topics over and over again. The ability to focus is reflected in the interaction of Jane (a young unmarried pregnant woman) with the nurse:

They continued to look at the birth atlas, the nurse explaining each picture and relating it to Jane. Jane followed with interest, asked some questions, and expressed surprise and amazement over some of the information....

Mrs. C, an elderly lady living alone, presents an example of inability to focus:

The patient did most of the talking. She rambled on at length about incidents in her past. The nurse had great difficulty getting a word in.... [The nurse] would ask a question and the patient would then take off nonstop for the next 15 minutes. The nurse would say, "Mrs. C, what you are saying reminds me of..." or, "What about that...." This would work fairly well — briefly. The nurse listened attentively but would frequently say, "Yes, I remember you told me that when I was here last."

4. *The patient's mood-response pattern.* Mood response refers to the nonverbal aspects of a patient's behavior. People with a positive mood response tend to have body mobility, a relaxed posture, changing facial expressions and tones of voice, and they show animation and sense of involvement. Persons exhibiting the negative aspects of mood response tend to have rigid postures, flat affect, a sense of distance or noninvolvement, and are generally immobile. Examples of some of the characteristics of mood response are:

She talked rapidly and constantly in a high, breathless voice. She sat tense, erect on the edge of the sofa during the whole hour-and-a-half visit. She was smiling almost constantly (whatever the topic), smiling with an unconvincing "everything is rosy" sort of smile.

She talked without hesitation — laughed, became serious, looked carefully at the calendar that she was to use to document the dates when her child had seizures, and seemed relaxed and involved.

ANALYSES OF FAMILY RECORDINGS

When recordings of each family visit were analyzed for these four factors, it was found that 28 of the 37 sample families had a consistent positive or negative pattern in these four factors that agreed with the nurses' judgments of their coping ability. For example, the ten families whom the nurses viewed as "noncopers" were all found to exhibit negative characteristics in these four phenomena. The 18 families who were identified as able to cope consistently exhibited positive characteristics in relation to these four factors.

The data regarding each of the nine discrepant families (those who did not exhibit a consistent pattern of these coping or noncoping factors) reveal that, almost without exception, the discrepant characteristics — whether positive or negative — could be explained in terms of factors or constraints that appear to be outside the patient's direct personal control. For example, Mrs. C, who couldn't "focus," was judged to be coping, since she had a positive score on the other three factors. This inability was considered the result of senility, and her conversation reflected this fact.

Depending upon the predicted magnitude and duration of these "outside" factors, a nurse can accurately judge the patient's actual coping ability within the context of the reality of his life. One might conclude, then, that when a patient exhibits a mixture of positive and negative characteristics relative to life style, entrée, focus, or mood response, the nurse should carefully analyze the patient's situation in order to make a sound decision regarding his actual coping abilities.

On the other hand, it might be said that in the absence of other critical and temporary situational factors, a patient who consistently exhibits positive aspects of the four factors might be considered able to cope with his usual, predictable problems. And a patient who exhibits a consistent pattern of the negative characteristics of these factors could be considered unable to cope with his problems. A detailed and complete analysis of such a patient or family would then be indicated in order to decide the most predictably effective nursing interventions. Similarly, when a family exhibits a mixture of positive and negative traits relative to the four coping factors, the nurse should analyze the family carefully before judging its actual coping abilities.

CONCLUSIONS

These coping factors are useful only as a gross screening device and are not a substitute for making a final decision about a family. They can, however, assist the nurse in setting priorities for her caseload, and may enable her to determine which families need intensive or immediate attention.

In addition, assessment of this cluster of factors may prove to be a reliable method of validating nursing assessments based on a longer, more detailed, or more subjective list of criteria. If so, it would be a quicker method, producing more accurate results, and one that would prevent variations of interpretation in appraisals made by nurses who represent a wide spectrum of values and backgrounds. However, these criteria must be field tested and standardized before we know their real value in patient care assessment.

REFERENCES

1. Freeman, Ruth B. *Community Health Nursing Practice.* Philadelphia, W. B. Saunders Co., 1970, p. 60.
2. U.S. Public Health Service, Nursing Division. *How to Study Patient Progress,* by D. E. Roberts and H. H. Hudson. (Publication No. 1161) Washington, D.C., U.S. Government Printing Office, 1964.
3. Simon, J. R. Systematic ratings of patient welfare. *Nursing Outlook* 9:432–436, July 1961.
4. Vickers, Geoffrey. What sets the goals in public health? *N. Engl. J. Med.* 258:589–596, Mar. 20, 1958.
5. McCall, G. J., and Simmons, J. L. *Issues in Participant Observation; a Text and Reader.* Reading, Mass., Addison-Wesley Publishing Co., 1969.

30

Quality of Care:
The Nursing Audit, Part A

Maria C. Phaneuf

What is a nursing audit and how is it conducted? What are its benefits and values to public health nursing agencies or other community nursing settings? These questions are answered in this chapter through a description of how one public health nursing agency used the nursing audit.

INTRODUCTION

Consideration of the quality of nursing care and problems of measurement are necessarily preceded by examination of one's beliefs about nursing care. Here are some of the major questions which I asked myself when I began to think about the nursing audit:

Are all people entitled to personalized, continuous, comprehensive family-centered health care? Can nursing, as a major component of health care, make the difference between life and death? Between rapid recovery and delayed convalescence? Between vigorous and marginal health? Between helplessness and rehabilitation? Between death in peace and dignity or death in fear and isolation? Are institutions and agencies which provide health care accountable to patients and families to other health professionals, and to the community for the nursing care they provide? Can the quality of nursing care given to people be measured? Are nurses responsible for measuring the quality of their care against standards and for the continuous voluntary raising of the standards?

My answers were affirmative and these beliefs therefore lie at the heart of the nursing audit. The beliefs, of course, are open to challenge. Health care is often provided with discrimination based on ethnicity, color, age, nature of illness, or life style of the recipients of care. Nurses are not fully agreed on the importance and influence of nursing as a major component in health care systems. The principle of accountability is not easily accepted, as illustrated by resistance to accreditation and certification of institutions and agencies. Some nurses say that quality of nursing care is an intangible, and therefore not subject to measurement. Fortunately, however, the thousands of nurses who have become interested in the audit are clearly agreed that, whatever the difficulties entailed, nurses themselves should take on the admittedly difficult responsibility of appraising the quality of nursing care.

One of the public health nursing agencies that took on this responsibility has given permission for a case presentation of its audit test run. This agency is listed among the 15 largest voluntary agencies in the United States and has a long and

From "Quality of Care: Problems of Measurement, Part I — How One Public Health Nursing Agency Is Using the Nursing Audit," *American Journal of Public Health*, Vol. 59, No. 10, pp. 1827–1832, 1969. Reprinted by permission of the publisher and the author.

distinguished record of community service. It is accredited by the National League for Nursing and is certified as a Home Health Agency under Medicare. The board of directors and the entire staff are committed to continued strengthening of the contribution of the agency to the community service and to public health nursing.

PHASE ONE – WORKSHOP

A consultant was invited to present the audit method at a two-day workshop in April, 1968. Participants included the executive director, the supervisors, members of the administrative staff, agency consultants, and selected staff members. During this workshop, the audit method was described and there was a practice session during which agency cases were examined in simulated audit-committee process. Three main points about the audit were emphasized.

What Is the Audit?

The nursing audit is a method for systematic written appraisal of the process of nursing care, which is made after the discharge of the patient through examination of the patient-care records. The appraisal is retrospective because this permits a view of the completed cycle of care.

Patient-care records are used because complex modern care cannot be given to complex human beings without use of the record *as a service instrument – as a means to service.* Without such use of the record, care cannot be personalized, cannot be safe, and will not be characterized by continuity which is an essential component of quality. In addition, the record is legal documentation of care, and records are available and easily accessible for audit. The method was designed for use in hospitals, public health nursing agencies, and nursing homes because the responsibilities of professional nurses for the care of people are not altered by the settings in which care is given.

What are the standards against which quality of care is judged?

The one dependent and six independent functions of nursing are used as the standards. Evaluations are based on broad measurement of the extent to which the functions are executed.

The functions of nursing are:

1. application and execution of physician's legal orders
2. observation of symptoms and reactions
3. supervision of the patient
4. supervision of those participating in care
5. reporting and recording
6. application of nursing procedures and techniques
7. promotion of health by direction and teaching.

Critical components for each of these functions have been identified and numerical values for them have been established on the basis of reasonableness.

There are a total of 50 components. The numerical value assigned to each nursing function is the sum of the numerical values of its components.

The audit for each record yields an over-all numerical rating computed from the points scored for each function. The score for each function indicates the degree to which that function is executed, i.e., it provides specific basis for action toward improvement or for satisfaction. The numerical values are stated in ranges and then translated into word judgments: excellent, good, incomplete (care is good as far as it goes but it does not go far enough), poor, or unsafe.

The audit report includes a summary of the over-all ratings for each case audited, and a summary of each of the seven categorical (function) ratings. In other words, the over-all rating yields a broad judgment of quality and the ratings of the functions pinpoint specific areas of strength and weakness.

Who Does the Nursing Audits?

Audits are done by audit committees which include an administrative representative, supervisors, head nurses, and staff whose clinical competence is recognized by the institution or agency in which the committee operates. Additionally, the committee should include nurses unaffiliated with the institution or agency. A hospital committee would include a public health nurse and one from a nursing home. The public health nursing agency committee would include a hospital nurse and one from a nursing home. A nursing home committee would draw on a hospital and a public health nursing agency for representatives. In this way, the pool of talent on the committee is augmented; nursing is unified in its striving for quality, which leads to closer collaboration in the interests of patients and community service; and nursing in the community is strengthened by the unity.

The hospital audit committee needs the cooperation of the medical records librarian who needs to know what requests will be made for charts and why; who is authorized to examine the charts; and who is responsible for returning them to the medical records library.

In *all* handling of the patient-care records for audit, it must be emphasized that audit forms and reports are *never* filed with patient-care records and these records should not show that they were audited. All audits and audit reports are filed with the nursing administration.

PHASE TWO — THE COMMITTEE IN ACTION

An Audit Committee of 11 agency nurses was appointed by the executive director after consultation with her staff. Because this committee represents the professional conscience of the agency, members were chosen for their clinical acumen and commitment to the care of people. The appointments therefore carried special prestige as well as responsibility.

The committee oriented itself to the purposes of the audit and acquired practice with the method. They developed a common philosophy about care and about auditing; they tested their clinical judgments with each other; and they learned to focus on the patient and his recorded care instead of centering on individual nurses who gave care, or making assumptions beyond what was recorded.

After this orientation, the committee members separately reviewed the cases assigned to them, made their judgments on each audit item for each assigned case, and made their quality judgments on the case as a whole. The committee then met to review the work done, to make decisions regarding moot cases, and to prepare an audit report for the executive director. A total of 60 cases was audited — 30 cases in which a cerebral vascular incident was the primary condition, and another 30 cases in which heart disease was primary.

Aside from workshop time, the committee work — from orientation through auditing of the 60 cases — required seven conferences lasting two and a half or three hours each. Time required for the average case review by individual members initially amounted to one hour or more; this was reduced from 15 to 20 minutes by the end of Phase Two.

Audit Results — Sixty Cases

The over-all findings for the 30 cerebral vascular incident cases were that one patient received excellent care; six received good care; eight patients received incomplete care (care was good as far as it went but did not go far enough); 11 patients received poor care; and 4 received unsafe care.

In the 30 cases where heart disease was the primary condition, none of the patients received excellent care; 3 patients received good care; 5 received incomplete care; 16 poor care; and 6 unsafe care.

From this, it would appear that, on the whole, the patients with cerebral vascular disease received better care than did the patients with heart disease (Table 1). The committee concluded that long-time agency emphasis on rehabilitation nursing and inclusion of physical therapy as a part of service accounted for the difference.

Table 1. Over-all audit results: quality judgment, 60 cases in two clinical groups

	Number of cases		
Quality judgment	Cerebral vascular incident	Cardiac disease	
Total	30	30	60
Excellent (161–200)	1	0	1
Good (121–160)	6	3	9
Incomplete (81–120)	8	5	13
Poor (41–80)	11	16	27
Unsafe (0–40)	4	6	10

Table 2. Audit results: quality judgments by nursing functions — 60 cases*

Nursing function	Excellent	Good	Incomplete	Poor	Unsafe	Total
1. Application and execution of physicians' legal orders	7	17	23	11	2	60
2. Observations of symptoms and reactions	6	5	13	22	14	60
3. Supervision of the patient	4	7	12	14	23	60
4. Supervision of those participating in care	5	5	12	20	18	60
5. Reporting and recording	4	7	12	15	22	60
6. Nursing procedures and techniques	2	8	26	21	3	60
7. Promotion of physical and emotional health	1	5	17	17	20	60
Quality judgments	29	54	115	120	102	[420]

*See appendix for comparison of quality judgments of the 60 cases by clinical group.

The committee realized that the over-all ratings present a broad view of quality, and that ratings of each of the seven functions for the 60 cases pinpoint areas of strength and weakness. Some examples from this categorical review are illustrative (Table 2). (The appendix table shows these quality judgments by nursing functions in each of the two groups of 30 patients.)

The analyses indicated that the best-executed function was the carrying out of physician's orders — the dependent nursing function. Weaknesses in execution of this function were also found. The major ones were lack of evidence of understanding of the pathophysiological processes, and failure to take the patient's health history into account in assessing needs and planning nursing intervention.

Observation of symptoms and reactions was found to be fragmentary, partly as a result of the previously mentioned weaknesses. One of the major problems also appeared to be the ignoring of significant secondary diagnoses — nearly half of the patients had such diagnoses.

Weaknesses evident in execution of the other nursing functions were judged to be related to two major points. Because the observations of symptoms and reactions were not sufficiently sharp, other responsibilities and opportunities for nursing intervention were not perceived.

Where care was judged to be good or excellent, it was obviously personalized, i.e., clearly individualized in accordance with the patient and his situation. On the whole, care appeared to be inadequately personalized.

The committee's mock-up audit report to the administration gives some indications of the potentials of audits for the improvement of care. The report included the tables which are a part of this paper and basic data such as sex and age distribution in the patient group, source of referral, status at the time of discharge by the agency, and other pertinent facts.

The recommendations for the agency included:

1. Use of the International Classification of Diseases in obtaining and recording primary and secondary diagnoses.
2. Increasing emphasis on obtaining orders regarding *all* medications used by the patient, whether or not they were administered by the nurse.
3. Exploration of reasons why nurse-to-physician communications are incomplete, and nursing judgments so seldom conveyed. (The committee had expected to find physician-to-nurse communications less than adequate; it was a surprise to find that nurse-to-physician communications were a greater problem.)
4. Increasing attention to assessment of vital signs, with recording and use of findings.
5. Establishment of the policy of requiring nursing assessment of the patient's physical and emotional condition at the time of admission and at the time of discharge.
6. Development of standards for charting, using the nursing audit schedule as a process guide.

PHASE THREE — THE COMMITTEE ASSESSES ITS WORK AND PLANS NEXT STEPS

The consultant met with the Audit Committee and the executive director who had not previously participated in committee proceedings. After consideration of experience and findings, the committee conveyed to the director its readiness to perform audits as a standard operating procedure; there was agreement that the procedure was necessary and feasible. It was decided that, because the agency discharges approximately 1,000 cases a month, review of a 10 percent randomized sample of the closed morbidity, maternity, and health supervision cases would suffice.

It was further agreed that the Audit Committee would not assume or be given responsibility for implementing the recommendations made in its report. However, individual members would participate in planning the continuing education program, and in other actions through which desired changes pertinent to quality care might be introduced. It was also agreed that the director would regularly advise the committee of action taken on its findings and recommendations.

Following this meeting, the committee presented its experience and findings to the supervisory group and the report was accepted. The supervisors planned to report the committee's work to their staff nurses. They interpreted the audit as one constructive tool that would be put into use in regularly appraising the quality of the agency's service to patients and families.

In the judgment of the consultant, this agency has effectively and efficiently initiated internal use of the nursing audit. Findings are comparable to those obtained in other settings.

COMMENT

Properly used, the audit is a detached, critical inquiry into quality. The question to be answered is, "What quality of care are we giving?" Strengths and weaknesses are to be expected wherever care is given to human beings by human beings. The point is to find out what the strengths are, and to build on them; to find out what the weaknesses are and to correct them.

Our work on the method continues, with a view to its refinement; and, as we proceed in the work, we heed individual and group suggestions generously given to us by nurses who do audits. We are particularly indebted to the agency that permitted its experience to be reported here.

Presently, we are experimenting to see whether a single nursing and medical audit instrument can be devised. Definitions will be refined and measurements of quality will be made more precise if this proves to be necessary and feasible. What will not be altered, however, is the focus on evaluation of care as rendered to patients. We will continue with a holistic view of the patient and emphasis on a holistic view of his care.

BIBLIOGRAPHY

Phaneuf, Maria C. Analysis of a Nursing Audit. *Nursing Outlook* 16,1:57—60 (Jan.), 1968.
Donabedian, Avedis. Promoting Quality Through Evaluating the Process of Care. *M. Care* 6,3:181 (May—June), 1968.

APPENDIX

Audit results: Quality judgments by nursing functions categories — comparison of 60 cases in two clinical groups

Nursing function		Excellent	Good	Incomplete	Poor	Unsafe	Total cases
1. Application and execution	A	2	9	12	5	2	30
of physicians' legal orders	B	5	8	11	6	0	30
2. Observations of symptoms	A	5	2	6	10	7	30
and reactions	B	1	3	7	12	7	30
3. Supervision of the	A	4	4	7	6	9	30
patient	B	0	3	5	8	14	30
4. Supervision of those	A	5	4	9	9	3	30
participating in care	B	0	1	3	11	15	30
5. Reporting and	A	2	3	7	8	10	30
recording	B	2	4	5	7	12	30
6. Nursing procedures	A	2	6	11	9	2	30
and techniques	B	0	2	15	12	1	30
7. Promotion of physical	A	1	4	10	9	6	30
and emotional health	B	0	1	7	8	14	30
Totals		29	54	115	120	102	[420] —

A = 30 cases, cerebral vascular incident.
B = 30 cases, heart disease.

31

Quality of Care:
The Nursing Audit, Part B

Avedis Donabedian

The preceding chapter described the use of the nursing audit as a means of assessing the quality of nursing care provided in one public health nursing agency. Dr. Donabedian comments on some of the considerations and problems inherent in this measurement approach; factors that must be dealt with in future assessment of the quality of patient care.

The task here is to call attention to certain issues of general import that are raised by the particular approach to the assessment of the quality of nursing care used in the preceding paper. This review will be brief because this author has dealt at greater length with these issues in other publications.[1-3]

RESPONSIBILITY FOR THE QUALITY OF CARE

Very properly, Miss Phaneuf begins with the need for assumption of responsibility for, and a commitment to, the quality of care. Without this foundation stone, the structure of quality assessment cannot be built.

Having accepted responsibility for the quality of care, there still remains a decision about the level and scope of agency concern. One may distinguish several steps in a progression of widening concern.

1. The care provided by a specified professional group (in this case, nursing) in a particular agency.
2. That portion of patient care provided by a particular agency, including the contribution of all professionals involved in the care of any given patient.
3. The total care of any given patient irrespective of the source of care.
4. The provision of health services for the community (however defined) as a whole.

It is necessary to explicitly specify the level and scope of concern because the aspects of care that require assessment may vary from level to level and so may the methods best suited for their assessment. For example, the degree of access to care is an essential concern at the community level; it is much less relevant when the question asked is whether a patient already under care receives quality nursing.

From "Quality of Care: Problems of Measurement, Part II — Some Issues in Evaluating the Quality of Nursing Care," *American Journal of Public Health,* Vol. 59, No. 10, pp. 1833–1836, 1969. Reprinted by permission of the publisher and the author.

APPROACHES TO EVALUATION

There are a set of issues that concern the selection among available approaches to evaluation. One may classify these approaches under three headings: structure, process, and outcome.

The evaluation of *structure* consists in the appraisal of the instrumentalities of care and of their organization. It includes the properties of facilities, equipment, manpower, and financing. It is the major approach used in drawing specifications for assessment, certification or accreditation by official and voluntary agencies. It assumes that when certain specified conditions are satisfied good care is likely to follow.

The evaluation of *process* consists in the appraisal of the care itself. The nursing audit is an example of this approach. It is not satisfied with the mere presumption of quality in any specified setting. It subjects to professional judgment the elements and details of care. It puts to actual test the assumptions that certain structural characteristics are related to certain levels of performance.

The evaluation of *outcomes* consists in the assessment of the end results of care — usually specified in terms of patient health, welfare, and satisfaction. The extent to which agreed-upon desired outcomes are achieved is the ultimate test of the assumptions inherent in the use of structure and of process in the assessment of care.

Among professionals, one finds much difference of opinion as to which of the three approaches one should use. In particular, there almost always appear to be two camps: those who favor process and those who favor outcome. Following are some observations concerning this division.

1. Whether one emphasizes outcome or process depends on the nature of agency responsibility and the questions that the agency feels required to ask. If the question is "Does the patient receive good nursing care?" the most direct answer would seem to derive from an examination of the process of care. If the question is "What good, if any, are we doing?" the answer is obviously to be found in the outcome of care.
2. The distinction between process and outcome is, to some extent, an abstraction. Between the initiation of care and its termination there are a number of completed tasks ("procedural end points") and states of the patient ("intermediate outcomes") that can be used as indicators of the quality of care.
3. A well-rounded system of quality appraisal would probably include concurrent or coordinate assessments of structure, process, and end results, to the extent that each of these is observable and measurable under the constraints inherent in any given setting.

SOME TECHNICAL ISSUES IN THE EVALUATION OF PROCESS

There are a number of technical problems and issues in the nursing audit that can be only briefly mentioned.

1. *The Record as a Source of Information* — One objection to audits, whether medical or nursing, is that they assess the quality of the record rather than that of the care actually provided. Skillful recording may give a false impression of quality, and omissions from the record may convey a false impression of poor care. The record is, of course, an indispensable tool of patient management and it is perfectly legitimate to evaluate the quality of recording. The doubts that are cast on the record as a true mirror of the care actually provided are probably exaggerated; but they have never been fully erased. There are a number of precautions that may be taken to minimize possible misrepresentation by the record. The most important are to devise appropriate records, to enforce reasonable standards of recording, and to allow for discussion of the findings with the person who has provided care.

2. *Definitions, Criteria and Standards* — It is extraordinarily difficult to define what quality is. Very probably quality is not a homogeneous property but a large bundle of characteristics. Certainly clients, physicians, and nurses may look for different characteristics as signifiers of quality and/or weight them differently. As a prelude to any evaluation it is necessary, therefore, to arrive at some agreement concerning what aspects of care are to be assessed and on what constitutes "goodness" in each aspect. The criteria and standards that embody these judgments are operational definitions of quality for any particular method of assessment.

Criteria and standards are implicit in any judgment of quality. The extent to which these are made explicit may, however, vary. Some authorities in medical audits favor explicit formulation of criteria and considerable specificity in standards. Others favor a more unstructured approach in which expert judges are simply guided by how they themselves would have managed a given patient. A cursory review of the nursing literature suggests that nurses are much more systematic and self-conscious in developing quality criteria. In contrast to studies of physician care that focus on purely technical performance, there is also greater attention to social and psychological aspects of patient management.

The nursing audit described by Phaneuf uses a framework of nursing functions to specify in considerable detail what the criteria should be. But it leaves to the reviewers to judge the extent to which nursing care has measured up to professional standards in each of the characteristics that are specified.

3. *Scales and Measurements* — Some students of quality have a preference for over-all ratings with a minimum of divisions such as "good," "fair," or "poor." Others have assigned numerical scores to elements of care and cumulated them to arrive at one over-all numerical representation of the quality of care. The nursing audit is an example of the latter approach.

In either case, but especially in the second, there are certain vexing problems of measurement. Since quality appears to include a multiplicity of elements or characteristics, the question arises as to whether the scores for these elements can be legitimately combined into one over-all measure and in what way. Such cumulation is made difficult for at least two reasons. First, performance in one aspect of care may not be independent of performance in another. For example, treatment depends on antecedent diagnosis. In extreme cases, performance in one element may be so bad that it cannot be compensated for by excellence in other elements, and the care must be rated "poor." Second, it is difficult to defend the weights (whether equal or unequal) that are assigned to different components or elements of care.

4. *Validity and Reliability* — We have already suggested that the validity of the assessments of process can be tested by determining the outcomes of care. This is the standard procedure in clinical research. It is seldom, if ever, used in quality assessments. The validity of assessments of care rests largely on agreed-upon professional judgment. The reliability or repeatability of judgments using any given method of assessment is easier to test and should be part and parcel of the development of that method. There is reason to believe that reasonably reliable judgments can be obtained through the audit of medical records. It is also claimed that reliability is improved by the prior specification of criteria and standards. Nevertheless, more attention needs to be given to establishing reliability in the assessment of patient care.

SOME OPERATIONAL ISSUES IN THE NURSING AUDIT

There are a number of issues that pertain to the implementation of professional care audits in general.

1. *Who Should Conduct Them and for What Purpose?* — There is general agreement that each profession is solely competent to judge the quality of care provided by its members. However, as the concern broadens to include the total care of individual patients it will become necessary to develop methods that require joint assessment by representatives of several professions.

A second question is whether the audits should be internal, conducted by agency personnel, or external, conducted by persons from outside the agency that is under examination. There is some evidence to suggest that external auditors tend to be more critical than are internal auditors. However, experience has shown that both internal and external audits can be effective. A "mixed" audit committee as proposed by Miss Phaneuf may combine the advantages of both.

The purposes of the audit are recognized to be primarily educational and constructive rather than punitive or destructive. Some authorities have suggested that this preferred orientation be institutionalized by confining the analysis to the identification of pervasive patterns of agency performance. Under this approach, individual physicians or nurses would not be identified or called to question, and the emphasis would be on altering general patterns of professional behavior. This proposal would seem to limit unduly the administrative usefulness of the professional audit.

2. *Implementation and Effectiveness* — There has been remarkably little study of the ability of professional audits to bring about lasting changes in professional behavior. There have been anecdotal accounts of remarkable success and of abject failure; but little is known about the circumstances that determine success or failure. There is urgent need for studies of the professional audit primarily as a complex social process rather than merely a technical problem of measurement.

3. *Cost, and Cost in Relation to Effectiveness* — Data on the cost of audits are almost nonexistent. Nor are there any data on cost in relation to effectiveness of audits or of alternative methods of appraisal. Such studies are sorely needed.

FINDINGS

The findings reported by Miss Phaneuf show significant weaknesses in performance even in a prestigious agency such as the one studied. These findings are in keeping with the more extensive reports of physician care. These have shown serious problems in almost every study reported. There have been significant failings in management even in university-affiliated institutions. Where technical error is considerably reduced, failures in the nontechnical dimensions of care become more salient. It is clear that the quality of care cannot be taken for granted. It must be carefully maintained and nurtured. Furthermore, as the prevailing levels of quality improve, the standards by which quality must be judged become more rigorous and demanding. To that extent, the quest for quality can never end.

REFERENCES

1. Donabedian, A. Evaluating the Quality of Medical Care. *Milbank Mem. Fund Quart.* 44:166–206, Part 2 (July), 1966.
2. _____. Promoting Quality Through Evaluating the Process of Patient Care. *M. Care* 6:181–202 (May–June), 1968.
3. _____. *A Guide to Medical Care Administration,* Volume II, *Medical Care Appraisal — Quality and Utilization.* New York: The Program Area Committee on Medical Care Administration, American Public Health Association (Aug.), 1968 (to be published).

VI
Communication

Communication is the exchange of information between individuals. From the earliest days of life we learn to communicate. Even the infant's cries and movements convey a message to its mother, and her touch and reassuring voice carry information in response. Within the first few years of life the normal child has mastered the complex rules of a language and can speak fluently by the age of six or seven. At the same time, children are acquiring the nonverbal skills of their culture, learning to interpret the meaning of facial expressions and gestures. Both verbal and nonverbal communication becomes a routine activity of everyday life, as natural and vital as breathing.

A great deal of communication occurs without much conscious thought. A patient describes symptoms and health professionals nod their heads to give assurance that the message is understood. A child asks for food and the mother responds. The questions asked are formulated quickly, almost as easily and unconsciously as breathing. For most people communication is a continuous process whenever they are with others, but one that is largely outside of awareness. Desires and needs are expressed, questions raised and feelings conveyed; these in turn are received, interpreted and responded to in a relatively unplanned fashion.

Communication skills are important tools for the community nurse, and they cannot be left to chance. Communication as a tool in community nursing is much more of a conscious, planned, purposeful process. The skillful use of words, tone of voice, silence and body movements are all required to convey meaningful, therapeutic messages. It requires proficiency in the art of attentive listening and expertise in questioning to encourage feedback and increase understanding between patient and nurse. This kind of communication does not happen automatically: it is only learned through conscious effort. The chapters in Part VI examine many facets of this complex process.

Because the way people communicate is learned, it is strongly influenced by culture. As the community nurse interacts with people from different backgrounds — the poor, Chinese-Americans or Afro-Americans, for example — the meaning of different communicative acts changes. A particular tone of voice or facial expression may denote grief, depression or sadness in one subculture but not in another. Silence on the part of a patient can have different meanings depending on the cultural background. The cultural aspect of communication was implicit in many of the articles in the preceding sections. It is discussed here in Chapter 34. Nurses must realize that culture influences both the messages they give and those they receive in the communication process.

32

What is Empathy?

Beatrice J. Kalisch

One essential element in any successful communicating relationship is empathy. It is the ability to borrow another person's feelings to understand them while maintaining one's own identity. Empathy provides a perspective of acceptance and insight coupled with objectivity in viewing the patient-family situation. The community nurse will find her therapeutic relationships greatly enhanced through skilled use of empathic communication. The nature of empathy, how it is developed, and how it is communicated are all cogently portrayed in this chapter.

Empathy is the ability to enter the life of another person, to accurately perceive his current feelings and their meanings. According to theorists of psychological therapy, it is an essential element of the interpersonal process. When communicated it forms the basis for a helping relationship between nurse and patient.

Empathy is the antithesis of the usual professional analysis and evaluation which prompts such comments as "I know what your problem is" or "I am aware of the psychological dynamics which make you act the way you do."

Important in the definition of empathy given above is the word current. Empathy must involve understanding the *current* feelings of a patient, not his feelings of yesterday or the day before. Expectations of behavior and feelings based on earlier experiences with him or similar patients can be misleading.

Previous perceptions can help in comprehending the feelings of a patient if they do not block understanding of what he is currently expressing. For example, on Monday his nurse knew Mr. Smith was feeling depressed. When she approached him on Tuesday, she expected him to be depressed and, so, was unable to recognize that he was now confused, not depressed. In short, approaching a patient with a preconceived frame of reference makes it very difficult to be in tune with his current feelings.

Empathy is of greatest value at the moment of confrontation. For example, if a nurse doesn't understand a patient's meanings and feelings until after a meeting with him, she cannot be helpful during the interactive process. Her understanding will be of limited value unless she has an opportunity to respond to the same theme at a later meeting.

In order to perceive meaning it is necessary to focus on what the patient "is" during the interaction rather than on the intellectual content of what the patient says. It is easy to interpret literally the verbalizations of a patient and ignore the deeper veiled and unspoken expressions of the person in the immediate present.

Another key point in the definition of empathy used here is that the perception of feelings must be accurate. Since a nurse is human and, thus, less than perfect, her perceptions will not always be accurately empathic with all of the patients all of the time. But if she at least communicates that she is making the effort to understand, she will be helpful to him. Rogers states it concisely:

> ...I am often impressed with the fact that even a minimal amount of empathic understanding — a bumbling and faulty attempt to catch the confused complexity of the client's meaning — is helpful, though there is no doubt that it is most helpful when I see and formulate clearly the meanings in his experiencing which for him have been unclear and tangled.[1]

Obviously, there is a danger that a patient might become more frustrated, angry, or hopeless if a nurse, over a period of time, continues to lack insight into his feelings. Indeed, if a nurse fails repeatedly in her interactions with a patient, ideally she should arrange for a replacement. She must be humble enough to provide the patient with another helper when she becomes convinced that she no longer is able to help him.

EMPATHY vs. SYMPATHY

What is the difference between empathy and sympathy, another type of human understanding?

In empathy the helper *borrows* his patient's feelings in order to fully understand them, but he is always aware of his own separateness. He realizes that the feelings of the patient are not his own.

Sympathetic understanding, on the other hand, involves a process in which the helper *loses* his own separate identity and *takes on* the patient's feelings and circumstances as if he were in his place, as if, for example, he were a diabetic as the patient is. This is sharing of feelings. Rogers underlines this difference when he points out that empathy is the ability "to sense the client's private world as if it were your own but without ever losing the 'as if' quality."[2]

There are several reasons why sympathy does not provide as much help to a patient as does empathy. First, when a nurse views a patient's feelings in terms of how she would feel if she were in a similar position (sympathy), she is not necessarily accurate in her perceptions, for the patient's reaction may be, and indeed often is, quite different from the response of the nurse. For example, a patient may be frightened at the prospect of having an injection, but the nurse may not be or *vice versa*.

Empathy, denoting a view of a patient "as if I were he," will generally yield a much more accurate perception of the true feelings of the patient than does sympathetic understanding.

Another reason why sympathy is not as helpful an interpersonal relationship as empathy is because the process of taking on the circumstances of the patient causes involvement of the self to such an extent that the nurse herself is then in need of help. In empathy, a nurse's realization that her identity is separate from the patient's enables her to be sufficiently free from the intensity of emotion to help the patient.

In sympathy, a nurse is preoccupied with her similarities to the patient, or those she imagines she has, and this interferes with her ability to concentrate on the patient and his point of view. In addition, sympathy denotes condolence with the patient's viewpoint whereas in empathy such agreement is not necessarily present. With empathy, a nurse can understand a patient's viewpoint and convey this understanding to him without agreeing with it.

COMMUNICATING EMPATHY

To be useful, empathic perceptions must be effectively communicated, both verbally and nonverbally, so that the patient experiences the feeling of being understood by the nurse.

Client-oriented therapists and others have called the communication of empathy a reflection of the patient's feelings. Ginott referred to this as an emotional mirror where an image of feelings (not a sermon) is reflected back without contortion.[3] Jourard underlined this point when he said that nurses could promote the "real-self-being" and self-disclosure of their patients by an empathic acknowledgment of what has been expressed.[4]

Examples of empathic expressions would be, "It seems as if you are very discouraged with physical therapy" or "It sounds as if you are quite concerned about whether you made the right decision." If you simply say "I know how you feel," a patient cannot be sure that you truly understand his real feelings.

Such reflections must not be rote or parrot-like but based on a genuine sensitive understanding of the current feelings of the patient. And if the unspoken aspects of these reflections do not convey empathy to the patient, they will be valueless. As Shlien explains:

At most points in communication where others would interpret, probe, advise, encourage, we reflect.... Reflection can be, in the hands of an imitating novice, a dull wooden mockery. On paper it often looks particularly so. Yet it can be a profound intimate, empathetically understanding response, requiring great skill and sensitivity and intense involvement.[5]

Empathic communications must be expressed in the language of the patient. If a nurse's expressions are foreign to the patient, he will not be able to experience the empathic understanding. Cameron points out that a helper:

...always adopts some of the patient's own terms in their communication, always being sure he does this without artificiality, condescension, or facetiousness. When a patient says approvingly, "you speak my language," this may well be a sign that the therapist is reaching the patient at a common sense, personal level.[6]

Moreover, the feeling tone used by a nurse must be that of the patient. In other words, if the patient is angry, the nurse's tone also is one of anger. Similarly, if a patient's expressions are sad, the nurse's feeling tone should be one of sadness. This does not mean that the nurse shares these feelings, she only borrows them. At first, it is usually difficult for a nurse to take on the feeling tone of the patient because this often seems rather artificial to her. However, with practice, this type of communication often becomes much easier and more natural and the results are rewarding.

Reflections of feelings should not take on a declarative tone which implies the nurse is telling the patient what he thinks and feels. It is so easy to communicate to a patient that one is the judge and jury of how he experiences the world! The reflections, instead, should be provisional, allowing and encouraging a patient to refute the nurse's perceptions of his feelings. Social and cultural conditioning often prevent a patient from telling an expert he is wrong. It is up to the nurse to interact with the patient in such a way that he feels he can say, "No, you're not right."

Sometimes, a patient is not ready to admit certain feelings; he needs to be allowed to deny them, at least for the moment. During interactions, it is wise to check with the patient to determine whether or not his true feelings and experiences are being correctly perceived. For example, a nurse might use the word "fearful" in describing the feelings of a patient, but to the patient they are more feelings of "anxiety" or "tension."

The patient who is free to correct a nurse moves onto a higher level of self-understanding, but the patient who cannot refute a nurse's reflections tends to build up defenses and withdraw, defeating the purpose of the facilitative relationship. One way of checking is to say, "If I understand you correctly, you feel quite angry about the whole business. Is this right?" However, if a nurse's tone of voice and attitude clearly indicate that her perceptions are of a provisional nature, it is not essential that she question every reflection. Because nonverbal evidence of empathic communication is difficult to learn, it is wise to have a tentative beginning when dealing with indirect, hidden, or below-the-surface feelings.

Many experienced helpers drop the third person "you" and substitute the first person "I" in their empathic acknowledgments once they have developed a relationship with a patient. Instead of saying "You really are feeling helpless" they might state "It's a helpless feeling" or "I feel so helpless." Even though on rare occasions this causes momentary confusion in the patient, it often facilitates empathic communication and helpers find it both more efficient and effective.

Research studies reveal that when a helper is active and responds frequently to a patient, the patient has a greater feeling of being understood. The helper stays in tune with the patient's feelings and provides him with a greater opportunity for fast correction of errors in perception. Again, careful balance is the keynote. It is a common mistake to interrupt a patient at very frequent intervals with "yes," "um hum," and other banalities. These not only distract but reveal an absence of true understanding.

Emphatic perception and communication must be reviewed in terms of levels or categories rather than as an "all or nothing" characteristic. The "Nurse-Patient Empathic Functioning Scale" [pages 279–281] is largely based on the scales of Bergin and Solomon, Truax, Carkhuff, and Reddy.[7,8,9,10] On this five-point scale, where category 0 denotes the absence of empathy, the second stage marks

The Nurse-Patient Empathic Functioning Scale

CATEGORY 0

The nurse ignores both the conspicuous, surface feelings and the deeper, hidden feelings of the patient. The nurse may be bored, apathetic, uninterested, indifferent, unconcerned, detached, thinking of other matters, giving advice, or offering examples from her own experiences but is definitely not communicating an awareness of the feelings of the patient. The nurse functioning at this level can be harmful to the patient and cause him to become *less* integrated or adjusted than he was before their encounter.

Example

N:	Good morning, Mrs. Smith. Here is your breakfast tray. (mechanically)	(Bored)
P:	No, you just go on and take that tray back. I'm not going to eat! (defiantly)	
N:	Well, Mrs. Smith, you'll never recover if you don't start eating. (sarcastically)	(Advice; ignoring feelings)
P:	I'm not going to eat. You need not try to make me because I'm not going to! (turns head to wall away from nurse)	
N:	(Glances at empty chair by bedside.) I wonder where your clean sheets are. Didn't they leave them? (casually)	(Disinterested; ignoring feelings)
P:	(Crying softly, turns toward nurse) Don't bother with me.	
N:	All right, forget it. (Leaves room with the tray)	(Unconcerned; ignoring feelings)

CATEGORY 1

The nurse sometimes communicates an accurate awareness of the conspicuous current feelings of the patient but at other times she is inaccurate in her perceptions of these surface feelings. She may misinterpret the essence (content) or strength (intensity) of the patient's expressions. The nurse ignores any feelings which are hidden and below the surface. In category 0 the nurse is completely ignoring the patient's conspicuous feelings; in category 1, she is *not able* to grasp their full meaning. The nurse classified in this category is still not helping the patient for she is not in tune with him.

Example

P:	Are you the nurse who will be taking care of my Eddy? (excitedly)	
N:	Yes. Why?	
P:	(Speaking rapidly) I don't know what I am going to do. Eddy with this, this, uh, sickness, and my husband is so upset, I, uh, I don't know what, what to say to him. (stammering). I just....	
N:	(Interrupting) Your husband wants to find out what's wrong with Eddy?	(Inaccurate identification of conspicuous feelings)
P:	Yes, he knows that it is something with the water....	
N:	Mmm.	

P: He was playing and came in and . . . (she starts to cry) . . . he said his tummy hurts and then he went to the bathroom and there was, was (crying harder) blood in his potty. I, I don't . . . (crying so much she can't continue talking).

N: I know how you feel, but Dr. Jones is a very competent urologist and I am sure he is going to do everything he can for Eddy. (gently, warmly)

(Inaccurate identification of the essence and strength of conspicuous feelings)

CATEGORY 2

This represents the mid-point of the continuum of empathic communication and is the stage where the nurse begins to be of help to the patient. The nurse is communicating an accurate awareness of the conspicuous current feelings and their meanings to the patient. She realizes the presence of hidden feelings but is not accurate in defining their essence or strength and does not know what they mean to this particular patient. The nurse does express an interest in understanding the patient's hidden feelings and communicates "I am trying to understand." The provisional nature of the reflections of those hidden feelings she does attempt to express allows the patient to refute the nurse's perceptions.

Example

P: The doctor told me I was going to be well enough to go home in a few days. (flatly)

N: How do you feel about going home?

(Fact-finding to get more information)

P: Well (pauses momentarily), they want me to go to a nursing home. (sadly)

N: Oh? (sitting down in chair beside patient's bed and looking at patient).

(Nonlinguistic communication of conspicuous feelings)

P: I've heard terrible things about nursing homes. They say they don't feed you right (pause), and, they, they, uh, don't treat you well. I sure don't want to go to a place like that.

N: You don't want to go there because you don't think you will be treated right?

(Reflects conspicuous feelings accurately)

P: Yes, they say if you don't want to eat at certain times you don't get fed at all! (pauses) And also they think you should do everything they want you to and besides you don't have much to do there anyway.

N: Are you worried about having enough to do to fill up the hours?

(Reflects conspicuous feelings accurately)

P: Yaah and, uh, (pauses), well, my children, uh, they, they don't come to see me very much, they are so busy, and I'll be, uh, uh, alone. (voice becomes almost inaudible)

N: You want your children to come see you, don't you, so you won't be so lonely? You wish they weren't so busy?

(Reflects conspicuous feelings accurately but inaccurate identification of hidden feelings)

CATEGORY 3

The nurse responds accurately to the current conspicuous feelings and their meanings to the patient. In this category, the nurse expresses an accurate awareness of hidden feelings in their appropriate essence and strength. These feelings are those which the patient has not yet conveyed or expressed. However, the nurse moves only slightly beyond the patient's conspicuous feelings and thus there are feelings present which the nurse is not aware of.

Example

P: I have always been dependent on myself only.

N: You're afraid you may have to go live with someone? Is that right?   (Reflects slightly hidden feeling)

P: Yaah, probably one of my sons and they really don't have room for me and I would be putting them out and making a hardship on them.

N: It sounds as though you feel that after a while they might come to resent you because you moved in.   (Reflects hidden feeling)

P: Um hmm. Very much so. Cause, like I said, they are working and have their own problems, and, ah, they don't need another one.

N: You feel that you would be more or less moving in, into their lives, butting in, so to speak, and this bothers you because, you think they would take you in out of an obligation rather than because they really wanted to?   (Reflects slightly hidden feeling; deepest feelings not reflected)

CATEGORY 4

The nurse communicates accurately without reluctance or uncertainty the current conspicuous and hidden feelings of the patient. She perceives and reflects in appropriate words, voice tone, and nonverbal behavior, feelings which are much below the surface, those that the patient has not been able to express himself, or was not able to before the interaction with the nurse. If the patient is exploring his deepest feelings already, the nurse is very much with him in these deepest moments. The difference between categories 3 and 4 is that in the latter, the deepest, most hidden feelings are understood and expressed by the nurse. In category 3 only those hidden feelings slightly beyond the patient's conspicuous feelings are understood. Also in category 4 the nurse is so infallibly in tune with the patient that she does not hesitate in her responses.

Example

P: I just don't feel like having a bath this morning. (flatly)

N: It really makes you mad to have people telling you what to do all the time, doesn't it! (emphatically)   (Reflects deep hidden feelings)

P: Yes! Someone comes in here every other minute telling me to eat breakfast, go to O.T., take a bath, and anything else they can pick out of their minds! (heatedly)

N: You wish to heck they would just leave you alone and quit treating you like you were a helpless child! (angrily)   (Reflects deep hidden feelings)

P: Yaah, that's right! (angrily) It reminds me of my mother, dear mother! (slight pause) Even when I was 16 years old she told me what clothes to wear, she even went out and bought them without me! She dictated where I went, I couldn't even go to the dances. (voice becomes softer and she begins to cry)

N: She really made you feel helpless and useless. (softly and sadly)   (Reflects deep hidden feelings)

P: Yes, as if I weren't capable of going to the bathroom by myself. (continues to cry)

N: And now the very people who are supposed to be helping you turn around and treat you the same way.   (Reflects deep hidden feelings) the first point where the nurse is helpful to the patient. Below that level a nurse's relationship with a patient can actually be detrimental. Conspicuous feelings refer to the most evident and obvious ones — those that the patient is able to express himself — while the hidden feelings describe the deeper, below-the-surface emotions, which a patient cannot express or could not prior to the interaction with a nurse. The patient may or may not be aware that these hidden feelings are his, but when the nurse communicates them verbally and nonverbally they are not completely foreign.

One may delve below the surface in terms of content or essence of the communications as well as the intensity or strength of feelings. For example, a patient may describe an event very calmly but actually may be quite angry underneath. The nurse who is highly empathic will reflect the patient's emotions in an angry feeling tone, thus permitting the patient to move on to greater self-realization and more accurate identification of his deepest inner feelings.

Several additional points are important. First, through empathic communication, a helpee receives "relief from experiential loneliness."[11] This overcomes, to some degree, a feeling of being isolated in the world with one's problems. Second, a nurse's willingness and desire to understand how the patient feels about his world implies that the patient's point of view is of value.

Third, emphatic understanding places the focus of evaluation within the patient rather than within the helper. The nurse does not offer advice or attempt to persuade the patient to think in certain ways when she is being empathic.

The Nurse-Patient Empathic Functioning Scale: A Schematic Presentation

Categories of nurse empathic functioning	Level of Patient's Feelings	
	Conspicuous current feelings	Hidden current feelings
Category 0	Ignores.	Ignores.
Category 1	Communicates an awareness which is accurate at times and inaccurate at other times.	Ignores.
Category 2	Communicates a complete and accurate awareness of the essence and strength of feelings.	Communicates an awareness of the presence of hidden feelings but is not accurate in defining their essence or strength. An effort is being made to understand.
Category 3	Same as category 2.	Communicates an accurate awareness of the hidden feelings slightly beyond what the patient expresses himself.
Category 4	Same as category 2.	Communicates without uncertainty an accurate awareness of the deepest, most hidden feelings.

Rather, she understands and accepts the patient's feelings without offering an evaluation of them.

A patient treated thus becomes less dependent on the opinions of others, values less his social self-concept, and values more his private self-concept. Empathic understanding is not a passive process and will not happen without effort. Rather, it is a very active experience which requires a high level of energy output and involvement. A nurse must concentrate intensely on the patient, on what he says, and what he doesn't say. This intense concentration allows the nurse little time to reflect on her own personal needs, values, and ideals, which, in turn, keeps her from inculcating her own judgments into the patient's life which would interfere with helping. It is similar to being so engrossed in a movie that all of one's attention, emotions, and thinking capacities are involved to such an extent that it is impossible to reflect on oneself. Of course, this heavy concentration makes errors by the nurse in perceiving the feelings of the patient less likely.

Empathy is a difficult and complex goal to achieve. All of us want to give reassurance or advice because this makes us feel as if we are doing something for the patient. We tell him about our own experiences in similar circumstances or with other patients in an effort to show that his problem is not unique to him. Or, perhaps, we may attempt to interpret his behavior to him or respond in ways other than trying to comprehend his world from his viewpoint and then let him know that we understand.

We long have been socialized to respond in these ways and it is difficult to break habits. Further, we have often been told that a helper should use communication methods he finds most comfortable. While this is true, it should not be the sole criterion for accepting or rejecting a communication mode. Any new response is strange and awkward at first, but becomes more natural with practice and use.

REFERENCES

1. Rogers, C. R. Characteristics of a helping relationship. *Personnel Guidance J.* 37:13, Sept. 1958.
2. _____. Necessary and sufficient conditions of therapeutic personality change. *J. Consult. Psychol.* 21:99, Apr. 1957.
3. Ginott, Haim. *Between Parent and Child.* New York, Macmillan Co., 1965, pp. 35–36.
4. Jourard, S. M. *The Transparent Self.* 2d ed. Princeton, N.J., D. Van Nostrand Co., 1971.
5. Shlien, J. M. A client-centered approach to schizophrenia: first approximation. In *Psychotherapy of the Psychoses,* ed. by Arthur Burton. New York, Basic Books, 1961, p. 302.
6. Cameron, Norman. *Personality Development and Psychopathology: a Dynamic Approach.* Boston, Houghton Mifflin Publishing Co., 1963, p. 769.
7. Traux, C. B., and Capkhuff, R. R. *Toward Effective Counseling and Psychotherapy.* Chicago, Aldine Publishing Co., 1967, p. 58.
8. Truax, C. B. A scale for the measurement of accurate empathy. *Psychiatr. Institute Bull.* (Wisconsin Psychiatric Institute, University of Wisconsin) 1:12, 1961.

9. Carkhuff, R. R. *Helping and Human Relations.* New York, Holt, Rinehart and Winston, 1969, Vol. 1, pp. 174—175.
10. Reddy, W. B. *The Effects of Immediate and Delayed Feedback on the Learning of Empathy.* Cincinnati, University of Cincinnati. 1968. (Unpublished doctoral dissertation.)
11. Van Kaam, A. L. Feeling of being understood. *J. Individ. Psychol.* 15:69, 1959.

33

Home Visit — Ritual or Therapy?

Marlene Mayers

*Visiting families at home provides the community nurse with a unique oppor-
tunity. The insights and understanding gained from interacting with the family
members in their own environment can form the basis for sound, comprehensive
nursing intervention. Why, then, are so many community nurses' home visits
ineffective or frustrating? The quality and focus of the communication between
patient and nurse are essential considerations and provides a partial answer
to this question.*

What do community health nurses and their patients talk about during a home
visit? What does each see as the purpose for the visit? Does each understand the
other's concerns? How do they interact? To find answers to these questions, I
conducted a study in which I observed 16 randomly selected nurses employed in
a metropolitan health department, during their visits to 37 families.

The nurses were interviewed after each visit to ascertain the nurse's purpose
for the visit, her long-range goals for the patient and/or family, and her perception
of the patient's or family's concerns and problems. Several patterns and themes
emerged from these observations and interviews. However, before I describe
these, it would be important to look at the population visited and the nurses who
made the visits.

CLIENTS AND SITUATIONS

Many visits were to persons living in the inner city who were hidden away in the
upstairs and back rooms of old hotels or street-level shops. Some lived in austere,
box-like, government-financed housing developments, while other visits took
place in small apartments in large old houses in the alleys along the periphery of
the downtown business district. Some interviews took place in the depressing
skid row area, with its dilapidated hotels, bars, and businesses and lonely, down-
and-out, unattached residents. Still other visits were made to homes that were
scattered over a large geographical area characterized by its contrast of private
dwellings and high-rise apartments.

The patients vividly reflected the international flavor of the city and included
Caucasians, blacks, Mexican-Americans, Chinese, American Indians, and Filipinos.
They represented ways of life, backgrounds, and origins that covered a wide and
varied spectrum.

Typical patient situations encountered daily by the nurses in this sample can
be seen in the following examples.

The nurse received a referral reporting that a woman in a hotel seemed very ill and needed checking. We found the place and were directed to the manager, who was an East Indian woman. She spoke no English so her son interpreted. After some hesitation, he took us to a small cluttered room where an elderly lady lay clutching a thin blanket up to her neck. She appeared flushed, thin, and weak. She seemed fearful and anxious and a bit suspicious. Both the manager and her son hovered silently near and listened to the conversation.

The nurse, visiting a young Filipino mother and her three small children, discussed several topics and then asked the woman about her husband — if he was working. The mother said, "Yes, he's at sea (a seaman)." The nurse asked when he would return. The mother replied "I don't know," and by her look and tone sounded very much alone.

NURSES' PROFILE

The public health nurses, themselves, represented the other fascinating dimension of the dyad. They comprised an ethnic mix — primarily Caucasian, black, Chinese, and Japanese, who ranged in age from 23 to 50 years. Each nurse had her unique interpersonal style, and shared with me her professional expertise, analysis of her families, candid reflections on the satisfactions and disappointments of her career, and hopes and fears for nursing itself.

A glimpse into the thoughts and feelings of the nurses is represented by one nurse's comment about the nurse-patient relationships:

Well, it's great when you see some progress in a family due to your efforts. That's really satisfying. What's disappointing is when you see some of these horrible situations and you can't make any changes. You're helpless because of the total social system — it's stacked against them (the clients). It's too big to buck.

THE FINDINGS

After analysis of my field notes taken during and after the visits, several findings concerning the content and process of the visits became apparent. These findings can be grouped into five categories: topics of conversations, unshared long-range goals, obscuring of legitimate concerns, nurse's interactional style, and ritualistic performance.

Topics of Conversation

When the subjects of conversation were abstracted and placed into categories, it was found that 17 topics were usually discussed. The most frequently mentioned was "general health or physical signs and symptoms." Medical care regimens and personal or family emotional problems were second and third in frequency, and the least commonly mentioned topics were such things as clothing, assistive devices, ambulation problems, and attendant care. It became evident that the conversations of the visits were dominated by nursing content material. This finding runs contrary to the commonly held belief that the roles of public health nurses and social workers are blurred and difficult to differentiate — a belief often expressed by the nurses in the sample.

However, an analysis of the data revealed that in the 195 instances of the 17 topics discussed, only 40 might also be considered in the province of social work. These include financial, 14; housing, 5; problems with living conditions, 7; clothing, 2; attendant care, 3; and jobs, 9. These findings are similar to those in a study conducted by the California Department of Social Welfare. Of the 36 "social goods" for which social workers would be expected to assume responsibility, eleven were identified as equally within the province of nursing.[1]

Unshared Long-Range Goals

Another phenomenon became apparent when the observed content and process of a visit were compared with the nurse's comments about the visit and the patient or family. The purposes of the visits (both stated and implied) were separated into two major categories: those stated or implied in the patient's presence, and those stated to the researcher after the visit. For example, the purposes made known to the patient were reflected in such phrases as: "I've come to see how you're doing," or, "You're ill and I can help." They were generally very specific and short-range in nature, whereas the implied goals represented a different level of abstraction. They reflect such purposes as: "to allow the patient to talk about specific problems"; "to give information about health"; or "to talk socially."

Often the goals stated by the nurses to the researcher referred to specific social and personal kinds of goals, such as: "help patient to achieve a sense of personal satisfaction and independence"; and "to adjust to or demonstrate a satisfactory parental role." But half of these purposes could not be detected, even as an implicit purpose, from the content of the home visits. This leads to some reflections about this phenomenon — the nurse's hidden agenda. It would seem that nurses might share their objectives more specifically with their patients, so that both might work more productively together in achieving the stated and agreed upon goals.

In addition, when the three categories of purposes were analyzed — case by case — there appeared to be varying degrees of agreement among the three. There seems to be more congruence in those cases where the nurse, in the post-visit interview, states her purposes in terms of specific, short-range goals. For example, it was found that when a nurse perceives her purposes as "get needed medical care" or "keep six-week appointment," then it was also quite apparent that the client also understood these to be their mutual purposes.

However, when a nurse stated her purposes to the researcher in terms of more abstract personal-social goals, such as "adjustment to new culture," "demonstrate satisfactory mothering role," or "achieve stable home life," there was seldom any evidence of the patient's understanding of these purposes. For less abstract purposes, patients seemed able to deduce from the content of the visit what the nurse's purpose was even if she did not explicitly state it.

Further analysis of the purposes of the nurse-patient relationship reveals that about half the purposes could be classified as relatively abstract and long-range in nature. This is not to say that in most nurses' judgments these abstract, long-range goals are not valid. They probably are, and some of these statements reflect important and probably much-needed changes in the family.

However, based upon the post-visit interview data, it can be deduced that half of the purposes of the visits were completely unknown to patients, since the nurses in the sample did not share their more abstract purposes for the visit with them.

Obscuring of Legitimate Concerns

Again, the concerns about the family expressed by the nurses to the researcher after the visit were not reflected in the content or process of the visit. A nurse would say, for example, that she was concerned about a patient's "mothering" ability, but that fact was generally obscured during the visit, so that the patient would never have guessed the nurse's concern.

One can understand a nurse's hesitancy to explicitly share certain concerns with her patient. It is useful, however, to question whether or not this obscuring of legitimate concerns should be quite so prevalent as the visits of this study make it appear to be.

Since nurses tend to operate on the premise that positive reinforcement is good, perhaps they also tend to overly obscure their concerns about a patient. They appeared, in the sample, to couch their statements in such a way that the patient was unlikely to be able to guess that the nurse had some very real concerns. Use of this "couching" tactic may have two important effects: it leaves the patient unaware of the nurse's real concerns and, perhaps more important, it leaves the patient unaware of the seriousness of his own situation or condition.

The findings suggest that a nurse carefully softens or obscures her fears and concerns when dealing with threatening areas to herself or to her patient. This "couching" tactic is reminiscent of the "awareness context" interactional phenomena discovered by Glaser and Strauss in their study of dying.[2] They developed a paradigm for analyzing the interactional properties of the awareness contexts of dying in relation to the dying person, his family, and his nurses and doctors. They found four types of awareness context which they called "closed, suspicion, mutual pretense, and open awareness." Each awareness context type, except open awareness, is a kind of obscuring phenomenon.

It is possible that a productive area for the further analysis of nurse-patient relationships in community health would be to study in a similar way the awareness contexts of the important and possibly threatening concerns that a nurse may have regarding a patient. Such research might lead to the discovery of interactional strategies which, when described and analyzed, could yield meaningful and vital data. This kind of data could help nursing to develop a theoretical basis for the refinement of nurses' interactional skills.

Nurses' Interactional Styles

After observations, interviews, and interactions with the 16 nurses, one impression became clear; each nurse has a basic, generally unchanging, interactional style. For example, if a nurse tends to be a nondirective listener, she tends to use that style in every client situation. If she is directive, she is consistently so. There were few exceptions to this general characteristic.

This finding — individualistic and consistent style — is important to nursing educators, whose goal is to educate a nurse to consciously use a variety of interactional strategies or skills as she perceives the varying and changing needs of her patients. All of the nurses in the sample were graduates of baccalaureate programs in nursing and all were exceptionally well-qualified by the usual public health nursing standards. Yet they tended to consistently use a single interactional style. It was as characteristic of recent graduates as it was of less recent graduates.

In her study of nurse-patient "give and take," Conant noted a similar finding: nurses have their own individual patterns of interviewing which remain generally unchanged from client to client.[3]

For a more "real life" presentation of the interactional styles of the nurses in this study, several excerpts from the field notes follow. Each excerpt describes a different nurse which reflects her characteristic style.

> The nurse was direct and concerned. She spoke clearly and used his name frequently to keep his attention.

> The nurse used many of the strategies of the nondirective method. She allowed long silences. She reflected feelings, most of which were of discouragement or depression. She also made statements that implied negative judgments. She gave no really perceptible positive support.

> The nurse was kindly but projected no real sense of concern by her expression or tone of voice. She used logic to overturn the patient's excuses.

To find out if there was a correlation between the nurse's interactional style and the client's response, a detailed cross-analysis of these factors was done that yielded no particular trends. It seemed to make no difference whether the nurse was consistently directive, nondirective, information-giving, or whether she had a combination of these traits. However, this cross-analysis did lead to a discovery concerning what I call in any case patient-focused nurses versus nurse-focused nurses.

It was found that some nurses seem to follow the patient's clues. Others seem to act primarily from their own perspective or to react to the patient's clues from their own frame of reference. For example, in a case where a patient was in trouble and unable to function, the nurse acted upon her own notion of solutions without consulting the patient. She was seen as nurse-focused. If she had perceptively attempted to understand the patient's view of his situation and his ideas regarding solutions, she would have been seen as patient-focused.

Regardless of the specific interactional style, the patients of nurses who were patient-focused consistently tended to respond with interest, involvement, and mutuality. The patients of the "nurse-focused" nurses did not. The patient-focused nurse projects a sense of concern, involvement, and personal interest. The nurse-focused nurse does not. The following examples will illustrate this difference:

The nurse looked at the patient directly and kindly and said, "You know, Mr. N, I believe that you are in bad shape, and I think you probably need to be hospitalized. I don't know whether your hip is broken or not, but it might be. Your doctor needs to check you over and decide what is best. I would like your permission to call your doctor right away. Now it's possible that he won't be able to come out here to check on you and so he may ask me for my opinion. I want you to know that I will tell him that I believe you are in very bad shape and that I believe that you need to be hospitalized. Now, Mr. N, may I go ahead and call Dr. K? The patient hesitated a moment and then said, "O.K., go ahead."

Although she was quite directive, she nonverbally projected a real sense of concern about him as a person. Her words also reflected concern for his rights and a respect for him as a human being when she candidly told him what she was thinking and what she would say to the doctor. She was patient-focused when she provided him with as much information as she had so that he could participate in the decision.

A nurse-focused intervention style is illustrated, as follows:

Mrs. F paused momentarily and then asked, "What do you think about my little one? He doesn't talk yet. He's two years old and he doesn't say anything."
The nurse asked, "Does he say any words at all, like 'mama,' or 'no'?"
The mother explained that he makes sounds, but no words — he just makes sounds and points. The nurse then said that a lot of kids don't talk when they don't have to, as when the mother anticipates everything and doesn't make him talk to get the things he wants.
"But," persisted Mrs. F, "my older boy learned to talk; why doesn't my little one talk?" Her voice belied her very real worry.
The nurse continued lightly, reiterating that "a lot of kids don't talk until after two years of age, and if they don't need to talk, they won't, but they do eventually learn."

This nurse did not respond to the mother's expressions of concern. She continued to reiterate her advice and to take lightly the mother's worry.

It seemed from the findings of this study that the apparently consistent interactional style of each nurse, regardless of the situation, and the high correlation between patient-focused interactions and positive patient response are more significant than the particular method used — directive, nondirective, information-giving, and so forth.

Ritualistic Performance

As the study progressed, I became impressed that what I was observing was a well-established, time-honored ritual. With few exceptions, nurses and their patients seemed to put little or no active thought into each developing phase of their dialogues. Each seemed to react to the cues of the other as if the lines had all been rehearsed many times before.

One cannot help but wonder why so many of the visits were so ritualistic. Are the nurses and their patients uncommitted to their task of being together? Are they both trying to "get through it" as effortlessly as possible? Do they feel hopeless about the value of their interactions? Does a nurse reach a point at which she makes another visit just because it's in her file, or the family lives nearby, or because she must make a certain quota of visits? Do the clients, often overburdened with public agency visitors, soon learn how to say and do the "right" things so that they can be rid of the visitor and get to other things?

Whatever the reasons, the nurse-actors portrayed their parts of the ritual with an impressive repertoire of skills, rationales, rationalizations, and interactional strategies. At the same time, the patient-actors played their roles with remarkable credibility — displaying acceptance, involvement, cooperation, game-playing, resistance, and token tolerance.

The discovery of hidden plots and purposes mentioned earlier led me to realize that the obvious and explicit elements of the ritual were like the top of an iceberg, deluding an unsophisticated observer or actor into a false sense of security and an inaccurate understanding of what was taking place.

CONCLUSIONS

Although one may question the sample size and observer-participant method of research used in this study, certain of the findings give all of us in community health nursing pause for thought. We might look more closely at how we conduct home visits, what purposes they serve — for ourselves as well as the patient — and then objectively decide if they are ritual or therapy.

REFERENCES

1. Social Welfare Department, State of California. *Primer for Counting Social Benefits and Gains.* Sacramento, Calif., The Department, 1970.
2. Glaser, B. G., and Strauss, A. L. *Awareness of Dying.* Chicago, Aldine Publishing Co., 1965.
3. Conant, L. H. One step beyond. What it means to be involved. In *An Exploration Study of Nurse-Patient Give and Take.* Proceedings of the fifth American Nurses' Association Nursing Research Conference, held at New Orleans, Mar. 3—5, 1969. New York, American Nurses' Association, 1970, pp. 56—62.

34

Sociocultural Factors:
Barriers to Therapeutic Intervention

Donna Aguilera

Communication and understanding between patient and nurse is basic to thera-
peutic intervention. However, sociocultural barriers that inhibit or distort
communication are often not considered. Individuals from many sociocultural
backgrounds come within the community nurse's purview. Awareness and
recognition of different cultural values and norms will enable the community
nurse to prevent these factors from becoming communication barriers. In the
following chapter the author illustrates this point through a situation of
counseling in crisis intervention.

INTRODUCTION AND SUMMARY

Traditional psychotherapeutic techniques have been developed from clinical
observations of the behaviors, attitudes and values of the middle-class culture.
The problems of translating them effectively to meet the needs of other class
cultures have been compounded by the fact that the majority of mental health
professionals are themselves from the middle class. This situation has created
persisting communication barriers in a treatment modality which emphasizes the
need for clear intercommunication.

This paper deals with the need for mental health professionals to be aware
that there are sociocultural barriers to therapeutic intervention. Never has this
been so important as in this current period of transition into community mental
health programs where they will be expected to meet the needs of many cultural
groups. Crisis intervention methodology is suggested as an effective technique of
brief, inexpensive therapy that has been successfully utilized in community
mental health programs. A case study is presented to demonstrate the technique
as used successfully by a nurse-therapist.

Every era has its own unique cliches and catch phrases: the '60s will probably
be remembered for introducing the terms "lack of communication" and "the
generation gap." The student protesters and the hippies say that the "establishment" doesn't understand them, that they don't speak the same language... in
essence, they can't communicate.

Today we live in a very verbal world; we talk, but are we communicating? we
hear, but are we really listening? What I am asking is: are we consciously aware
of what the other person is trying to tell us, not only by his words, his gestures,
his behavior but the gestalt — the *total* verbal and nonverbal messages he is sending? Or, do we consciously or unconsciously create barriers to understanding by
"recoding" the message received to fit our own cultural values and norms?

From *Journal of Psychiatric Nursing*, Vol. 8, No. 5, pp. 14–18, 1970, Charles B. Slack, Inc.,
6900 Grove Road, Thorofare, New Jersey. Reprinted by permission of the publisher.

When an individual with a problem seeks help from someone in the mental health profession his *ability* to make his needs understood can often be the key factor in his receiving the kind of help he needs, wants and understands. The inability to communicate needs and feelings to others can lead to misunderstandings, and the individual's problem remains unresolved. Since psychotherapy is considered primarily a verbal process, communication and understanding between the patient and therapist is essential. If this is lacking, mutual suspicion may be aroused, *with the therapist feeling that the patient isn't trying to solve his problem and the patient feeling that the therapist isn't trying to help him solve his problem.*

It is not the purpose of this paper to discuss *specific* ethnic and cultural factors but rather to explore certain sociocultural factors that can create barriers to therapeutic intervention. As nurses we work with individuals and patients from various sociocultural backgrounds. And perhaps more than others in the helping professions, we are aware of some of the problems that we are confronted with daily. With more understanding and knowledge of how some of the barriers begin we can be more effective nurses.

SOCIOCULTURAL FACTORS

The inability to understand and accept the attitudes and values of those individuals who are not in our same educational, economic and ethnic group is one such barrier. We forget or fail to recognize that the behavior and values that are acceptable and valued in one cultural group may be unacceptable and considered of little value in another, or that what is seen as normal in one would be abnormal in another.[1]

We are all familiar with the codes of ethical conduct that we instill in our young at a very tender age. Certain behaviors are considered acceptable and appropriate and others unacceptable and inappropriate. If two young boys who are considered members of a "middle-class" socioeconomic group have an argument over whose ball or toy it is, they are expected to settle their disagreement like "gentlemen." In other words, they must talk over their differences, learn to share, learn to compromise. This is acceptable behavior in their group. In a lower socioeconomic group the same argument might be settled with a rousing fistfight — with the winner getting the ball or toy. This would not be considered unacceptable or inappropriate behavior for this group.

If we have a patient who has been injured in a fist-fight or street-fight do we immediately stereotype or make a value judgment that this person has been using inappropriate behavior? This could create a barrier to understanding and communicating with members of different cultural groups.

One criticism of traditional psychiatric treatment methods is that its theories and techniques have been developed by professionals who come predominantly from the middle class and, therefore, identify with its cultural values and goals.

Freud's psychoanalytic theories were based on his observations made in a middle-class, continental culture. One of the basic assumptions was that a patient would have enough *time* and *money* for a long course of private therapy sessions.[2]

Studies by Heine (1960), McMahon (1964), and Meyers (1968) were made in an effort to identify those individuals who might be likely to "succeed" in psychodynamic-based therapies. The conclusions reached were that the individual (1) feels a strong need to relate to people, (2) is psychologically oriented, (3) has the intellectual capacity to deal with abstracts, (4) is sophisticated in the jargon of psychiatry, (5) has some idea of the values and goals of psychotherapy, (6) is introspective in nature, (7) is highly motivated to find out why he feels the way he does, and (8) places a high value on self-control. These characterological traits reflect many of those also reported for the middle-class culture. It is for these reasons that individuals of this group will accept the lengthy time and money spent in therapy sessions.[3]

What, then, is left for those individuals who need help with emotional problems but, for any number of reasons, would not meet the above criteria? Let's look at the other end of the continuum and see what this group of individuals might expect, based on the realities of their past experiences, when in need of psychiatric help.

According to the Hollingshead and Redlich (1958) study and the follow-up study by Meyers (1968), the lower sociocultural groups (which they term Class IV or Class V), (1) could not invest the time or the money for extensive psychotherapy; (2) their lower educational level would limit their understanding of psychiatric jargon and psychotherapeutic goals; (3) they are inclined to be more concrete and direct in their thinking; (4) they are not particularly introspective; (5) if they seek help they want it immediately, not six months from now; and (6) they are inclined to view authorities with suspicion and dislike and will only seek their help as a last resort.[4]

The ethnic, racial and occupational groups of people who live in the culturally and economically lower margins of society have been categorized as "lower class." Much of what has been written about them tends to have a negative connotation. In socioeconomic programs there seems to be more interest in what can be done *for* them rather than *with* them. This is particularly true of those programs which have tried to effect a change in their ways of life, since apparently little confidence has been expressed in their ability *to* change. Recently, however, emphasis has been placed on a new theme — that of recognizing their *strengths* rather than their *weaknesses;* of going into their communities and working with them to make changes that *they* feel are necessary.[5]

Currently, Federal legislation has made funding available for the development of community mental health programs and facilities, and professional disciplines have shifted the focus of their activities to include the sociocultural components of mental illness. As a result of the increasing number of programs being maintained by state and local governments, more individuals from the lower sociocultural groups are having their first contact with mental health professionals.

Community psychiatry is, even now, emerging as a new, broad, fluid field. Currently, more emphasis is being placed upon short-term, reality-oriented psychotherapy than on long-term psychoanalytic therapy.

CRISIS INTERVENTION

One type of short-term therapy that has evolved and is rapidly gaining recognition is *crisis intervention*. It is based primarily on the theoretical framework of Caplan (1961) and Lindemann (1956). In brief, their theory is: a person is usually in a state of emotional equilibrium or homeostatic balance. In a crisis, this balance is upset by some precipitating event that has occurred in the individual's life. It could be a situational event, such as a divorce, loss of job, death of a loved one, physical illness, etc.; or a maturational event, such as adolescence, menopause, old age, etc.; or it may be a combination, compounded by the other. For some reason or reasons, the individual is unable to cope with the stress; he becomes immobilized and unable to solve his problem and seeks help.

Therapeutic intervention based on the crisis model is sharply time-limited: the individual is usually seen for no more than six sessions and the focus of the therapy sessions is on the "here and now." The therapist is direct in approach and concentrates on relieving the symptoms of stress as soon as possible. Crisis intervention is directed toward helping the individual solve a specific problem. Major characterological and behavioral changes are not expected, nor are they dealt with in the therapy sessions.

Crisis intervention techniques are not restricted to those of the lower sociocultural levels; however, because of certain inherent factors, it is felt that its techniques are more effective for those at this level than the techniques of other types of therapy. A community mental health center serves individuals from many different sociocultural levels. Psychotherapy for an extended period of time may be too expensive for an average middle-class family and there may be no need if only a crisis situation exists.[6]

Crisis intervention usually involves four phases. The first is the assessment of the individual and his problem. In this phase it is important to find out why the individual came for help at this time. The crisis-precipitating event usually occurs two weeks to several hours prior to the request for help. Questions to be asked are, "What has happened in your life that is different?" "When did it happen?" "How do you feel?"

In this phase it is important to determine if the individual is suicidal or homicidal. Again with direct questioning you ask: "Are you planning to kill yourself?" If so, "how?" "Do you have a specific plan?" "When?" "Where?" If he *does* have a specific plan, time and method available — and it appears lethal — he is referred for hospitalization.

Following the assessment, intervention is planned. In this second phase you determine how the individual perceives the event. Is he being realistic or has he distorted the meaning of the event? How does he see this as affecting his future? . . . his job? . . . his family? You would find out what coping mechanisms he has used in the past to solve his problems — and why they aren't working now. You would also determine who is available as a situational support: Who does the individual trust — someone he feels close to — a friend, a member of his family, someone at work, etc.?

The third phase is the actual intervention. The approach may include any number of techniques and is only limited by the flexibility and creativity of the therapist. It may mean helping the individual to view the crisis in more realistic terms, or to express and ventilate his feelings of anger, guilt, etc. Or it may mean helping him through the grief process if he has had a loss of a significant relationship. It could also mean helping the individual find better and more effective methods of coping with stress.

The final phase is resolution of the crisis and planning with the individual the methods for coping with future stressful events. If he has increased his problem-solving skills while resolving the crisis, he should be functioning at a higher level of equilibrium than he was prior to the crisis.

As a nurse-therapist at the Benjamin Rush Center in Los Angeles, a community mental health center that uses crisis-intervention techniques, I have found them to be an extremely effective treatment modality. The following case study illustrates how I helped a mother and her daughter resolve their crisis, using these crisis-intervention techniques, even though we were from different sociocultural backgrounds.

CASE STUDY

Mrs. D (age 42) and her teen-age daughter Becky (15) came to the center upon the recommendation of a neighbor and asked for help with a problem. Mrs. D looked much older than her years and was obviously extremely depressed. She walked slowly into my office, sat with slumped posture in the chair, and would not maintain eye-contact with me. Her appearance was one of dejection and hopelessness. Becky was a slim, attractive young girl who seemed alert and intelligent, but it was obvious that she was uncomfortable, tense and nervous.

When I asked Mrs. D why she and Becky had come to the center she looked at Becky and began to cry. She lost complete control and kept sobbing. She was finally able to say that Becky wanted to leave home and live with her Aunt Marge. I could get no further information from Mrs. D, as she was unable to control her crying and talk coherently. I said to Mrs. D that I wanted her to see the doctor at the center; that he would give her some medication to help her control herself. I said Becky could stay and talk with me and perhaps she could tell me what had brought them to the center.

I took Mrs. D for a medical consultation with the doctor on call; he gave her a mild tranquilizer. I then took her to the restroom so she could wash her face and lie down in the lounge afterwards while I talked with Becky. (Therapist's note: This maneuver served two purposes: first, it showed Mrs. D that I was concerned for her and that I wanted to provide some immediate help; and, second, it indicated that I was accepting her behavior, thus establishing a basis for rapport.)

When I returned to talk with Becky I asked her why her mother was so upset. She replied, "It's probably me — I had another fight with my stepfather last night." She added rather defiantly, "He isn't really my stepfather; they aren't married — he just lives with us." I asked what had started the fight. She said she was in the kitchen with her mother, drying the dishes and trying to talk with her. She was trying to explain that the reason she wanted to go to live with her Aunt Marge was that she could go to a different school. Her "stepfather" walked into the kitchen and told her to open him another can of beer. She said, "In a minute . . . I'm talking to Mom. He said, "I want it *now!*" and then he slapped her. She hit him back and then ran from the house. When she came back her mother was crying and said, "I don't understand you, maybe someone else can." She then called the crisis center and was told to come in with Becky the next day.

I asked Becky *why* she wanted to go to a different school. She hesitated briefly and then began to explain. She said her older brother, Steve, 17, and her sister, Linda, 16, went to the same school. This was Becky's first year there and both Steve and Linda had very bad records at school. Both had had problems at school — Steve because of drugs and Linda because of drugs and "boys." I asked Becky what she meant about "boys"; she said that Linda had had one illegitimate child and one illegal abortion — that she was "just wild." She went on to say that "Everyone at school . . . the teachers and the kids . . . all look at me and treat me as if I were just like Linda and Steve! I'm not! I'm *me!* I don't want to be like Linda, but it's so hard . . . with everyone thinking and expecting me to be!"

I asked why she wanted to live with her Aunt Marge, explaining that she could transfer to another school and start "fresh" and still live at home. She said, "It's my stepfather — I can't stand him, he's made passes at me, tries to touch me . . . I'm afraid of him." I asked if she had told her mother this and she said, "Yes, but she doesn't believe me — she doesn't want to believe me." She added, "But it isn't only him — I don't want to be around the crowd Steve and Linda have at the house."

I asked if her Aunt Marge had room for her and wanted her to live with her. She said, "Yes! She is younger than mother; she only has one son, Bob, 10 years old; she has a nice house and she is a good Catholic. You can ask her — she told me she wants me to live with her."

I told Becky I wanted to see how her mother was feeling to see if she could come in for the remainder of the session. Mrs. D was much calmer and apparently in control of herself, so she rejoined us.

I explained to Mrs. D what Becky had given as the reasons why she wanted to leave home and asked if she felt these were valid reasons. Mrs. D sighed, wiped her eyes and said, "Yes — what she told you is true. I guess I've failed all my children. I've been a terrible mother; I don't blame her for wanting to live with my sister."

I asked if her sister wanted Becky to live with her and she answered, "Yes, I just don't want to *give* Becky up . . . she is the only one that hasn't given me any trouble." I said, "You wouldn't really be giving her up — you would just be giving her a chance to maybe turn out differently from Steve and Linda."

I asked how far apart they would be if Becky were to live with her sister. Mrs. D said about thirty minutes by bus. I asked Becky that if she did live with her aunt would she still visit her mother on the weekends and holidays. She very flatly answered, "No, I just want to get away." Mrs. D began to cry again and, since the hour was up, I told them that somehow we would have to arrive at some kind of compromise. I told them that before they came back the following week they should try to talk *with* each other rather than *at* each other, and then maybe when we met again we could find a solution to their problem. They agreed. Mrs. D left with medication to last her until the next therapy session, and the exchange number where she or Becky could reach me at any time if an emergency arose.

The next week Mrs. D and Becky came to the center accompanied by her Aunt Marge. Both Becky and her mother seemed to be more relaxed. Marge was an attractive woman in her middle thirties. I told them how pleased I was that they had thought to include her in our session, since she too was involved in solving their problem.

I asked how their week together had been, and if they had been able to come up with any ideas we could work on together. Surprisingly, Mrs. D started talking first and said, "I know I was being very selfish last week . . . trying to keep Becky with me. I know she is growing up, and that it *isn't* good for her at our house . . . but she is my daughter and I love her. But Marge *can* do more for her now than I can. I'll give her up." Marge immediately spoke up, saying, "Anita, you aren't *giving* her to me . . . you are only letting her live with me for awhile. She is *your* daughter! It is just that I love her and she deserves a decent break . . . I understand how she feels."

I spoke up in order to refocus on the problem and to end a possible "debate." I looked at Becky and said, "Becky, how do *you* feel right now?" She looked at me with tears in her eyes and said, "I know Mom loves me; for the first time I *know* she loves me. I know she doesn't understand me . . . but she loves me. I'll call her every day if only she will let me live with Aunt Marge!" I then asked her, "Becky, do *you* love your mother?" For the first time Becky looked directly at her mother and said, "Yes, I love you — but I don't understand *you*, either!"

Needless to add, tears began to flow — from mother, daughter and Aunt Marge. I will also admit that my eyes weren't too dry at that moment. Objectivity is necessary — it's true, but maybe sometimes we *should* become emotionally involved with our patients — in order to see their world, their life, as *they* live it.

I too am a mother and I can imagine how I would feel if one of our sons told me he wanted to leave our home because he was unhappy. Mrs. D was experiencing a loss; I would also experience a loss. Would I be able to withstand the stress . . . or would I go into crisis? No matter what sociocultural background we are from we must always look at those three critical factors that can decide the outcome of a stressful situation: One, how does the individual perceive the event; Two, does he have adequate coping skills; Three, are there available situational supports?

To be able to help those individuals from a background dissimilar to ours we must try to understand that, though they may look differently, talk differently or have different cultural values and standards — as nurses, if we are aware of these differences, perhaps we can overcome some of the barriers and learn to *communicate* with them . . . instead of just *talking* to them.

REFERENCES

1. Aguilera, Donna C., Messick, Janice M., and Farrell, Marlene S. *Crisis Intervention: Theory and Methodology.* St. Louis: The C. V. Mosby Co., in press.
2. *Ibid.*
3. *Ibid.*
4. *Ibid.*
5. *Ibid.*
6. *Ibid.*

ADDITIONAL REFERENCES

Caplan, Gerald. *An Approach to Community Mental Health.* New York: Grune and Stratton, Inc., 1961.

Hollingshead, A. B., and Redlich, F. C. *Social Class and Mental Illness.* New York: John Wiley & Sons, Inc., 1958.

Lindemann, Erich. "The meaning of crisis in individual and family." *Teachers College Record,* Vol. 57, No. 3 (1956).

Meyers, Jerome K., Bean, L. L., and Pepper, M. P. *A Decade Later: A Follow-up of Social Class and Mental Illness.* New York: John Wiley & Sons, Inc., 1968.

35

The Interview

Whether in the home, clinic, school or other setting, interaction between patient and nurse must be purposeful and therapeutic. These conversations require structure and planning to avoid the pitfall of haphazard and fruitless communication. A basic tool to accomplish this is the interview, which, if used skillfully, can facilitate effective data-gathering, assessment and evaluation. This chapter offers a pragmatic approach to the principles and practice of interviewing.

"If interviewing were an art, it could spring fullblown from instinct and impulse. But it is a professional skill, about which a body of knowledge exists, which can be learned and creatively adapted in individualized ways to serve a variety of purposes."[1]

The interview is a significant part of the health discipline, as well as of other areas of professional contact with the public. Some of the basic tenets of interviewing are appropriate to public health, and their application can help in building skills for the nurse and other workers who judiciously employ them in the day-to-day conduct of their jobs. Though space limitations prohibit an exploration in depth, an examination of some of the more salient aspects of interviewing is offered in the belief that the subject is always of timely interest.

Definition. Among various commentators on the subject there appears to be consensus on definition. It is perhaps best stated by Greenhill,[2] who indicates that interviewing involves a purposeful process of communication between individuals and that communication is "the act of transmitting facts, feelings, and meanings by words, gestures or other action."

This concept goes beyond the more-or-less classic view of interviewing in which a series of preplanned questions is followed in methodical order to achieve a given end. While a place may still exist for such — in opinion or rating polls for instance — the interview as conducted by a professional health worker is considered a much more personal activity. It carries with it a responsibility not only to faithfully pursue the objective, but to establish and perpetuate a close patient-professional relationship as a foundation for future service.

Further, it is not always a one-time effort, but often a continuing operation requiring days or even months to realize goals. However, each segment of the interview may be treated much like the entire process in that basic components of interviewing and elements of communication may be effectively applied.

COMPONENTS OF INTERVIEWING

Purpose. Every interview has a purpose or goal, whether immediately apparent or not. The professional seeking information has a definite goal in mind. The

From *Currents in Public Health,* April 1966, Ross Laboratories, Columbus, Ohio. Reprinted by permission of the publisher.

professional offering service may quickly establish a need on the part of an individual for which a goal of information or action is desired. A patient may present himself with a problem and, in stating it, establish a purpose. It is most often the responsibility of the professional to guide the interview toward realization of the goal.

Setting. A choice of setting is not always available. Frequently, effectiveness is decimated by unavoidable distractions as are found, for instance, in the home. Efforts toward reducing the possibility of interruptions and distractions should be made before interviewing commences. A room which can be closed off or even an automobile will sometimes provide all the privacy that is needed.

In the health department there are often facilities where interviewing may proceed more formally and without interruption. This formal atmosphere seems to produce more valuable interviews. Greenhill comments, "the more the formal setting is approximated, the better are the returns."[2]

Objectivity. The understanding of meanings, instead of simple recording of words or responses, is the interviewing skill some call objectivity. It entails a conscious effort and is one of the important elements acquired through experience. It is tempered with a refusal on the part of the interviewer to permit his own attitudes, beliefs or prejudices to influence the objective interpretation of responses or comments.

Objectivity includes an effort to pursue a subject until the meaning is clear in the interviewer's mind. If such is not feasible, due to time limitations or possible deleterious effect on the course of the interview, interpretation for the sake of entering notes should be avoided. If any doubt exists, objectivity would be better served by recording that an interviewer was uncertain of meaning.

Rapport. Successful interviews are nearly always marked by a degree of rapport built mainly on mutual consideration and respect. The professional must develop it individually with each interviewee. In addition to a friendly greeting, courtesy during the discussion and sincerity throughout are other ways in which essential rapport may be achieved.

"The client must be seen as a unique individual, not as a stereotype. It is not the 'unwed mother,' the 'delinquent,' the 'VD case,' the 'hard-to-reach,' the 'mental case,' whom we see in an interview. It is a person with a name who must be understood not as a 'case,' or a statistic, but as a human being who has certain problems which exist for good reason."[1] Thus, there is a personal aspect to the interview, involving consideration and respect for the individual and for resolution of his problem.

Confidence in the interview process, and in the interviewer, assists in achieving rapport. One of the jobs of the professional is to convey, through skillful use of words and actions, "the idea that the interview has a structure or plan aimed toward a problem solving resolution and is not just a haphazard conversation."[1]

Additionally, consideration and respect are fostered by obtaining and providing sensible information. To put it another way, "Information given or asked for should be only that information which will clarify meaning, focus content and contribute to accomplishing the purpose of the interview."[1]

Attitude. Wolff[3] states that attitude is an important component of the interview and "that in any study of interviewing skills, we need to take a thorough and detached look at our own attitudes." She makes the point that because attitudes are so much a part of each individual, the individual may feel that they are the only valid attitudes for others as well as himself.

The threat to objectivity by the professional worker's projecting attitudes into an interview is self-evident. While professional aloofness, or dismissing the possibility of one's attitudes becoming involved, may lessen the chances of injecting them, it is an unrealistic practice and often holds more serious consequences by weakening rapport. Self-examination and an awareness of attitudes are necessary to achieve objectivity and to avoid incorporation of the professional's attitudes into the interview.

Beginning, Middle and End. A successful means of initiating an interview is often simply allowing the person interviewed to talk out his feelings or to state a problem his own way. The early portion of an interview should also establish an endpoint to that segment. Progression toward this ending is facilitated if it is in the minds of both parties.

The middle is used to pinpoint a problem or issue, and suggest ways in which it can be handled. Quite often a problem is too comprehensive for resolution within the limits set. In these cases, attempts should be made at identifying a part of the problem and attacking it, thus rendering manageable at least one portion of a problem which seemed entirely unmanageable at the outset.

When the initially established termination point has been reached, it is best to try to end that segment of the interview. Going beyond frequently leads to confusion on the part of the interviewee and may tend to decrease the value of the interview itself. Acknowledging new or additional thoughts, and indicating that they may be discussed at a definite future time, can be effective in meeting this situation.

The summation is a useful tool with which to terminate an interview segment. Summation allows both parties opportunity to review what has been discussed, fortifies comprehension of results, and sets the stage for future interviewing.

ELEMENTS OF COMMUNICATION

In order that facts, feelings and meanings may be transmitted, an interaction of communication between at least two persons must occur. Most authorities believe that there is a science to this interaction, with attendant skills which can be learned and successfully applied to the interview process.

Initiative. Initiative is given to the interviewee by prompting him to begin the discussion. Interruptions, except for assistance in word finding or otherwise urging continuance, are avoided during this time. The interviewee is provided every opportunity to express a problem or state a situation in his own words.

Approach. Mainly, an indirect approach is utilized through open-end or non-leading questions and statements. Leaving the way open for an interviewee to express himself is an important device. It encourages his greatest contribution to the communication interaction. The nonleading question or statement has its obvious benefits in that it elicits only the interviewee's own thoughts.

Specificity. In most cases, an interview is concerned with specifics — certain problems, situations, happenings. The professional should lead the interview where necessary along specific lines, avoiding what the individual usually does, or what his general feelings are.

Singleness of Idea. Covering only one idea or thought at one time is a logical procedure within the interview. It provides an orderly process in the elucidation of facts and feelings, and assists in determining meanings clearly. Questions involving two or more thoughts would require two or more answers, with the result that just as many pathways would be opened. Phrasing questions within the reference of one answer is important in effective communication.

Language. Language differences present a whole new set of problems to the professional. An interpreter is usually the only recourse in this situation. But even when the participants speak the same language, there are important considerations to be made. A fine line appears to exist between acceptable use of the vernacular and personal affront to the interviewee. Adopting local or ethnic words and phraseology may possibly seem to be the best maneuver in promoting understanding. Usually, however, the professional is from a different background which is immediately apparent and it would thus be unnatural and possibly patronizing to assume such liberties. Under these conditions, the best of intentions could result in a disaster of misunderstanding. Until a high degree of rapport exists, the use of common, simple language is preferred.

Handling the Pause. The course of most interviews is marked by pauses, especially in the early portion. As interviewer and interviewee try to understand each other, consider ideas and thoughts, and seek to become involved in the communication interaction, there are invariably periods of silence. The interviewer must learn to treat these as a necessary part of the process and not be uncomfortable in them. If the pause occurs while the client is expressing himself or responding, it is usually followed by clarification of thought and valuable additional information. Interrupting the silence would destroy the opportunity to obtain this material. On the other hand, if a pause is after a question or remark by the interviewer, it may be that the client did not understand. This calls for rephrasing or restatement to assist him, but again not of the type that attempts to supply answers for the client.

In any event, verbal activity for the sole purpose of filling a void in the interview should be avoided. Meadow and Gass[4] suggest that "if the 'talk-ratio' is not decidedly in favor of the [interviewee] it is more than likely that the interview may have little significance. When the interviewer is able to relax, allow the interviewee time to think and tolerate the necessary pauses, productive material will start to flow."[4]

PUTTING PRINCIPLES INTO PRACTICE

There are innumerable ways in which the basic principles so far discussed may be put into practice. Some suggestions and examples may be helpful in illustrating their application.

Verbal Techniques. In beginning an interview, the interviewee is encouraged to express himself freely. If, for instance, the purpose of the interview is to offer prenatal clinic services, an opening might be "Do you have any questions about pregnancy or labor that I may help you with?" This provides the client with an opportunity for expression and establishes a base for bringing out needs and wants. On the other hand, a statement such as "I'm here to enroll you in our prenatal clinic," offers no such opportunity. It presupposes a need, which the interviewee may resent, and may place her on the defensive.

Once the interviewee has talked about her condition, clues as to her needs and desires may be picked up, thus developing a more complete picture. The person may have made reference to a pain. The professional notes this and later says, "Tell me about your pain." The open-ended statement as used here permits the initiative to remain with the client, and usually additional information is obtained. If the professional would have said, "Where is this pain?" or "Is it bad?" or similar remarks, the client would have been directed to a simple, or yes or no reply, and the professional would have had to restart the interview. Also, consider how confused the client would have been if the interviewer had said, "How often do you have this pain and does it seem to come on in the morning or evening or after meals?" This would have required that the interviewee sift through her past experiences and come to some conclusions, which may not be representative of her true condition, just to try to answer the question.

With elucidation of the client's feelings, a next step could be to suggest that a doctor's advice would be helpful. The interviewee would probably agree and this would provide the opening to introduce the clinic services.

A statement such as "Perhaps by the end of our time today we can discuss how the prenatal clinic can help you," would set the limits of the interview.

Vander Zanden and Vander Zanden[5] offer another example of putting principles into practice. They state, with respect to the leading question concept, that there are degrees of subtlety in this area. For instance, the question, "You feel better now after your medicine, don't you?" is obviously leading. Some, attempting to avoid directing a reply, might phrase it in this manner, "Would you say that you are feeling better now after your medicine?" But this is also a leading question. "By answering *yes,* the patient is merely agreeing with the language of the question in that it subtly suggests that an affirmative answer is anticipated and that he is expected to feel *better.* It would be more difficult to reply *no* since this would seem to contradict the question."[5] One way to render this query nonleading is to ask simply, "How are you feeling after taking your medicine?" This form promotes the desired non-directed response and assists in ascertaining the patient's true feelings.

Greenhill[2] suggests that "interviewing should be as open-ended as possible." With this method, statements by the interviewer do not seem to be closed off or appear to sound final. The client is encouraged to continue if such interjections as "You were saying," or "You said" are utilized instead of complete sentences which tend to fill in facts for the client. "Open-endedness," Greenhill adds, "seems to break down most often when the interviewer seeks to reassure the patient by saying, 'You're going to be all right,' or 'You've got a good doctor,' or 'After a few more treatments things will be all right'." While indeed these may be reassuring comments, they often make it difficult for a client to reveal what he is anxious or concerned about.

If reassurance is desirable, it can be done without thwarting the progress of an interview. "In following the principle of open-endedness, the nurse might better say, 'After a few more treatments it ought to go better, but let's talk about it. . . .' Thus, the way is left open."[2]

Attention must be given to attitude and objectivity if the interview is to be successful. But they can be readily overlooked when a type of statement utilized is one prefaced by phrases such as these: "I can understand how you feel, but . . ." and "You're right, but don't you think. . . ." Wolff,[6] in characterizing this approach, says that "kindness of manner and intent is not enough, it must be supplemented by a willingness to understand, an effort to help the patient express his concern, an attempt to see matters as he sees them." It would be easy for the interviewer's attitudes to creep in with remarks of this nature, and objectivity would consequently suffer. Better perhaps are lead-ins such as "Tell me about . . ." or "Is there anything further you would like to say about . . ." when attempting to explore subjects more completely.

Nonverbal Techniques. Little has been written concerning nonverbal techniques. Many of these fall into the area of good sense and courtesy, their appropriateness possibly unstated because they are not solely a part of interviewing. Such things as clean, neat attire and punctuality could certainly have no adverse effect on the course of an interview. Being at ease in the surroundings, and creating the same atmosphere for the client by being natural and showing true concern are valuable aids to a successful session.

Note-taking, a necessary part of most interviewing, should be as brief as possible. Lengthy entries tend to creat suspicion on the part of the interviewee that what he is saying may be recorded *verbatim*. He may then become more guarded in responding or expressing himself. Copious note-taking also requires that the interviewer's attention be focused away from the interviewee.

Other nonverbal techniques such as leaning forward to show interest, looking directly at the person while talking or listening and not permitting attention to be diverted by distractions occurring during the interview are all part of putting principles into practice.

The Intangible Aspect. Most authorities agree that interviewing skill and techniques can be taught and learned. It is through their meaningful application, though, that the interviewer reaps the most benefit from them. The value of any acquired skill often depends on the knowledge of when to apply it. Such knowledge is best gained through study and experience. The capacity for "words, gestures and other action" develops in the individual worker as experience is gained with exposure to the complexities of interviewing and as he becomes a student of that science.

In connection with the latter, the following bibliography has been compiled and presented here as a suggested reference list to those who would explore the subject further in text. Though admittedly incomplete, it represents much that is known about one of the professional worker's most important tools — the interview.

BIBLIOGRAPHY

Bingham, W. V., and Moore, B. V.: *How to Interview*, 4th rev. ed., Harper, 1959.

Fenlason, A. F.: *Essentials in Interviewing*, rev. ed., Harper & Row, 1962.

Bermosk, L. S.: *Interviewing in Nursing*, New York, MacMillan Co., 1964.

Fenlason, A.: *Interviewing in Psychiatry*, New York, Harper & Row, 1962.

Sidney, E., and Brown, M.: *The Skills of Interviewing*, Tavistock Publications, 1961.

National Opinion Research Center: *Interviewing for NORC*, Denver, 1947.

Russell Sage Foundation Library: Interviewing & Case Recording, *Bulletin #127*, New York, October, 1934.

Hyman, H. H.: *Interviewing in Social Research*, Chicago, University of Chicago Press, 1954.

Rogers, C. R.: *Client-Centered Therapy*, Boston, Houghton Mifflin Co., 1951.

Brady, D.: *Counseling*, Washington, D.C., Catholic University of America Press, 1954.

Payne, S. LeB.: *The Art of Asking Questions*, Princeton, Princeton University Press, 1951.

Counseling and Interviewing Adult Students, Washington, D.C., National Assoc. of Public School Adult Eductors, 1960.

Kahn, R. L.: *The Dynamics of Interviewing, Theory-Technique and Cases*, New York, John Wiley & Sons, 1957.

Narramore, C. M.: *Psychology of Counseling*, Zonderman, 1960.

Tyler, L. E.: *The Work of the Counselor*, ed. 2, Appleton, 1961.

Arbuckle, D. S., in *Counseling, An Introduction*, Allyn, ed., Prentice Hall, 1961.

Trout, B. E.: *Interviewing for Staff Selection in Public Welfare*, Washington, D.C., U.S. Dept. of Health, Education and Welfare, Social Security Administration — Children's Bureau, 1956.

Richardson, L. A.: *Interviewing, Its Forms and Functions*, New York, Basic Books, 1965.

Barrett, A. M.: *Interviewing, Its Principles and Methods*, New York, Family Welfare Association of America, 1960.

Newman, R. G.: *Interviewing in Psychiatry*, Washington, D.C., Washington School of Psychiatry, 1964.

Family Service Association of America: *Interviews — Interviewers and Interviewing in Social Case Work*, New York, Family Welfare Association of America, 1931.

REFERENCES

1. Weissman, I. G.: *Calif. Health* 22:201, May 15, 1965.
2. Greenhill, M. H.: *Amer. J. Nurs.* 56:1259, 1956.
3. Wolff, I. S.: *Nurs. Outlook* 6:267, 1958.
4. Meadow, L., and Gass, G. Z.: *Amer. J. Nurs.* 63:97, 1963.
5. Vander Zanden, J. W., and Vander Zanden, M. V.: *Nurs. Outlook* 11:743, 1963.
6. Wolff, I. S.: *Nurs. Outlook* 6:320, 1958.

36
Talking to Patients about Death

Jeanne Quint Benoliel

Grief, loss, pain, helplessness, hopelessness, life, death — these are matters that concern patients and their families, yet are topics that are often difficult for the nurse to discuss. Death, in particular, tends to be an uncomfortable subject and one that many nurses would rather avoid. In the hospital and at home the patient and family need help in facing and dealing with death. The when and how of communicating with patients about death is presented practically and concisely by this author.

The nursing literature in recent years has emphasized the need for nurses to listen to patients and families and talk with them about matters of serious concern. Death is one such topic, but knowing when and how to talk about death with a patient presents a problem to many nurses. Of the several reasons for the difficulty, perhaps the first and foremost one is the fact that people in our society have in general not learned to talk about personal death with any degree of comfort.

Although fear of death is probably as old as mankind, in modern industrial societies (perhaps especially in the United States) human death has come more and more to be regarded as a phenomenon to be controlled, denied, or hidden. As the dying have been progressively segregated from the remainder of society, the living have had little opportunity to become psychologically prepared for death, either their own or that of someone close to them. More than that, the living have learned that death is a subject to be avoided in conversation and, if it is discussed at all, euphemistic terminology such as "He passed away" is required. As a result of these societal customs and practices, nurses and patients come to their interactions with each other without much experience in talking openly about the meaning of personal death.

When a nurse and a patient try to talk together, they are likely to find that conversation about dying precipitates unexpected emotional reactions such as sadness or fear or anger. To their surprise, and sometimes their embarrassment, these unanticipated feelings cannot always be controlled and may even be expressed in behaviors that are personally disturbing to one or both of them. Thus the lack of an adequate socialization for talking about death, in combination with the high value attached in this society to keeping emotions under tight control, serves to prevent the nurse and the patient from moving easily and comfortably into open conversation about the patient's death and the many meanings it may carry for him.

In addition to the inhibitions that come from a general cultural conditioning, open talk about dying carries a personal threat of extreme importance for anyone

From *Nursing Forum*, Vol. 9, No. 3, 1970, pp. 255–268. Reprinted with permission from Nursing Publications, Inc., 194-B Kinderkamack Road, Park Ridge, New Jersey 07656.

whose span of time has been foreshortened by an illness that is life-threatening in nature. The reported finding that patients being monitored by cardiac pace-makers are prone to deny any fear or apprehension about having heart disease makes a good deal of sense when one recognizes that these people are constantly being reminded that the threat of death is never far away.[1] This finding is in keeping with Ross's observation that the use of denial by patients tends to occur whenever the threat of death is close and real for them, whereas, if given the opportunity, they can often talk quite openly about the subject during periods of remission.[2] Ross also notes that individuals with strong needs to control their lives experience a high degree of psychological threat from fatal illness and respond with increased efforts to control the environment, usually alienating other people in the process.

Although loss of human existence is the primary threat carried by fatal illness, it is also true that diseases are psychologically disturbing because they are associated with specific types of dying. According to one study forty-nine out of eighty children with juvenile diabetes mellitus reported fears about having insulin reactions, and twenty-eight of them said specifically that they were afraid of becoming unconscious and of dying because help might not be available.[3] Bard makes the point that persons with cancer must be regarded as people under a special and severe form of stress because the disease is perceived as loathesome, pain-producing, and progressively disabling.[4] He believes that whenever cancer is suspected or found, the individual's responses include a reactivation of unresolved issues many of which are unconscious, and there follows a reorganization of psychological defenses such that the individual establishes a belief-system to explain why this terrible event has happened to him. The two commonly observed patterns are self-blame and projection, that is, blame of others or outside forces.

That the diagnosis of cancer leads to pervasive anxiety was clearly evident in my investigation of the processes by which women adjust to having a breast removed because of malignancy. The findings also showed clearly that anxiety about cancer is not limited to those for whom the diagnosis has been made; the anxiety permeates all of us. One important consequence is that the person living with cancer often finds himself in a kind of social isolation during a time when he is most in need of human relationships.[5] The feelings of pessimism felt by the public about cancer are shared by doctors and nurses and, in the case of nurses, may be heightened because they have more direct and frequent exposure to cancer patients for whom cure is no longer a possibility. It was clearly evident in the mastectomy study that by talking openly with persons who have cancer a person is brought close to his own fears about malignancy. To experience this kind of emotional discomfort is not easy, and this reality may well be one of the crucial factors that prevents nurses from engaging in conversation about delicate and tension-producing subjects.

In addition to personal threat, the nurse is often hampered in conversation because of the professional threat imposed by a patient's dying. A nurse's

avoidance of personalized interactions with dying patients is readily understandable when one recognizes the stresses and strains that are imposed by attempts
to meet simultaneously the two somewhat conflicting goals of practice — to provide personalized comfort and relief from suffering and to prolong and protect
life. This threat is especially high in any setting where the work requires nurses
to deal with death on a more or less regular basis.[6] Moreover, many nurses have
not had educational experiences that would have helped them to develop constructive ways of coping with this difficult dilemma. The recent emphasis in
schools of nursing on the psychological care of patients has made the younger
generation in nursing sensitive to the problem, but many of this group have not
learned to cope with conversational difficulties any more successfully than have
other nurses. One reason is that educational programs in nursing vary widely in
the caliber of training that is offered for professional conversation about topics
that cause the nurse to experience emotional conflict affecting both personal
and professional values.[7]

Despite the problems involved, there are growing numbers of nurses who are
skilled in talking in meaningful ways with patients and families as they live
through the many psychosocial crises associated with living and dying. The guidelines that these nurses use in deciding when and why to talk with patients about
death come from the expanding body of literature concerned with the psychosocial meanings of illness, grief, and adaptation to change.

Common to many of these writings is the recognition that physical disorder,
social change, or serious illness requires a psychological reorganization of the
individual's perception of himself. Such a reorganization of identity takes place
through stages, and the process of grieving is one component of the adaptation
that is required.

Nursing publications in recent years have given much attention to the stages
of grief as they have relevance for nursing actions and interventions in the care
of those in the terminal stages of living. The process of adaptation to having
cancer quite obviously includes the need to mourn for oneself, but so does the
adaptation to any chronic illness. Crate suggests that the adaptation to any
chronic disease takes place through five stages: (1) shock and disbelief during
which denial is a commonly seen pattern of behavior; (2) gradual awareness of
the reality of the changed condition by expressions of guilt and anger; (3) reorganization of relationships with other people; (4) resolution of the loss through
active grieving; and finally, (5) a reorganization of identity to incorporate the
changes that have taken place.[8] Crate proposes that the patient's adaptation to
his illness can be facilitated if the nurses who are providing his care can modify
their patterns of interaction to allow him to experience the emotional impact of
each stage in a nonjudgmental way.

Butler has suggested that although death is a significant feature in the psychology and psychopathology of the elderly and also in younger persons with
fatal illness, we know very little about this phenomenon largely because

psychiatrists and psychologists, unable to deal with their own unconscious concerns about death, have essentially avoided the area.[9] He proposes that the biological fact of approaching death, a reality tied to the process of aging, provokes the individual to engage in a process of thinking he calls the "life-review" — a reorganization of past events into some kind of gestalt in anticipation of forthcoming death.

Ross proposes that dying in the psychological sense takes place in five sequential, though overlapping, stages.[10] By understanding these stages and the behaviors that are likely to appear during each of them, the nurse has available a general guideline with some indicators as to when patients are likely to want to talk about death and when they are likely to avoid such discussion.

While in denial (the first stage), the patient's words and manner convey the message that he is not going to die even though he may have been told that he has a serious illness. With the second stage of anger comes a shift in reaction and behavior from that of "It isn't true" to a more hostile manifestation of "Why me?" The first stage is relatively easy for nurses because the patient does not want to talk about death and usually behaves as though everything is fine. In sharp contrast, the second stage tends to be difficult for nurses because the patient displaces his anger freely and generally finds fault with everything and everybody, often for no apparent reason. Next comes the stage of bargaining, during which the individual tries to make a deal with God (or sometimes with the doctor) to have his death postponed until a certain time or until a certain purpose is achieved.

The fourth stage begins when the person starts to sense his many losses and to assimilate the reality of what is happening. Psychologically speaking, the person with terminal illness has to cope with two kinds of depression — a reactive one in response to past losses, including his inability to function in important social roles, and a preparatory depression that must take account of the total loss that lies ahead for him. The reactive depression is a mixture of sadness, guilt, and shame, and the person can be helped to deal with these reactions in constructive ways by being allowed to talk about what is happening and to find solutions for the real problems that concern him. In contrast, the preparatory depression tends to be characterized by sadness and silence, and it is here that touch and quiet presence may be more helpful to the patient than efforts to engage him in conversation. Sitting quietly with him and holding his hand, even for only a few moments each day, may be a tremendous comfort to him. In the hospital, the nurse may serve another important function by protecting the patient from visitors who try to cheer him up instead of allowing him to go through the inner experience of coming to terms with the successes and failures of his life.

The stage of acceptance comes when the patient reaches a point of being almost devoid of feeling and when he draws quietly into himself and waits for death to come. Not all individuals reach the point of acceptance. In the case of some, the need to control is so strong that they must fight until the very end has come. Other individuals do not reach acceptance because they are prevented by other people from experiencing the full emotional impact of fear, rage, and sadness and of assimilating the reality of forthcoming death into their personal realities. Social isolation is another deterrent. Butler suggests that for those persons who are deeply affected by being cut off from social ties severe affective and behavioral consequences appear to occur when the process of life-review takes place in social isolation.[11]

Children and young people with life-threatening illness are especially prone to severance from meaningful relationships because those around them (parents, siblings, friends, doctors, and nurses) are unable to cope effectively with their own anxiety and feelings of helplessness and hopelessness. In a very real sense, the young person with a terminal illness is in double jeopardy because he so often loses the intimate relationships that he needs at a time when he is losing the most precious of his possessions — life itself. When placed in a context of social isolation, he is also effectively blocked from expressing and dealing with the reactions of sadness, guilt, shame, anger, and hostility that are part of the process of grieving. Here is one example of the consequences. A five-year-old boy was in the final stages of leukemia. His mother was obviously upset and spent most of the time crying while she was with him. On one occasion while she was out of the room, the boy told the nurse that he wished that his mother did not cry so much. In his words, "When she cries all the time, it doesn't give me a chance to cry."

It seems clear to me that if we as nurses want to be maximally helpful to patients with life-threatening illnesses, we must learn how to talk with people who are sometimes angry and guilty, sometimes withdrawn and sad, and sometimes happy and carefree in manner. Talking with cheerful patients usually is not difficult because they so often give us the approval we need. Hostile patients are much harder to work with because they so freely dispense disapproval instead of praise. We are often deterred from making the effort to talk with depressed patients because moods are contagious, and we try to avoid situations that trigger us into our own (often unresolved) feelings of loss and grief and sorrow.

If we truly want to find out what is on the patient's mind at any moment, we must be willing to risk being confronted with our own feelings of discomfort and dismay and to learn positive ways of coping with our negative feelings. Instead of denying our anger or running away from our helplessness, we should recognize and accept the reality of these feelings in ourselves. More than that, we need support and understanding and guidance from another helping person as we go through the experience of developing our conversational skills. Especially is this kind of help needed when the nurse is trying to learn how to carry on conversations with patients who talk about death in ways that cause her to feel helpless or panicky. I would be remiss if I were to convey the impression that conversing with patients at the level of their basic concerns is an easy matter.

When a patient unexpectedly asks the nurse, "Am I going to die?" a multitude of reactions and thoughts are triggered in her. With panic comes the thought,

"What shall I do or say?" With helplessness comes the notion, "I just want to get out of here." With fear comes the thought, "What if I say the wrong thing." Let me offer some observations about this type of situation and some suggestions for coping with it.

Any time that a patient spontaneously introduces the topic of his dying, whether by a question or by a statement, he is telling you that he desperately needs to establish communication with another human being and that he needs help in coping with what is happening to him. He is not really asking you to answer his question; rather, he is pleading with you to listen because something is bothering him. When students ask what they should do when they find themselves in such a situation, I offer the following suggestions.

If you are standing, draw up a chair and sit down. This action serves several positive functions. It provides you with support if you feel as though your legs are about to collapse. It also provides the patient with support because you are now in the position of being two human beings trying to cope together with his problems, instead of you being the professional towering over him and taking control. The action also tells him that you heard his call for help and are sufficiently concerned to take the time to listen.

If you do not know what to say, do not say anything. Usually the person who has spontaneously introduced the topic of his death will continue to talk freely because something is on his mind that is troublesome. If he has trouble getting started again, a simple open-ended question can often serve as an opener — for instance, "Mr. Jones, you seem upset by something. What is the matter?" It may be that he is worried about his family or concerned about money, or he may not understand what the doctor said and may want additional information. Only by taking time to listen to him can you find out what the problem is from his point of view.

The stage of illness, the patient's knowledge about his disease, and his accustomed pattern of engaging in conversations all influence what he is likely to mention about himself and his future. Commenting about persons with cancer, Craytor notes: "Soon after a diagnosis is made, the patient may talk freely of cancer and his treatment. If metastasis is found later, he may no longer be able to call his disease by name."[12] She makes the point that conversation between nurse and patient is probably most helpful when the patient is allowed to set the pace of talking about the gravity of his condition.

In my judgment, the nurse who is an effective conversationalist with patients has a fine appreciation of timing and is sensitive to verbal and nonverbal cues that the patient is ready to talk about a delicate matter of personal concern. There are certain times when a person seems to have a need for a verbal sounding board against which to talk about his reactions to what cards fate has dealt him. This need seems very strong during the period after the doctor's announcement that the individual has a dread disease or is faced with major surgery. In a sense, many people need to handle the psychological shock of "bad news" by talking over and over again about their bad luck; the experience of talking seems to function as a mechanism for coping with the high level of anxiety that has been generated. I have observed the same need in people who have been exposed to death for the first time or who have just been through an experience that shocks their sense of decency. These people, too, will ventilate freely if they encounter a good listener.

For the person who is living with a life-threatening illness, there are many critical points when his level of tension goes up even though he may not be able to talk openly with other people about his deep concerns. If we want to make ourselves available to such a person in the event that he wants to talk, it is helpful to know when to expect these moments of heightened concern. Every trip to the physician's office for a medical checkup is a tension-producing experience for the patient. Every new admission to the hospital raises the question in his mind, "Am I really okay?" Any subjective sensation that conveys the idea that he might be getting worse is a source of tension and worry. Any time he becomes aware of discrepancies in what other people tell him he begins to wonder.

People do not necessarily want to talk openly about their fears about death on these occasions when tensions are high, but they do appreciate having a concerned person available should they want to make that choice. They also appreciate talking with someone who can clarify their misunderstandings and assist them in finding other resources to help with other problems that arise. Nurses are often in position to be that concerned person, but they can only do so if they are willing to risk the uneasy feelings that come with personal involvement. To open to patients conversational doors of this kind, the nurse must come to grips with her own feelings about pain, grief, loss, helplessness, hopelessness, life, and death.

The nurse must also recognize that to provide this kind of opportunity to patients means moving into a different kind of working relationship with physicians and other authority. The nurse's problem with respect to physicians is epitomized in the comment, "I cannot sit down and talk with Mrs. Smith because the doctor has said that she is not to be told her diagnosis." I take the position that talking with a person to clarify what he thinks is happening or to understand his worries is not equivalent to telling him his diagnosis; rather, it is the one way to learn what is on his mind. It may be that he already knows his diagnosis but recognizes that his family and doctor need to play the illusion-game. It may be that he desperately wants to talk with his doctor, and when the nurse learns this, she can begin to negotiate with the physician on behalf of the patient. The point is that to keep the patient in a form of social isolation by placing the burden of responsibility on the physician is to deny the patient an opportunity to make his wishes known and to participate in the final decisions affecting his life.

The building of regular supports into the health-care system is a necessary and crucial step if the nursing staff is to be able to offer personalized care of patients on an ongoing basis. A discussion of that important issue has not been the focus of this paper but has been discussed elsewhere.[13,14] The primacy of life-saving values is clearly evident in hospitals and other health care institutions, and open conversation about death is extremely threatening to people who define their professional identities primarily in terms of ability to prolong life. This being the case, nurses who try to make dying a personalized experience for the patient are likely to find themselves in conflict with the system.

Any nurse who is truly concerned about personalizing patient care through her own efforts must reckon with the reality that to do so means a willingness to "rock the boat" of the health-care system as it presently functions. It means learning to function without the social rewards of approval from the many other workers who want to maintain the status quo. It means accepting responsibility for altering the psychosocial environment in ways that maximize the well-being of patients. It means helping to revamp the traditional authority-responsibility pattern of doctor-nurse working relationships into one that leads to a better understood division of labor and to better care for all concerned.

Making such a choice is not an easy route to take, but it is a personally reward-ing one. And the opportunity to make the choice exists. We nurses have a lot of power to function for or against the best interests of the patient. The choice is ours — not the physician's.

REFERENCES

1. Browne, Ivor W., and Hackett, Thomas P., "Emotional Reactions to the Threat of Impending Death: A Study of Patients on the Monitor Cardiac Pacemaker," *Irish Journal of Medical Science,* April 6, 1967, pp. 177–187.
2. Kubler-Ross, Elizabeth, *On Death and Dying,* New York: The Macmillan Co., 1969.
3. Buckman, Wilma, Olney, Mary, and Simpson, Ellen, "The Child's Adaptation to Diabetes," unpublished paper presented at A.M.A. Clinical Convention, Las Vegas, Nevada, November 29, 1966.
4. Bard, Morton, "The Price of Survival for Cancer Victims," *Trans-action,* Vol. 3, March/April 1966, pp. 10–14.
5. Quint, Jeanne C., "Institutionalized Practices of Information Control, *Psychiatry,* Vol. 28, May 1965, pp. 119–132.
6. Quint, Jeanne C., "The Threat of Death: Some Consequences for Patients and Nurses," *Nursing Forum,* Vol. VIII, No. 3, 1969, pp. 287–300.
7. Quint, Jeanne C., *The Nurse and the Dying Patient,* New York: The Macmillan Co., 1967, pp. 77–112, 163–200.
8. Crate, Marjorie A., "Nursing Functions in Adaptation to Chronic Illness," *American Journal of Nursing,* 65, October 1965, pp. 72–76.
9. Butler, Robert N., "The Life Review: An Interpretation of Reminiscence in the Aged," *Psychiatry,* Vol. 26, February 1963.
10. Kubler-Ross, *op. cit.*
11. Butler, *loc. cit.*
12. Craytor, Josephine K., "Talking with Persons Who Have Cancer," *American Journal of Nursing,* 69, April 1969, p. 748.
13. Quint, Jeanne C., "Nursing Services and the Care of Dying Patients: Some Speculations," *Nursing Science,* Vol. 2, December 1964, pp. 432–443.
14. Quint, Jeanne C., "The Threat of Death: Some Consequences for Patients and Nurses," *Nursing Forum,* Vol. VIII, No. 3, 1969, pp. 287–300.

37

Solving Health Problems
through Small Group Action

Barbara Osborne Henkel

*An increasing number of the community nurse's activities take place in groups —
patient groups, families, work groups, team conferences. Some groups function
for the purpose of problem solving, others for sharing, support or teaching.
Whatever the reason and whether the nurse acts as leader or member, the use of
basic knowledge about individuals functioning in groups and group dynamics
will facilitate group process and ultimately community health.*

$\mathbf{M}$uch work on health problems in the community is accomplished through
group activity — study groups, health councils, committees, clubs, conferences,
and conventions. Participation is more productive in these groups when we
know: how people behave in a group setting, how to plan for constructive
action, and how to participate as a member of a group.

BEHAVIOR IN A GROUP SETTING

Group behavior is more than a composite of what each member does; it is the
result of interaction between personalities. Some personalities will complement
each other, some will cooperate, some may be uncooperative, and some will act
at cross purposes. Mix all of them together and in time a behavior pattern typical
of the group will emerge. The group will have its own personality. Like the individual, it will develop its own attitudes and values. It will strive to maintain its
own integrity and will resist forces that threaten it.

Needs of Group Members

The needs that each has as an individual affect behavior when working with
others — needs for new experience, security, response, recognition, altruism,
fair treatment, freedom, and creativity. The process of meeting these needs can
promote or interfere with group achievement. When a number of people meet
for the first time to solve a problem through group action each may feel insecure,
may have doubts about what is expected, and may wonder if any good will come
of this. These are some of the concerns or worries:

Who is who? Who are the other people? Why are they here? Will I like them?
Are they like me in terms of background, occupational level, education, and
status in the community?

Will I fit in? What am I supposed to do? Can I do it? What are the others
supposed to do and are they able to do it?

From Barbara Osborne Henkel, *Community Health,* 1970, Allyn and Bacon, Boston. Reprinted with permission. Only the second section of the chapter is reproduced.

What is expected of me? What am I to do during the meeting, listen or talk? Do I take part in setting the goals or is this all arranged ahead of time? How long will the meeting last?

What will the leader do? Will the leader really run the show? Will he share and distribute leadership responsibilities? What can he offer in terms of background, knowledge, and assistance? What kind of guy is he?

What is the purpose? What are the *real* goals and objectives? Are there hidden agendas? Are the goals and objectives entirely predetermined or can they be altered? Is this a short- or long-term project?

Will I feel at ease? Since any new situation produces some fears, doubts, and anxieties, the members of the group need to feel accepted and wanted as soon as possible; they want to feel that they are part of the group.

Will this be of value to me? Members of the group will want to feel that the program has value for them as individuals, that they have a place in it, and that they will miss something important by not being involved on a continuing basis.

Will this be mentally stimulating? In addition to personal and emotional acceptance, members should have at least one challenging and stimulating mental experience during the first session. They should not only be talked to about what they will do, but they should also do it.[22]

There are some behaviors that interfere with group progress which relate to needs for security and recognition. If these go unchecked they can seriously impede productivity. People may overdo the following things:

1. Talk about their broad background of experience to establish status and gain recognition.
2. Try to dominate the discussion and keep it on the "right track."
3. Try to make peace at any price and avoid controversial issues.
4. Avoid contributing or making decisions by acting bored, acting as if this is beneath them, saying nothing, sulking, leaving early, or suggesting that a committee be appointed.
5. Take over the meeting by answering all questions and by outtalking or speaking louder than others.
6. Refuse to do anything until there is an expert to give advice.[23]

Refusing to act until there is an expert to advise or appointing a committee to study the matter in detail before making a decision can be rationalizations for doing nothing. Dale describes these in his article "Good Reasons for Doing Nothing."

[22]*Conducting Workshops and Institutes* (Chicago: Adult Education Association of the U.S.A., 1956), 20–21.
[23]Dorothy Nyswander, "Behavior in Groups — Some Principles of Group Process," *The Voluntary Health Agency — Meeting Community Needs, Continuing Education Monographs No. 1* (San Francisco: Western Regional Office, A.P.H.A., 1961), 35.

"This proposal would set a precedent." Change is threatening and may be uncomfortable. This statement can be reversed to "there is no precedent to guide us."

"We have not yet conclusively proved that the old method can't be made to work or that the proposed new one can." Other similar evasive techniques are, "let us get all the facts, or make another survey."

Maybe "the time is not ripe." This rationalization might be phrased as "the public is not ready," "why hurry so much," or "let's lay a firm foundation."

"The situation is hopeless." Others have tried to cope with this problem and failed, why should we be any luckier? Maybe we should wait until we are sure of some success. After all, no one would expect us to do anything about a hopeless situation. "We can't afford it" is a stock answer frequently given without any realistic appraisal of whether it can be done or not.

Often used today is "it is a controversial issue." This immediately closes all avenues of investigation. Any new program involves some controversy and "serious, sustained discussion on these controversies reveals whether we are dealing with a man-sized issue or with a piddling enterprise unworthy of anyone's important time and thought."[24]

Some of the probable *real* reasons for doing nothing are fear of change, the insecurity of changing to new patterns of behavior, or the discomfort and energy required to reorganize present ways of doing things. But these are not the reasons we give, or the reasons others will give us when new programs are suggested. As we work with others we should try to evaluate what is going on. If someone is interfering with action, is it because the group has not taken all the preliminary steps, or is it because of one of the "reasons for doing nothing"?

PLANNING FOR CONSTRUCTIVE ACTION

Attention to the physical setting, to social needs, and to orienting participants as to what will happen assists in getting meetings or projects off to a good start. The chairman, sponsor, or coordinator has this responsibility.

Physical Arrangements

Physical arrangements can contribute to making any meeting more successful. Such things as lighting, ventilation, acoustics, and comfortable seats are important. If the meeting is to last for more than an hour, there should be a break to permit people to move about. Everyone should be able to see speakers and visual materials clearly and without strain, and audio equipment should be pretested to insure that it is in operating order. Failure to provide for these things can create annoyances that only the most highly motivated person will overlook. If the group is small, it is helpful if each person is seated so that he can see all the

[24]Edgar Dale, "Good Reasons for Doing Nothing," *The News Letter,* 26:1–4, December, 1960.

others. If the group is large, twenty or more, it is wise to plan to divide into smaller groups to work on a phase of the problem, or to talk things over.

Orientation

At the initial meeting orientation should include opportunities for participants to learn about each other; a general definition of the objectives or problems facing the group; an explanation of the function of the group, such as fact finding, policy deciding, or implementation of programs; and a tentative assignment of responsibilities or future course of action.

Since everyone has a desire to be regarded as a person of some worth, considerable energy will be expended at first to gain recognition and status. Until this is achieved, little may be accomplished. Starting with a social hour where people mingle informally is effective and popular. Name cards stating occupation and other identification are widely used. Other techniques for giving recognition to members include, introduction by the chairman, self-introduction or, in large groups, allowing persons to tell their immediate neighbors about themselves.

Many meetings fail to get off the ground because no one knows what is expected of them. There has to be some agreement on what is going to happen. The first step is to develop a common set of perceptions and to define a common set of purposes. The chairman or sponsor needs to be prepared with some definitions of the problem and some suggestions for proceeding. Concrete proposals give people a starting point. In all probability, the group will modify and amplify, or even reject the first proposals, but the members will become ego involved.

Groups, committees, or councils have different functions. These must be carefully defined or people may be at cross-purposes, and they will be dissatisfied with what goes on. The orientation should clearly spell out functions or responsibilities. Fact finding groups are concerned with surveying needs and defining problems. Policy making and advisory groups determine objectives and outline means of achieving goals. When the purpose of the group is implementation, members assume responsibility for doing the job. For example, a group of citizens might be disturbed about a health problem. They accumulate evidence of this need and present their findings to the city council or city fathers. This policy making group decides what can be done about the problem and what agency or group should be responsible. The agency or group in turn plans how this responsibility can be met and meets it. A committee may have more than one function. Not only must members know the main purpose of the committee, but they must find satisfaction in their designated role. Some people like the role of advisor, others like to implement. Participants should be selected for the role they are to fulfill.

Action

The chairman can use the "scientific method" or "steps in problem solving" as guidelines to get things started. If he follows each of these steps everyone will have clearer concepts of what is going on; people will be more apt to develop common perceptions; there can be opportunities for individual participation; and many will probably experience some feeling of success. These steps should be taken cooperatively with the group, but the chairman or leader must keep things going.

1. Define and briefly explore the extent of the problem or problems.
2. Choose one or several problems for consideration.
3. Plan how more information can be gathered. Shall resource people be brought in, shall subcommittees investigate specific facets and report back to the group, or shall each person investigate on his own?
4. Redefine and clarify the problem on the basis of the additional information accumulated.
5. Decide whether or not the group can or should work on the problem. Not all problems can be resolved.
6. Make specific plans about how to proceed if the group decides to tackle the problem.
7. Assign responsibilities to people to carry out or implement plans for procedure.
8. Evaluate the results. Methods for evaluation should be incorporated into procedures, and appraisal should be continuous to enable replanning.

When a particular problem is solved or project completed, the group should formally decide to terminate or choose another project. Sometimes groups disintegrate in such a manner that members develop "feelings of lack of success," and such a feeling of failure may interfere with future community participation on the part of those involved.

PARTICIPATING AS A MEMBER OF A GROUP

Participation with others in a committe or in a meeting is a skill that can be learned. These attitudes or beliefs are basic: each individual has a contribution to make, even though human abilities and potentialities differ; the belief in human dignity and worth is the foundation of democratic action; and in all groups there is diversity of interests, backgrounds, points of view, temperaments, and ways of working together. Experience shows that groups can contribute to finding better solutions than when the decision is vested in only one individual. Of course the basis of this process is the concept that people can work together and come to a common agreement about the solution of a problem which *they* define and wish to solve.

We must also be aware of what happens in group action. Change takes place among people at varying rates, and some people will be slower than others to grasp ideas and see relationships. Differences will exist and cannot always be reconciled, but this need not interfere with progress. Members of the group must move toward their goals as rapidly as possible, but slowly enough to keep people from feeling insecure and losing identification with the problem. Working either too slowly or too rapidly creates dissatisfaction. Then, too, an objective set by a group is not necessarily fixed, but may change.

People assume different roles when they work with others. Someone must lead or direct, and others must follow. In some situations a role is assumed for the length of a specific project, and other times in the course of a particular meeting the same person may sometimes lead and sometimes follow. We should know how to be a leader and how to be a follower. As chairman, moderator, or leader, you can help people work together when you

1. Keep group attention away from personalities.
2. Channel the thinking of the members toward common goals.
3. Reflect questions back to the group or to the experts for answers.
4. Are alert to points which need further clarification (observation of people's faces may give clues as to whether or not they understand).
5. Repeat a statement that is not heard by everyone, using the words of the author.
6. Involve as many people as possible, but not necessarily everybody present.
7. Remember that people can disagree without being disagreeable.
8. Briefly summarize the points that have been made during a discussion.
9. Bring to the attention of the group any digressions from the original topic; ask them whether or not they wish to continue along that line.
10. Prevent a few members from taking too much time by noticing how frequently people participate.
11. Make sure that different points of view concerning the problem are presented and sympathetically understood.
12. Guide the discussion away from mere contention by occasional humor (not sarcasm) to relieve tension, or summarize both sides calmly.

The role of participant is not one that comes naturally. It, too, requires understanding and development. You can contribute to successful relationships when you

1. Try to distinguish between the *intent* of the person speaking and *what* he says. (People may be so filled with their own *intents* that they do not "hear" what others say.)
2. Let the more slow-speaking members have a chance to contribute, and *listen* to them.
3. Try to state your own points briefly and clearly.
4. Avoid wrangling over details and technicalities.
5. Challenge matters you cannot accept.
6. Ask for clarification of the points you do not understand.

7. Be willing to delay if necessary until correct and authentic information is secured to avoid poor decisions.

8. Refrain from impeding progress by using such reasons for doing nothing as "it is controversial, get an expert, the time is not ripe, we can't afford it, or, it would set a precedent."

The checklist "Self-Appraisal for Group Participation" on [this] page is a device for self-evaluation that can help you improve your skill.

Self-Appraisal Check for Group Participation

	Poor	Fair	Good
1. Was I an active participant?			
2. Was I an enthusiastic participant?			
3. Was I an active listener?			
4. Did I avoid dominating the group?			
5. Did I avoid straying from the point under discussion?			
6. Did I express my point of view?			
7. Did I select facts pertinent to the problem?			
8. Did I support my point of view with adequate, relevant facts?			
9. Did I use reliable sources of information for my facts?			
10. Was I opinionated?			
11. Did I respect the point of view of others?			
12. Was I willing to listen to all sides of the issue before making a decision?			
13. Did I avoid becoming emotional?			
14. Was I interested in hearing what others had to offer?			
15. Was I willing to compromise if necessary?			
16. Was I willing to defend my own stand?			
17. Did I do clear thinking on issues or rearrange my prejudices?			

Source: Adapted from "Student Check List for Self-Appraisal," *Learning Through Group Discussion* (Wesleyan University, Middletown, Connecticut. Publishers: The Junior Town Meeting League, 1949), p. 30.

SUMMARY

Committees, councils, conferences, and other similar groups of people work together to solve many problems. Members of these groups will accomplish their objectives more successfully when they apply knowledge about how people react in a group setting, how groups proceed in problem solving, and how individuals function in leadership and participant roles.

Some health problems can be prevented or alleviated through education of the public. In order to promote worthwhile educational programs we need to observe the principles of learning, understand what makes people "ready" to act, and know how to use the forces which are apt to stimulate desirable health behavior.

BIBLIOGRAPHY AND SUGGESTED READINGS

Texts

Cohen, Arthur R. *Attitude and Social Influence.* New York: Basic Books, Inc., 1964.

Goerke, Lenor S., and Stebbins, Ernest L. *Mustard's Introduction to Public Health.* New York: The Macmillan Company, Inc., 1968. Pp. 399–415.

Katz, Alfred H., and Felton, Jean Spencer. *Health and the Community.* New York: The Free Press, 1965. Pp. 799–811, 838–852.

Knutson, Andie L. *The Individual Society, and Health Behavior.* New York: Russell Sage Foundation, 1965. Pp. 357–511.

Lippett, Ronald, Watson, Jeanne, and Westley, Bruce. *The Dynamics of Planned Change.* New York: Harcourt, Brace and Company, 1956.

Ross, Murray G. *Case Histories in Community Organization.* New York: Harper and Row, Publishers, 1958.

_____. *Community Organization, Theory and Principles.* New York: Harper and Row, Publishers, 1955.

Warren, Roland. *Studying Your Community.* New York: Russell Sage Foundation, 1955.

Periodicals

Griffiths, W., and Knutson, A. L. "The Role of Mass Media in Public Health," *American Journal of Public Health,* 50:515–523, April, 1960.

Havighurst, Robert J. "The Learning Process," *American Journal of Public Health,* 51:1694–1699, November, 1961.

Hochbaum, Godfrey M. "Effecting Health Behavior: The Professional and the Lay Side of the Coin," *International Journal of Health Education,* 10:171–179, October-December, 1967.

Jenkins, C. David. "The Semantic Differential for Health," *International Journal of Health Education,* 10:132–141, July-September, 1967.

MacGregor, Gordon. "Social Determinants of Health Practices," *American Journal of Public Health,* 51:1709–1715, November, 1961.

Sehgal, B. S. "Health Behavior: How Much Influence Does Knowledge Have?" *International Journal of Health Education,* 10:60–67, April-June, 1967.

Swinehart, James W. "Voluntary Exposure to Health Communications," *American Journal of Public Health,* 58:1265–1276, July, 1968.

Volkart, Edmund H. "Motivation in Small Groups," *Health Education Monographs,* No. 6, 1959, Society of Public Health Educators, Inc. Pp. 14–28.

Young, Marjorie A. C. "Review of Research and Studies Related to Health Education Practice (1961–1966)," *Health Education Monographs,* No. 26, Society of Public Health Educators, Inc., 1968.

VII
The Family in Community Nursing

Community nurses work with families. Nursing service may be focused on one individual but the nurse must remember that individuals are members of families. The interrelationships between family members considerably influence how each person thinks, feels and acts. For example, an authoritarian parent will affect how the child responds to authority figures in other settings. Frequently, individuals make decisions that influence other family members. A mother decides not to attend the well-child clinic and, as a result, her child's diabetes goes undetected. The family's physical and emotional health has an impact on each member. When one person is ill it affects the normal roles played by others. Additional strain may be felt physically, emotionally and financially; roles may be redefined, relationships may be changed.

The community nurse has two major reasons for focusing on the family. First, the whole family needs service. Family health is largely determined by the dynamics of interaction among members. How well is the family functioning? What are its interrelationships? What is its stage of development? The nurse must be able to assess these dynamics. Knowing family developmental stages and tasks then enables the nurse to develop measures for preventing problems and promoting family health.

The second reason for focusing on the family is that the community nurse works through the family to reach individuals. This enables the nurse to view the individuals in perspective, in their total context. Also, every member is then considered and none is overlooked. For instance, a home visit aimed at rehabilitating a woman after a stroke may disclose her husband's problem of alcoholism. Measures can be taken toward regaining his health as well as hers.

The cultural dimension is another important element in family nursing. Every family has its own cultural values and practices. These influence the way family members eat, dress, live and believe. Practices that negatively affect health may be firmly entrenched in the family's cultural value system and not easily changed. For example, a child severely injured in an accident needed a blood transfusion. The parents refused because receiving blood from another person violated their belief system. The community nurse must determine the family's cultural orientation. This will increase

323

the nurse's understanding of the family and make nursing care planning more appropriate.

Various aspects of family-centered community nursing are considered in Part VII. Each chapter describes a different facet of family care. Each is geared to increase the nurse's understanding of families and, in turn, the effectiveness of the nursing service offered.

38

The Nursing Process in Family Health

Jayne Anttila Tapia

Every family must accomplish certain tasks to achieve normal, mature functioning. Families differ in their ability to carry out these tasks. Because they are all not operating at the same level, consequently their responses to community nursing service will vary. Jayne Tapia presents a model for the community nurse to use in assessing the family's level of functioning. At the same time she describes the nursing activities that are most appropriate for each level.

Public health nurses have long believed that the family is the unit of community nursing service; there is nothing new about this concept. What *is* new, however, is that more and more nurses are beginning to realize that they are not always able to describe accurately what nursing service to the family means, nor have they been able to render this kind of service consistently.

Yet, the need for coordinated, ongoing, comprehensive health and illness care for all members of the family, as a group and as individuals, is all too evident today in our fragmented health delivery system. Community health nurses can and should play an important part in providing this type of care in the newly emerging health delivery systems. But, to do this, they must have a clearer idea of what they mean by working with a family, rather than just with individual members.

They must be able to diagnose specific health problems of the family, prescribe a nursing approach to the family, carry it out, and evaluate its outcome just as they now do with individuals. Their goal should be to help the family grow in its ability to meet its needs and fulfill its functions in a more healthful way, while, at the same time, using their own talents and time most effectively.

PAST DEFINITIONS

Several attempts have been made to clarify and define family nursing service. Mickey described it as being called for in situations in which an individual or a family has a health problem requiring nursing assistance of the kind that might include therapeutic care, health teaching, counseling, or guidance.[1] The assumptions underlying this definition were that the family did not have prior knowledge or competence to meet the situation and that the provision of nursing service would produce change.

Freedman and Lowe devised a form to systematize the process by which a nurse judges family nurse competence, and Lee and Frazier tried to differentiate family group service from such concepts as "the family as a unit of service" or "family health service."[2,3]

I propose another means of determining family nursing needs and related nursing activities: the study of the tasks of the nuclear family and the family's ability in accomplishing these tasks. According to Feldman and Scherz, the four main tasks of the nuclear family are to provide for security and physical survival, emotional and social functioning, sexual differentiation and training of children, and growth of individual members.[4] Families, however, differ in their ability to carry out these tasks and, thus, have different levels of family functioning. In order to provide nursing service appropriate to the needs of a particular family, the community health nurse must be able to assess the family's level of functioning.

Using the above tasks as guidelines, I have developed a model for family nursing based upon a continuum of five levels of family functioning. Level I is the chaotic family — at the infancy stage of development; Level II is the intermediate family — at the childhood stage; Level III is the normal family with many conflicts and problems — at the adolescent stage; Level IV is the family with solutions to its problems — the adult stage; and Level V is the ideal independent family — at full maturity.

Nursing services and activities appropriate to each level of family functioning can also be put on a continuum. The major focus of the nurse's work with a Level I family is to develop a trust relationship; with a Level II family, to help the family begin to define problems; a Level III family will require a complex of nursing skills; and prevention will be the point of emphasis in working with a Level IV family.

All of these nursing activities are inherent in the nursing process, but they will be more effective if the nurse can concentrate her efforts on the nursing activity appropriate to the family's level of functioning. In doing so, the nurse will initiate nursing measures that are meaningful and economic in time and effort, and this in turn will lead to greater success in helping families reach their highest level of functioning.

Since the family's level of functioning is an indication of its state of health, any change in that functioning level also indicates a change in its health status. Thus, the degree of family movement from one level to another can serve as a yardstick whereby the nurse can measure and evaluate the effect of her nursing intervention and service.

INFANCY OR CHAOTIC FAMILY

The lowest level of family functioning is characterized by disorganization in all areas of family life.[5] The family barely meets its needs for security and physical survival; members are characterized by their inability to secure adequate wages or housing, to budget money, or to maintain adequate nutrition, clothing, heat,

MODEL FOR FAMILY NURSING

Nursing Activities	Trust	Counselling	Complex of Skills	Prevention	None
Continuum of Nursing Skills	Nurse and Family-Partners	Partnership	Partnership Stressing Family's Ability	Nurse—Expert and Partner with Family	Family Independent / Nurse not Needed
	Acceptance and trust, maturity and patience, clarification of role, limit setting, constant evaluation of relationship and progress.	Based on trust relationship, uses counseling and interpersonal skills to help family begin to understand itself and define its problems. Nurse uses honesty and genuineness, and self-evaluation.	Information, coordination, teamwork, teaching; uses special skills, helps family in making decisions and finding solutions.	Anticipated problem areas studied, teaching of available resources, assistance in family-group understanding, maturity and foresight.	Ideal family, homeostatic, balance between individual and group goals and activities. Family meets its tasks and roles well, and are able to seek appropriate help when needed.
Continuum of Family Functioning	Nurse-"Good Mother" to Family	Nurse and Family-Siblings	Nurse-Adult Helper to Family	Nurse—Expert and Partner	
	Chaotic family, barely surviving, inadequate provision of physical and emotional supports. Alienation from community, deviant behavior, distortion and confusion of roles, immaturity, child neglect, depression-failure.	Intermediate family, slightly above survival level, variation in economic provisions, alienation but with more ability to trust. Child neglect not as great, defensive but slightly more willingness to accept help.	Normal family but with many conflicts and problems, variation in economic levels, greater trust and ability to seek and use help. Parents more mature, but still have emotional conflicts. Do have successes and achievements, and are more willing to seek solutions to problems, future oriented.	Family has solutions, are stable, healthy with fewer conflicts or problems, very capable providers of physical and emotional supports. Parents mature and confident, fewer difficulties in training of children, able to seek help, future oriented, enjoy present.	
Family Levels	I Infancy	II Childhood	III Adolescence	IV Adulthood	V Maturity

and cleanliness. This family lives from day to day without orientation to the future.

These lacks increase the family's inability to provide for healthy emotional and social functioning of its members, and this is reflected in the family members' apparent alienation from the community. They distrust outsiders, are unable to utilize community resources and services, and become hostile and resistant to offers of help. The immaturity of the parents is shown in their inability to assume responsible adult roles — a factor that often results in socially deviant behavior, including child abuse and neglect.

The children suffer in other ways, too, because their parents are unable to act as the role models that the children need if they are to mature into capable, socialized, adult men and women. There is consequently much distortion and confusion of roles in the family. The children, sometimes at a young age, may even have to take over many of the tasks and roles of their nonfunctioning parents. Such situations perpetuate the family's pattern of chaos and disorganization into the next generation.

This type of family also fails in providing for support and growth of its individual members. The family exhibits depression and a feeling of failure, with no hope of success either for individual members or the family group. The basic insecurity of the family members prevents change: defensiveness and distortion are used as devices to keep people from getting near enough to cause change.

Establishing a trusting relationship with this type of family is the most important nursing activity in the therapeutic process, yet a most difficult one. The nurse must develop a caring, freeing relationship with one or more members of the family and help the family to feel that she cares about them, accepts them as they are, and understands their difficulties. If she cannot establish this relationship with them, she cannot help them to grow. While this activity is basic for a level one family, it is difficult for them to accept because of their fear and distrust of people outside of the immediate family.

The task will demand much of the nurse — maturity, patience, endurance, limit setting, and clarification of her role. The family will see the nurse as a good mother and will test her for consistency and try to be dependent on her. The nurse, seeing herself as a partner working with the family, cannot allow the dependency to go beyond the trust relationship. She must be constantly alert to the factors operating within herself, the family, the community, and environment in order to evaluate progress toward the development of mutual trust. When the nurse has ascertained that this relationship is developing, and that the family, like the newborn infant, has had its need for security met within an interpersonal relationship, she and the family can then move into level two activities.

CHILDHOOD OR INTERMEDIATE FAMILY

The second level of family functioning is characterized by a somewhat lesser amount of disorganization than the first level family. Members are slightly more able to meet their need for security and physical survival. Although still alienated from the community, they have more ability to trust and, subsequently, have more hope for a better way of life.

The parents are immature, and socially deviant behavior may occur. Distortion and confusion of roles exist but the parents are more willing to work together for the benefit of the whole family. The children are not neglected to the extent that they must be removed from the home, as is often the case in a level one family.

However, this type of family is still unable to support and promote the growth of its members. Members appear unable to change, are defensive and fearful, and lack the resources to gain a sense of accomplishment. This family does not seek help actively and requires much assistance before the members are able to acknowledge their problems realistically.

With this level two family, the nurse will continue to maintain the warm accepting support of the trust relationship, but now she uses it as a stepping stone to help the family begin to understand itself more clearly. Because of the trust established between the two, the family can begin to venture forth in self-discovery, with help from the nurse who will clarify and reflect their words, actions, thoughts, and responses. The nurse is honest in sharing her observations and personality with the family in order that they may feel more willing to be honest with themselves. By her actions, she demonstrates various roles and tasks to the family and uses these actions to further increase the family's understanding of itself.

This counseling relationship demands even more of the nurse than the previous trust relationship, as her interpretations and diagnoses must be accurate, her behavior consistent, and her concerns genuine. She must understand her feelings and relationship with the family very accurately. Her goal is to help this family grow to the point (level three) where they can work on solutions to some of their problems.

Progress is seen when members begin to feel more like a family and experience the nurse as a sibling — that is, they will vacillate between dependence and independence and compete for attention and control. The nurse, acting as a partner with this family, helps them to understand that she shares her thoughts and actions with them so that they may further understand themselves and their interaction as a family group.

ADOLESCENT OR FAMILY WITH PROBLEMS

The level three family is essentially normal but has more than the healthy and usual amount of conflicts and problems. As a unit, it is more capable of physical survival and of providing security for its members, but these abilities may vary greatly. Socially and emotionally, this family functions better than either previous types. Members demonstrate greater trust in people, have the knowledge and ability to utilize some community resources, and are less openly hostile to outsiders. Usually, one parent is more mature than the other, and the children have less overall difficulty adjusting to changes in the family, school, and environment.

This family, however, may have more difficulty in the task of providing sexual differentiation and training of children, than they have in the first two tasks. Although the children are cared for physically, there may be more emotional conflicts, resulting in much confusion for the children. In addition, because one parent may be quite immature, difficulties for one or more of the children may result. Very often individuals in the family experience successes and achievements outside the family, and members may even deliberately seek outside achievements to replace some missing satisfaction within their family life.

On the positive side, this family shows an increasing ability to face some of its problems and to look for solutions. They may seek and use outside help much more effectively and appropriately than a level one or two family. Members are future oriented even though the present may be painful.

A complex of nursing activities is required to help the level three family solve its recognized problems. The nurse assists them by providing teaching, information, coordination, referral, team-work, or special technical skills such as those involved in performing complicated nursing care activities. Often she must move backward to a previous level of nursing activities and then forward again as more and more difficulties are looked at and worked on. In order to facilitate success, the family should be encouraged to start with the easiest of the most pressing problems.

Working with this family demands of the nurse a wealth of technical and interpersonal skills as well as knowledge of community resources and the ability to lead, coordinate, and cooperate with other team members. The nurse is seen by the family as an adult helper with expertise in the solution of problems. The nurse provides the needed teaching, referral, and coordination to assist the family, but she continually emphasizes the importance of their making their decisions; she helps them to do so, to try out their decisions, and to evaluate outcomes. Thus, she helps them improve their ability to manage their roles and tasks as they proceed from one problem to another.

ADULTHOOD OR FAMILY WITH SOLUTIONS

A family at this level may be described as normal, stable, healthy, and happy with fewer than the usual number of problems or conflicts. This is because they are able to handle most problems as they arise. This family capably provides for physical security and emotional and social functioning. The parents are usually quite mature and confident in their roles as mates, parents, wage earners, and members of society. They have fewer difficulties in providing for sexual differentiation and training their children.

Their main problems center around stages of growth and various developmental tasks. If problems in this area arise, very often the parents refer themselves to outside sources for help. However, they may show excess anxiety over these problems. Individual members and group needs and goals are usually brought into harmony by this family. Although crisis may immobilize this family, they have the ability to adapt and change, enjoy the present, and plan for the future.

The main nursing activity with this family is preventive health teaching to enable the family to maintain its health. The nurse helps the members to antici-pate problem areas, to work through possible alternatives, and then to study the consequences of these alternatives. As she stresses prevention, she teaches the family about all the resources that are available in time of crisis or need. The nurse is also in a unique position to help this family grow and to increase the members' self-understanding and effectiveness in group functioning.

Such nursing activity requires much maturity, foresight, and experience. If the nurse is able to serve the family at this level, she knows that they will be functioning on a higher level than previously, and that they will use community services more appropriately when there is a need. This family sees the nurse as an expert teacher and partner and is able to utilize this partnership until it moves to level five.

MATURITY OR IDEAL FAMILY

This is only a short step above level four. Here the family can be described as truly homeostatic, with a healthy balance of individual and group goals, activities, participation, and concerns. All tasks are met by this family, and all supplies are provided. The only exception is in times of extreme or multiple crises, when the family is immobilized but can still ask for help from appropriate sources and use it.

Nursing activity is not necessary for this family unless there is a crisis, and at such times the family would seek help from the appropriate community source. If nursing services are required, the nurse would probably use nursing activities appropriate to the situation — either level III or IV — in assisting the family to regain its equilibrium.

The proposed model of family nursing attempts to explain how community health nurses view and work with families, what goals they set for the family, and what skills and attributes they need to accomplish their objectives. The model is based on an existential philosophy of man and the concept that health is a dynamic term which encompasses all aspects of a person's life and being — phys-ical, psychological, emotional, social, environmental, spiritual, and cultural.

REFERENCES

1. Mickey, Janice E. Studying extrahospital nursing needs; a preliminary report. *Am. J. Public Health* 48:881, July 1958.
2. Freeman, Ruth B., and Lowe, Marie. Method for appraising family public health nursing needs. *Am. J. Public Health* 53:47—52, Jan. 1963.

3. Lee, M. J., and Frazier, D. M. Recognition of family-group problems by public health nurses. *Am. J. Public Health* 53:932—940, June 1963.
4. Feldman, F. L., and Scherz, F. H. *Family Social Welfare; Helping Troubled Families.* New York, Atherton Press, 1967, pp. 68—71.
5. Geismar, L. L., and La Sorte, M. A. *Understanding the Multi-problem Family.* New York, Association Press, 1964.

39

The Impact of Illness
on Family Roles

Robert R. Bell

Two significant factors must be considered in family nursing. First, because of present trends in health care delivery, more sick persons are being cared for at home. This places greater demands on family members. Second, the usual roles of each family member will be influenced by having a sick person in the home. In the following chapter, Robert Bell describes these roles and how illness affects them. An understanding of these factors can facilitate community nursing action.

The twentieth-century American family has been influenced by numerous changes which are complexly interrelated with the broad social changes characteristic of modern American society. This paper focuses on some social changes related to family patterns for dealing with the illness of a family member. Since one of the major changes in the American family has been a shift from a large extended family to a small conjugal one, illness to one family member leaves fewer immediate family members to care for him. If the husband or wife becomes ill the other spouse usually must take on many new role obligations.

The concept of role is used here to refer to the range of expected behavior attached to a social-group position. It is assumed that every role has certain counterroles; thus any significant influence on one role within a complex of interrelated roles implies alterations or adaptions in related roles. Furthermore roles do not remain static; they may change over time, both in role prescriptions and as these prescriptions are actually filled by individuals. For example, the role prescriptions of mother today are different from the past, and individuals filling the mother role find that their rights and obligations change over time.[1]

In the following discussion we shall examine: (1) some changes in the family, with particular relevance for family adaptations to illness; (2) the changing nature of the patient role; and (3) how certain family and patient roles are interrelated.

FAMILY ROLE CHANGES

Rather than attempt to discuss the many changes in the American family, we shall direct our comments primarily to some changes in the family roles of women. This stress appears justified because many of the most significant changes in the modern American family have been related to the changing roles of women. Also, since our interest is in the impact of illness on the family, our female stress

From Jeanette R. Folta and Edith S. Deck, eds., *A Sociological Framework for Patient Care*, pp. 177—190. Copyright © 1966, John Wiley & Sons, Inc. Reprinted by permission of the publisher.

seems further justified because women's roles generally are more affected by illness (both as patient and nurse) than are other family roles.

In the past the role of the woman was clear and relatively simple — her primary adult role was that of wife-mother. She met certain needs of the husband, had the main responsibility for the care and the rearing of children, and maintained the home. Although she might have had some frustrations and dissatisfactions in filling the traditional wife-mother role, the role was generally accepted as the "natural" behavior pattern for women. "It was 'natural' because it was what women had been doing for centuries, and few other significant adult roles were being filled by women to indicate any alternatives."[2]

Today the vast majority of women undoubtedly enter marriage with a strong desire to fill most of the role demands of the traditional wife-mother. As in the past most women want children and want to maintain a home of their own, and in many cases the marriage will seem to be lacking if these traditional role expectations are not achieved.

Compared to the past, the difference today is that the woman often wants something more. This does not necessarily mean that she loves her husband, children, and home any less; but because of greater time and more greatly developed capacities for other interests, she often has other strong desires that seek fulfillment.[3]

The changing nature of family role demands by the modern woman is reflected in a number of social changes. Yet the new role interests of the woman are not at the expense of less interest in marriage — a greater proportion of women today are married than in the past.

In 1900, 2 out of 3 women in the total population had been married at some time in their lives; now this is true for 4 out of 5 women.[4] Furthermore women are entering marriage at younger ages; between 1890 and 1962 the median age of marriage dropped from 22.0 to 20.3 years for women.[5]

Another important change is that the modern woman lives in a world where increasingly the pattern is for her to live her older years without a husband. For example, "at ages 65 and over there now are 1276 women per 1000 men; by 1980 this ratio will be 1403 per 1000."[6]

The relative improvement in longevity of females is particularly striking because it has increased the disparity in expectation of life between the sexes. The average duration of life has increased by 19.32 years for white males and 23.11 years for white females.[7]

The greater life expectancy of women also is reflected in the increasing responsibility of women as family breadwinners. For example, the proportion of women who head households increases from 11 percent at ages 40—44 to 36 percent at ages 65 and over.[8]

Other important alterations of the woman's role are related to changes in education and occupational opportunities. In the United States today 66 percent of the women now under age 30 are at least high-school graduates. By contrast, of women now age 65 and over only 24 percent completed high school.[9] Furthermore the number of women pursuing higher education is increasing rapidly. The number of women earning B.A.'s was 5237 in 1900, 76,954 in 1940, and 145,514 in 1961.[10]

One of the most important changes in the woman's role has been entrance of a large number into the work force. In 1962 there were 23 million women in the work force and the forecast is for 30 million in 1970.[11] About 60 percent of all women workers are married, or, to put it a different way, among married white women about one-third are working.[12] The kinds of occupations that women enter are partially related to their age; for example, in the "clerical and kindred worker" category are 48 percent of the employed women in the 25—29 age grouping, but only 15 percent of the employed women of age 65 and over.[13]

A common statistical picture of the modern American woman indicates that she enters marriage at a young age, has a long period of married life, and often finds herself in the role of widow in her later years. Her increased educational background and occupational involvement is reflected in her participation in adult roles beyond the traditional wife-mother role. A greater importance is given to the family roles of the young woman in the maintenance and direction she provides for her family whether she works or not. This results in part from her husband working away from home and because his occupation is often his major adult role commitment. Also because of geographical mobility the modern wife-mother has fewer relatives to turn to and must herself make the major adjustments to new communities. For many modern women this means participation in the traditional wife-mother roles plus other roles. In the recent Report of the President's Commission on Women it was stated that "women's ancient function of providing love and nurture stands. But for entry into modern life, today's children need a preparation far more diversified than that of their predecessors."[14]

A great deal of controversy has arisen over the personal significance of the traditional roles performed by women in the modern family. Part of the trend for giving these roles greater significance has been the attempt to "professionalize" the wife-mother role.

By professionalization is meant the development of a set of rationales for an intellectual and emotional commitment to the functions of being a modern wife and mother. The new belief is that being a "good wife" and mother today calls for dedication, knowledge, and a sense of creativity similar to that found in professions.[15]

For example, although the health of the child has always been of vital concern to the mother, she was usually anxious about the child's physical health; today she is more likely to be anxious about psychic dangers.

Concerning oneself with the psychological health of a child revolves a greater intellectual commitment than simply worrying about his physical health. Child rearing takes on certain professional overtones with the woman who has been educated, and she keeps herself informed about various writings in regard to personality development.[16]

A part of the "professionalization" of the wife-mother role has been changes in her functions as family "nurse." In the past the wife-mother cared for the ill members in her family, but she did it primarily through "folk" wisdom. Medical remedies and suggestions were often acquired from older women who also frequently were available to help out when family illness occurred. Often the woman could put goose grease on the patient's chest, feed him chicken broth, and thus fill the role of family nurse. Today, however, the modern woman does not rely on "folk" knowledge but turns to medical experts. This means that the wife-mother is often the intermediary between the patient and the medical expert. Because medical knowledge is so complex and technical the wife-mother must be greatly concerned with correctly following the prescribed medical course. This is often true even when the diagnosis of the illness is not particularly serious because of the constant threat that it will develop into something more dangerous. It is ironical that as medical knowledge has alleviated many problems those problems that remain have often become even more frightening. That is, for the wife-mother the fear of not doing the right thing because of potential medical dangers is often greater than the actual medical problem involved. Thus new problems may be created.

Another related social trend that places increasing demands on the nursing role function in the home is the growing medical pattern of sending patients home from the hospital during the recovery period (and sometimes when there is little or no possibility of recovery). This often means that the woman must have knowledge and even some medical skills in taking care of the family member. The development of home-care programs appears to be on the increase. "The advantages of care in the individual's own home, provided adequate medical nursing and other needed services are available, is generally accepted in theory today."[17] That the home-nursing function is believed to be a part of the female role is also indicated in the Report of the President's Commission:

Modern family life is demanding, and most of the time and attention given to it comes from women. At various stages, girls and women of all economic backgrounds should receive education in respect to physical and mental health, child care and development, human relations within the family.[18]

Although the increasing care of some ill members may be argued as a function of the family, there is evidence that some general social values may not support the argument. For example, Farber found that

the community of "normal" families is not supportive of the revised norms of child care that must be established by families with a severely handicapped child. In effect, the norms and values regulating participation in the community of "normal" families are hostile to the demands made upon the parents of severely handicapped children.[19]

In general it is our contention that in the middle-class family a part of the "professionalization" of the modern woman's role includes her caring for ill members, but in her role of caring for the ill she is not the decision maker but rather has her "nursing" role defined by the medical community. Furthermore, with the home-care movement she will be called upon increasingly to fill a nurse function within the family, but defined for her from *outside* the family. This means that she will function in a mediating role between the impersonal, rational role decisions of the medical expert and the application of those decisions within the highly emotional context of her relationships to her husband or children. The psychological implications of this mediating role are great for both the woman and the ill member in the family. It might also be added that the shouldering of this mediating role function by women will contribute to a further extension of the impersonal relationship between the medical authority and the patient.

CHANGING PATIENT ROLES

The general observation that roles in American society have been undergoing significant change is also true with regard to the various roles related to illnesses. Within the limits of this paper we can focus only briefly on some of the changes in patient roles with particular reference to family members in the patient role and other family roles as related to the family member patient. That is although the changing role of the patient has many implications, we are primarily interested in how this role change is related to the family.

Becoming ill means that the individual is assigned a new and special role, that of the patient. "In this role he exchanges freedom, autonomy, and self-direction for control, but at the same time he gains protection, freedom from responsibility, and care."[20] One of the most important changes with reference to the patient role has been its expansion to include more persons with more different types of medical problems. The most obvious illustration has been the twentieth-century acceptance of the mentally ill patient. Jessie Bernard suggests that the inclusion under the patient role of "many persons formerly viewed as wicked or as criminal is one of the major results of an age of abundance. We can afford to treat them as medical rather than moral or legal problems."[21]

We must place a further restriction on our discussion because we cannot comprehensively discuss the range of physical and mental illnesses as related to the patient role. It is clear that there are differences in having a mental patient versus a physically ill patient in the family. There are differences in both the development of mental illness in the patient and the perception and understanding of that illness by others. On this point Rusk and Novey write:

Despite the progress in public understanding of the amoral nature of emotional and mental illness, there is still likely to be a greater feeling of failure and shame in such cases than when physical and organic illness occurs.[22]

In the family, which depends for efficient operation on the congruency of role relationships, any significant changes in roles may be difficult for other family members to accept and adapt to. But entering a patient role is generally one that other family members can accept as a condition of life because it is not a role change seen as deliberately entered, but rather as beyond the control of the individual. Although family members may sometimes find the means of adaptation to the patient role difficult, they generally see it as something they must attempt to adapt to. This is also true because a state of illness is partially and conditionally legitimized. "That is, if a person is defined as sick, his failure to perform his normal functions is 'not his fault,' and he is accorded the right to exemption and care."[23]

The process of family adaptation to illness is closely linked to the family's definition of the event as a family crisis and what they see as their alternatives for future action. In general, a family crisis calls for new family role procedures because it

is an event which strains the resources which families possess, cannot be solved by the repertory of ready-made answers provided by the mores or built up out of the family's previous experience with trouble, and requires the family to find new (and usually expedient) ways of carrying on family aspirations.[24]

The definition of and adaptation to the crisis of illness of a family member is influenced by the patient's and other family members' perception of the illness for the future. Farber suggests that "the existence of a family crisis depends upon the extent to which the family members regard an event as changing present or future family life in an undesirable way."[25] An important part of a crisis definition may be the extent of significant alterations that the family members see for their family roles. For example, if the man is chronically ill it may mean his leaving his occupational role, requiring his wife to enter that role. This implies for the man the loss of a highly significant role and for the woman the addition of another highly significant role to those she already fills. As Farber has pointed out, this crisis adaptation does not necessarily mean family disorganization, but rather an alteration of family roles and patterns of behavior.[26] Waller and Hill have suggested that

at least three variables help to determine whether a given event becomes a crisis for any given family: (1) the hardships of the situation or event itself; (2) the resources of the family: its role structure, flexibility, and previous history with crisis; and (3) the definition the family makes of the event; that is, whether family members treat the event *as if it were or as if it were not* a threat to their status, goals, and objectives.[27]

The role adaptations of the family to illness are often of a temporary nature with a return to "normal" family roles when the illness is corrected. In this kind of situation, role adaptations generally are easier because they are seen as temporary with a foreseeable return to the usual family roles. Of course, what may

initially appear to be temporary role adaptations may last far longer than anticipated. There may also be an unwillingness to return to the pre-illness family roles.
For example, a woman who temporarily becomes the breadwinner because of her
husband's illness may want to stay in her occupational role even when her husband has recovered and returned to his job. Or it may be that the ill family member may desire or be induced to stay in the patient role. It has been pointed out,
for example, that sometimes patients released from mental hospitals may be so
"protected" by their families that they feel no need to improve and thereby leave
the patient role.[28]

In the following discussion we shall look at some implications of illness for
both marital and parental role relationships. Before doing so, however, it should
be made explicit that our discussion and its impact on family roles is restricted
almost entirely to the middle class. The values and patterns of behavior often
found in the lower class lead to different family adaptations to health problems.
This means that the attitudes toward health presented by the middle-class medical
profession often have limited impact on the lower class. Rainwater has pointed
out that in the lower class

people will be inclined to slight physical difficulties in the interest of attending to more
pressing ones such as seeing that there is food in the house, or seeking some kind of expressive
experience which will reassure them that they are alive and in some way valid persons. The
same kind of medical problem will stand out much more sharply in the middle-class person
because he tends to conceive of his life as having a relatively even and gratifying tenor; his
energies are quickly mobilized by anything which threatens to upset that tenor.[29]

Many lower-class homes are one-parent, mother-head families and therefore
the mother has many family responsibilities with often little time to devote to
illness — whether it be her own or that of a child. When the illness is her own she
may have little time or inclination to seek medical help.

The attitude toward illness (even when it becomes chronic) in this kind of a situation is apt
to be a fairly tolerant one. People learn to live with illness, rather than using their small
stock of interpersonal and psychic resources to do something about the problem.[30]

Because of the limited family resources, Rainwater goes on to point out, "we
observe lower-class parents seemingly relatively indifferent to all kinds of obvious
physical illnesses that their children may have — particularly infections, sores,
colds, and the like."[31] Therefore most of the following discussion of illness in
middle-class families can have only limited application for lower-class families
and their role adaptations to illness.

ILLNESS AND MARRIAGE ROLES

In this section the focus is on some of the consequences of illness for the husband-
father and the wife-mother. As previously suggested there are differences in

consequences for the patient role and the other family members roles as related to whether the illness is physical or mental. We cannot take the space to explore many of the differences but we shall try to indicate from available research some of the implications related to physical versus mental illness for the family members. In general we suggest that there is often some personal and social stigma attached to mental illness, both for the patient and for other family members; whereas with physical illness both the patient and other family members are almost always absolved of any personal responsibility because they are seen as victims of circumstances beyond their control.

The stigmatic nature of mental illness for a family member is reflected in the common resistance to defining the member as having a mental-health problem. In many marriages the observable level of mental illness in a spouse necessary for overt recognition by the partner may vary greatly. In a study of mentally ill husbands, Yarrow suggests that the wife's recognition of illness may come when she

can no longer manage her husband; in others when his behavior destroys the status quo; and, in still others, when she cannot explain his behavior. One can speculate that her level of tolerance for his behavior is a function of her specific personality needs and vulnerabilities, her personal and family value systems, and the social supports and prohibitions regarding the husband's symptomatic behavior.[32]

There are several implications of recognizing that a spouse has a severe mental-health problem. First, there is the emotional drain of identification with the person and his problem; that is, the many consequences for the emotional interaction between two closely linked persons. Second, there are implications of altered roles for the future. Yarrow points out that for a wife of a mentally ill husband is is not only threatening to recognize his mental illness and her own possible relationship to its development but also that she may have "to give up modes of relating to her husband that may have had satisfaction for her and to see a future as the wife of a mental patient."[33]

In severe illness, whether physical or mental, the major implication for the family is that basic roles can no longer be adequately filled by assigned family members. Therefore one basic adaptation by the family to illness must be the redefinition of role responsibilities, which usually means an expansion of role by the unafflicted adult. Yet the role problems and attempts at solutions are bound to have important differences depending on whether the wife or husband is ill and the nature of the illness.

When the husband is seriously ill this generally means that he is no longer able to function in his major role as breadwinner. For him this results in his being removed from the interactional setting of his occupation and being placed in the very different physical and social setting of the hospital or the home. When he is in the home as a patient he is not functioning in the same past role setting where he was usually in the home during the evenings and over the weekend.

That is, in the past his role involvement in the home was limited in time and involved activity in his husband-father roles. With illness he may be spending almost all his time in the home in the new role of being a patient. Therefore for many male patients the home may appear to be a prison in the sense that they must stay there and be passively cared for rather than be away from home in the different and active role performance of their occupations.

Although the husband must make adjustments to his new patient role and the loss of his occupation role, his wife must adapt to him in his husband-patient role and she must often take on his previous breadwinner role. One common consequence is that the wife takes on the added roles but must do so within a restricted economic setting. She must often adapt to a lower income and greater medical expenses because of her husband's illness. If the husband is hospitalized she often has the added time problem of getting to and from and visiting with him in the hospital. Most of the time the wife has few guides to turn to for her new roles and must usually "play it by ear." Deasy and Quinn suggest that

the wife of a man who has been hospitalized as a mental patient for the first time finds herself in an anomalous position — she has not been prepared by personal experience to play this role, she probably has few role models within her immediate purview, and in most instances she feels constrained not to talk about the situation.[34]

It would also appear that when her husband is physically ill the wife may more easily turn to others for moral support and physical help than when her husband is suffering from mental illness. If this is true then the role responsibilities of the wife with a mentally ill husband are carried on with more isolation than a wife with a physically ill husband. The isolated world of the wife with an institutionalized mentally ill husband is clearly suggested in one study.

According to the wives' report, 50 percent of the patients in this study had no visitors outside the family during all the months of hospitalization, 41 percent had only a single or a very occasional visitor, 9 percent had frequent visitors. Friends telephone the wife to inquire about her husband, with vague promises of "wanting to see him" which never materialize.[35]

It would appear that mental illness often leads to loneliness for both the patient and the family. The patient and his family cannot escape the illness but others can and very often do. Because illness is something to be avoided in American society, the patient often finds that he suffers from a stigma which results in the loss of many persons with whom he had previously interacted. The stigma of the husband's illness also may alter the wife's interpersonal relationships with relatives and friends. Farber points out that "not only is she a 'single' person but she also becomes 'special' because of her problem"[36]

When the wife rather than the husband is the ill partner there are different implications for family roles. If the wife is hospitalized she, like the ill husband, is removed from the environment in which she performs her major roles — the home. This generally means the removal of the most significant family role member. Yet she is generally in contact with her husband who tells her about their home and family events, whereas the male who is ill often has little knowledge about what is going on in his occupational role setting. When the wife is ill and in her home, however, her role frustration may be even greater than when hospitalized because she is physically a part of her family setting yet unable to fill her usual family roles.

The husband may have to broaden his role participation when his wife is ill, but probably to less extent than the wife with an ill husband. This is suggested because the husband may often hire someone to do the chores normally done by his wife. Also the economic problems are relatively less when the wife is ill because even though the medical expenses are added the income level of the husband is not usually affected. And often the husband can acquire volunteer help from relatives and friends to help take care of the home. The wife with an ill husband is less likely to receive the kind of voluntary help she needs. This may be a reflection of the belief that men are often incapable (or unwilling) of taking care of many of the tasks necessary for running a household. Also the role of caring for a home is common to women and one may take over the chores of another in essentially the same way she performs those roles for herself. Yet the reverse of this, a man willing and able to substitute for the ill husband by taking over his breadwinner role, is far less common.

The hospitalized wife-mother may be greatly agitated by her withdrawal from domestic roles, especially from her mother role. If she is hospitalized, and has young children, it may be very difficult, because of hospital rules, for her to see her children. One study of wives hospitalized because of mental illness found they were "uniformly concerned with their abilities as mothers and with the possible effects of separation from their children." The medical solution "was handled by emphasis on the necessity of hospitalization and its function in preparing them to be 'better' mothers (and wives)."[37]

Because the role of being mother to her children is held to be so important, the conditions for her removal from the home must be justified. In the case of both mental and physical illness the hospitalization of the mother is legitimized by the medical decision. In the case of mental illness the medical decision to hospitalize removes the burden of decision making from the husband. One study of hospitalized wives with young children found that "for most husbands, the hospital's acceptance of their wives as patients was enough to confirm the legitimacy of separation and to suppress overt reproaches of abandonment."[38]

The hospitalization of a spouse for reasons of mental illness may also provide a rationale for redefining the marriage relationship. That is, the hospitalization of the spouse tends to put marriage and family roles in a state of suspension, rather than dissolving past family roles. This is particularly important with regard to the impact of mental illness on marriage roles. In many marriages the history of the mental illness prior to diagnosis and hospitalization may have been one of conflict between the marriage partners. Yet the hospitalization of a spouse for reasons of mental illness redefines the situation. For example, in the study quoted above it was found that "husbands who had been planning to separate from or divorce their wives met legal obstacles. Besides these, they experienced moral constraints, from within and without, which often moved them to reconsider their decision."[39]

In a study of husbands hospitalized for mental illness it was found that some of the wives had considered ending their marriage but that none actually did so. This study

hypothesized that a recurrence of the husband's illness, especially if it produces the same traumatic developments as were involved the first time, is likely to represent the "last straw" for some of these wives. It appears, however, that complete rejection of the patient is not very frequent after a single relatively brief period of hospitalization.[40]

One important consequence of serious illness for the marriage relationships may be the altering or ending of the sexual relationship. In American society, which gives approval only for sexual relations between marital partners, the inability of one spouse to sexually participate means that both partners are expected to end their active sexual life. For one physically incapable of engaging in coitus there is the added burden of guilt about his inability to meet the sexual needs of the spouse. Even if the well partner thinks about seeking out other sexual partners he would often be restrained by feelings of guilt toward the physically incapable partner.

Our main stress has been on the impact of illness on marriage roles. Of course marriage roles often overlap with parental roles. When one of the parents is ill the well partner must translate and mitigate adjustment as much as possible for the children. The well partner must often try to translate the altered role of the ill parent to the children. In the case of a parent suffering from mental illness the other parent may try to protect the children from the stigma of the parent's illness. One study found that in interpreting the father's mental illness to young children:

almost all the mothers attempt to follow a course of concealment. The child is told either that his father is in a hospital (without further explanation) or that he is in the hospital suffering from a physical ailment (he has a toothache, or trouble with his leg, or a tummy ache, or a headache).[41]

The same study found that adolescent and adult children share with the mother the problems of the father's illness more than any other group of persons. Many times, however, the mother is left on her own because the reactions of adolescent and young adult children are about equally divided into two patterns:

(a) Either the children visit their father regularly and assume much of the same role and attitude toward the illness as their mother or (b) they refuse to visit, expressing openly a great deal of hostility toward their father.[42]

There is little research with regard to the possible effects of a parent's illness on the family roles played by children. When one parent is physically or mentally incapacitated and the well parent has to fill the combined roles, the children may respond in several different ways. Some children may see the care directed at the patient, especially if the well parent is the mother, as threatening to their relationships with their mothers. One consequence might be the regression of the child resulting in another added burden for the mother. On the other hand some children may react to illness of a parent by maturing rapidly insofar as taking on added responsibilities in helping the well parent. This may be particularly true for daughters because of the high identification with their mother and her roles. There is some evidence in studies of working mothers that daughters take up some of the responsibilities of their mothers when they have other role demands. Douvan found that the proportion of girls who carry major responsibilities is larger where the mother works either full time or part time than in homes where the mother is not employed.[43]

One other factor of marriage as related to illness impact occurs as the married couple grows older. Many times when serious illness of one of the spouses (most often the husband) first occurs is when the conjugal family unit has been reduced to only the husband and wife. This is the period of the postparental years when the last of the children have left home. Fifty years ago marriages ended through the death of one of the parents about the time the last child was leaving the parental home. But today's married couples have an average of about 15 years to share together after their youngest child has left home.[44] That the woman is most often the marriage partner who survives and who has filled a nurse role for her husband's terminal illness is reflected in the statistics of life expectancy. Slightly more than one-fifth of all the American women at age 55 to 64 and more than half of those at 65 and over are widows. "There are currently about 8½ million widows in the U.S., two-fifth of them under 65 years of age."[45] That increasing rates of illness are related to increasing age is obvious. For example, "while persons over 65 accounted for only one in twelve of the total population in 1955, one-fifth of the patients occupying hospital beds were in this age group."[46] Therefore women can increasingly expect to perform some nursing roles to their husbands with increasing age, and when the husband is not hospitalized the care often will take place in the home with no members other than the husband-patient and the wife-nurse.

PARENTS AND CHILDREN

In this last section we shall look briefly at the impact of illness on the parent-child relationship. When both parents are present the illness of a child usually places the greatest role demands on the mother. In general this is a part of a greater commitment to the parental role by the mother than by the father. One study found that where there were retarded children they tended to highlight parental role differences. "The findings tended to support predictions that fathers would be more vulnerable to social stigma and extramarital influences such as children's physical appearance and sex."[47]

An important difference with implications for role relationships occurs when an adult in contrast with a child is ill. Although in both cases we assume strong emotional involvement, when the child is ill there is added his dependency and immaturity. There is a dimension of "unfairness" in seeing a child ill because he appears so vulnerable and helpless. Therefore the parent responding to a sick child is responding to both the sickness and the helpless dependency of the child. Even though many of the serious illnesses of childhood have been alleviated, middle-class parents generally take a preventive medical approach to children. This approach not only protects the child from possible illnesses but it also helps protect the parents from the emotional drain of coping with sick children.

Yet even with the great medical advances with regard to children, the parents (especially the mother) have a new nursing role with regard to their children. As pointed out earlier the mother today finds herself constantly turning to medical experts for instructions in dealing with an ill child, and she is kept constantly aware of the potential dangers of mental illness for children. Because of the dependent and vulnerable nature of the child she is particularly sensitive of doing the "right" thing in treating her child, both for his health improvement and for her own reassurance that she is being a good mother.

There is some evidence that certain types of illness, particularly those that indicate long-term physical disability, have a variety of implications for parental roles. There is often a resistance to the fact that a problem really exists. For example, in a study of families with physically disabled children it was found that parents showed "an active resistance to the medical reality, which delayed the initiation of necessary treatment and the beginning of realistic adjustment."[48] The illness of the child may lead not only to new definitions within the family setting but also be altered role patterns for the parents outside the family. Farber points out that

investigations consistently indicate a tendency for parents of handicapped children to be less sociable and more withdrawn, and for these mothers to be less likely than other mothers to take employment outside the home.[49]

CONCLUSION

In this paper the main purpose has been to look at some changing roles in the family, especially the role of wife-mother as related to illness. It appears that increasingly the family is expected to handle a greater amount of illness and that increasingly this is becoming a part of the "professional" role of the wife-mother. For the most part the family's involvement in the care of its sick members is seen as meeting medical needs with little concern with how this affects the overall needs of the family.

The home-care movement is supported by funds and agencies for increasing facilitation of their beliefs about the care of the ill. The assumptions and aims of this are well illustrated by programs to return the mentally ill to their families. Vincent writes,

the family is expected to adapt to the return of its mentally ill or emotionally disturbed members, just as it was expected to adapt to the return of the parolee member of the family several decades ago. The family will also be expected to adapt to the intrusion of the mental-health personnel concerned with the rehabilitation of the patient, just as it has adapted to the intrusion of the parole and probation officers, the judge of the juvenile court, and the social worker.[50]

Given the emotional involvement of family members with one and another it is not difficult to persuade them as to their "responsibility." As Vincent puts it:

Given the mores of our society how could the family maintain its ideological image if it refused to accept one of its members convalescing from mental illness or rehabilitating from crime or delinquency?[51]

It appears that the primary concern in research has been with how the family may be used in the care of its ill members. That is, the family is seen as a means for facilitating medical decisions. But rarely is the question asked: what does the involvement of the ill do to other family roles? A second related question rarely asked is: does the family really provide a more effective setting for the handling of illness, or is this often primarily a means of resolving some of the problems of the medical authorities? Although we have suggested some possibilities for answering these questions, further exploration is needed. From the perspective of the sociology of the family we need to know far more about the implications of what the family is being asked to do medically for the family itself and its impact on society in general.

REFERENCES

1. See Robert R. Bell, *Marriage and Family Interaction*, Homewood, Ill.: Dorsey, 1963, pp. 16–23.
2. *Ibid.*, p. 255.
3. *Ibid.*, pp. 259–260.
4. Margaret Mead and Frances B. Kaplan (Eds.), *American Woman*, New York: Scribner, 1965, p. 80.
5. *Ibid.*
6. "The American Woman," *Statistical Bulletin*, New York: Metropolitan Life Insurance Co., February 1965, p. 1.
7. "United States Life Tables: 1959–61," Washington, D.C.: U.S. Department of Health, Education, and Welfare, 1964, p. 5.
8. "The American Woman," *op. cit.*, p. 3.
9. *Ibid.*, pp. 3–4.
10. Mead, *op. cit.*, p. 91.
11. *Ibid.*, p. 45.

12. *Ibid.*
13. "The American Woman," *op. cit.*, p. 2.
14. Mead, *op. cit.*, p. 19.
15. Bell, *op. cit.*, p. 261.
16. *Ibid.*, p. 262.
17. George Rosen, "Health Programs for an Aging Population," in Clark Tibbetts, *Handbook of Social Gerontology*, Chicago: University of Chicago Press, 1960, p. 536.
18. Mead, *op. cit.*, pp. 32–33.
19. Bernard Farber, *Family: Organization and Interaction*, San Francisco: Chandler, 1964, p. 314.
20. Jessie Bernard, *Social Problems at Mid-Century*, New York: Dryden, 1957, p. 191.
21. *Ibid.*, p. 192.
22. Howard A. Rusk and Joseph Novey, "The Impact of Chronic Illness on Families," *Marriage and Family Living*, May 1957, p. 195.
23. Talcott Parsons and Renee Fox, "Illness, Therapy, and the Modern Urban American Family," *Journal of Social Issues*, 1958, pp. 32–33.
24. Willard Waller and Reuben Hill, *The Family*, New York: Dryden, 1951, p. 456.
25. Farber, *op. cit.*, p. 409.
26. *Ibid.*, p. 392.
27. Waller, *op. cit.*, p. 459.
28. Donald A. Hansen and Reuben Hill, "Families under Stress," in Harold T. Christensen (Ed.), *Handbook of Marriage and the Family*, Chicago: Rand McNally, 1964, p. 809.
29. Lee Rainwater, "The Lower Class: Health, Illness, and Medical Institutions," mimeo, March 1965, pp. 2–3.
30. *Ibid.*, p. 5.
31. *Ibid.*, p. 9.
32. Marian R. Yarrow et al., "The Psychological Meaning of Mental Illness in the Family," *Journal of Social Issues*, XI, 1955, p. 18.
33. *Ibid.*, p. 22.
34. Leila C. Deasy and Olive W. Quinn, "The Wife of the Mental Patient and the Hospital Psychiatrist," *Journal of Social Issues*, XI, 1955, p. 49.
35. Marian R. Yarrow et al., "The Social Meaning of Mental Illness," *Journal of Social Issues*, XI, 1955, p. 44.
36. Farber, *op. cit.*, p. 397.
37. Harold Sampson et al., "The Mental Hospital and Marital Family Ties," in Howard Becker (Ed.), *The Other Side*, New York: Free Press of Glencoe, 1964, p. 145.
38. *Ibid.*, p. 144.
39. *Ibid.*, p. 146.
40. John A. Clausen and Marian R. Yarrow, "Further Observations and Some Implications," *Journal of Social Issues*, XI, 1955, p. 62.
41. Yarrow, "The Meaning of Mental Illness," *op. cit.*, pp. 40–41.
42. *Ibid.*, p. 40.
43. Elizabeth Douvan, "Employment and the Adolescent," in E. Ivan Nye and Lois W. Hoffman, *The Employed Mother in America*, Chicago: Rand McNally, 1963, p. 146.
44. Mead, *op. cit.*, p. 89.
45. "The American Woman," *op. cit.*, p. 1.
46. Rosen, *op. cit.*, p. 527.
47. Irving Tallman, "Spousal Role Differentiation and the Socialization of Severely Retarded Children," *Journal of Marriage and Family*, February 1965, p. 42.
48. Thomas E. Dow, Jr., "Family Reaction to Crisis," *Journal of Marriage and Family*, August 1965, p. 363.
49. Farber, *op. cit.*, p. 313.
50. Clark E. Vincent, "Familia Spongia: The Adaptive Function," *National Council on Family Relations*, Toronto: October 1965, p. 13.
51. *Ibid.*

40
Nursing Care of the Infant in the Community

Marguerite W. Bozian

The infant is part of a family unit. Nursing care of the infant is not complete unless the other significant family members are also included. In addition to assessment of the infant's physical well-being, the family's physical, emotional, social and cultural status must be considered. Using the nursing process, Marguerite Bozian outlines the steps for community nursing care of the infant. In her discussion she emphasizes the family and also continuity of care between hospital and home.

Nursing, by virtue of its emphasis on the individual and its closeness to people, occupies a key position among the health care professions. The potential for quality family nursing care is present in our society.

THE NEED FOR CHANGE

It is time for the various areas of nursing to dispense with giving lip service to the continuum of health care and assume their roles in community health. Community nursing care can no longer be limited to those people who wear the appropriate uniform; it is the responsibility of each individual nurse to build the bridge into the community for the continuation of nursing care. It will be the sum total of all nursing efforts that will enable citizens of a community to obtain preventive, continuous, and comprehensive nursing care.

Public health nursing swims in a sea of nostalgia which has a high saline content and aids in keeping this specialty afloat. The public health nurse must lessen her grip on forms, rote procedures for tuberculosis, venereal diseases, etc., and put a little thought process into working with families. All the technical knowledge is to no avail if the mother sits there and says, "Yep. Yep. I understand." The only thing that she understands is that, if she says "yes" to everything, the public health nurse will go away sooner than if she says "no."

A new emphasis is needed and this emphasis must lie in the direction of motivating people to seek and use health care for the maximum health and welfare of the family. This emphasis necessitates concentration upon an understanding of normal growth, normal behavior, and basic needs and attitudes of people. Through this understanding will come indicators that a public health nurse can use as a foundation for formulating nursing plans for maximum effectiveness. Instead of telling people what to do, the nurse seeks to aid the family in defining their needs and stimulates the family to obtain and utilize health care.

From *Nursing Clinics of North America*, Vol. 6, No. 1, pp. 93–101, 1971. Reprinted by permission of the publisher and author.

THE NEWBORN AT HOME

Nursing care of the newborn in the community necessitates preventive, continuous, and comprehensive attention to all aspects of health care for the family. This is not in contrast to but an extension of the health care utilized by parents during the prenatal period and the period of hospitalization during and after the birth of the baby. Ideally this care extended as far back as premarital counseling or earlier.

The physical and emotional aspects of the growth of a newborn might be viewed as a "funnel" movement. The excitement of the role that a nurse plays in helping people create sound foundations for babies during the newborn period is further heightened by the contemplation of the future ramifications of this small beginning.

Several examples could be given to illustrate this. If, for instance, the nurse can help a mother understand the need for the newborn to begin developing a sense of trust in himself and his environment from birth on (the first task of an infant according to Erickson), then perhaps a personality deviation will be averted. To reduce this to dollars and cents to a community, it costs approximately $5000 per year to provide education for one child with an emotional learning problem in contrast to approximately $562.00 per child in regular school.[4] If an infant does not receive measles vaccine and becomes ill with measles with resultant blindness or deafness, this one child will cost the community approximately $1500—$3000 per year. Actually the Bureau of Handicapped under the Office of Education will allow up to $15,000 per year for the education and rehabilitation of *one* person who is blind and deaf.[3] These figures do not include indirect costs such as loss of manpower and productivity and loss of taxes from potential income, nor do they include the human hurt and pain felt by the individuals and their families.

The Infant and His Family Unit

Each infant is born into some type of a family unit. In 1970 many nursing visits are made to families where the person giving primary care to a newborn may be an aunt, a grandmother, a sister or a foster mother. Most of the newborns will have had contact with nursing care before being brought home to their own special environment. Usually, too, the family unit has received nursing attention before the birth of the baby and, therefore, the continuum of nursing care will most likely have been started prior to the birth of the baby.

A newborn infant is discharged from the hospital when the appropriate medical officer deems the infant is in a condition to maintain life and grow satisfactorily in his home environment. In some instances, nursing will have played a part in this decision; in others, it would have been desirable to consult nursing before discharge. Whether the newborn infant has had a normal hospitalization or has been ill, he is in need of essentially the same care. The infant with a physical disability is differentiated from the normal newborn only in relation to the additional care dictated by his specific illness or convalescent period.

For the nurse going into the home to make a visit, the concept to keep uppermost in mind is that the *basic* physical and emotional needs at this particular point in time are essentially the same for all infants. However, the anxieties, problems, and expectations are different for each mother and father. As the parents are the providers of care for infants, their concerns directly influence the execution and depth of care that will be provided to nurture and promote the optimal growth and development of each individual infant.

Based on this concept, it is essential to turn first to the mother and/or father and obtain an expression of concerns and difficulties that they are encouraging in relation to their own physical and emotional needs. It is ideal to have the father included, but it is realistic to recognize that this is a rare situation. Often, the nurse will be working with the mother only (or the grandmother or other adult). From verbal and nonverbal communications, information may be gleaned that is suggestive of the kind of support and guidance that will be appropriate during this emotionally and physically disturbing postpartum period. After all, the mother has had nine months for her emotions and body to accommodate to the growth of new life within her; it is logical to expect tremendous physical and emotional difficulties to occur in her accommodation to the new life now outside the body after an abrupt exit.

It is through the helping relationship that the nurse forms with the mother that relief comes for some of the mother's concerns. Carl Rogers defines a helping relationship as one "in which at least one of the parties has the intent of promoting the growth, development, maturity, improved functioning and improved coping with life of the other."[5] In other words, it is by the therapeutic use of self that the nurse is hoping to create more expression and more functional use of the mother's resources, strengths, and capabilities. It is the challenge of the nurse to help the mother identify and actualize them.

Special Needs of the Newborn

Once a beginning relationship has been formed with the mother and/or the father, the nurse can then focus attention on the newborn. Margaret Adams published an excellent article in the *American Journal of Nursing* on the inspection of the newborn in the hospital which is equally applicable for use in the home.[1] This program of inspection can be used for all infants. Modifications are made in relation to whether the infant is full term, premature, ill, or convalescing from illness. The basic concept is that the infant is joining the family unit and the family in turn will accommodate itself to his specific needs. Thus, an infant who was born prematurely will receive, in essence, the same care as a full-term baby, differing only in the special attention to specific needs dictated by his prematurity.

Premature infants make up the largest group of infants who have special physical needs. These needs are the consequence of incomplete intrauterine development. The thin, fragile skin and the decreased amount of subcutaneous tissue necessitate special handling and clothing. The need for warmth is further accentuated by the instability of the mechanisms for regulating body temperatures.

Muscular development is often delayed, and this results in weak suckling and rooting reflexes. Therefore, feedings should be more frequent, probably less in volume, and more regularly scheduled than for a full-term baby on a self-demand schedule. Since the stomach is tubular and sphincters are poorly developed, the infant regurgitates easily. The formula must be modified to accommodate the decreased ability to digest fat and the increased needs for protein and iron. As with normal infants, the babies should be fed in an unhurried manner, cuddled and loved. Thus a lifetime stage is set: dinnertime is the time for enjoyment and interaction among loved ones in a family setting where dinnertime is important. (The act of eating has psychologic implications for all groups. To deprived groups, eating may have been a matter of sheer survival.)

Since premature infants possess relatively fewer antibodies than full-term infants, special emphasis is needed in relation to the physical environment. Cleanliness and temperature are important factors in this environment. Because of a thin skin and immature hepatic function, the premature will bleed more easily, which necessitates careful vigilance for sharp objects. Since urine will be more concentrated, rubber pants are not used. Handling is limited to adult members of the family during the first months, and visitors are limited and should be screened for colds, sore throats, etc.

These nursing care measures are specifically designed for premature babies. However, one may logically perceive that they also apply to full-term infants, the difference lying only in the degree and intensity of the application of specific procedures.

Facilities for Health Care for Infants in the Community

The emphasis in health care is being placed on the prevention of illness and disabilities. This movement has been given impetus by the direction of federal spending. Many research projects are under way for studying the prevention of intrauterine defects. Much attention also is centered around prevention of prematurity, which is the principal cause of neonatal deaths. The need for parental counseling during pregnancy is becoming more evident. New developments in the field of genetics are exciting in that they indicate that congenital abnormalities can be predicted and prevented.[2]

Health centers are becoming more and more family-centered. These are being sponsored by OEO or under the auspices of combinations of agencies such as "model cities," various health departments, medical schools, urban renewal projects, etc. Each individual community has its own myriad of health care facilities and the community health nurse must be fully aware of them.

It is gratifying to note that more private medical facilities are shifting their emphasis toward total family needs and prevention of illness. Examples of these are the prepaid medical care plans such as that of the Kaiser Foundation and the New York City Health Insurance Plan.

THE NURSING PROCESS

Nursing Assessment

If the nurse has had contact with the family before the birth of the baby, there will have been some assessment of the social and emotional status of the family. In the initial visit, some data will be collected to determine the attitudes of the family toward the baby. These attitudes set the stage for the total care of the baby. The perfect physical care of a newborn is incomplete without love. The triad of physical, social, and emotional care is needed for depth and soundness.

A beginning evaluation as to the mother's base-line knowledge of infant care should already have been in process. If the information has not been volunteered the nurse should ascertain the type of health supervision the infant is receiving. The nurse continues the assessment during her physical inspection of the baby.

A checklist is available that was devised as a tool for students of nursing to use to enable them to be thorough in their examination of the newborn. Using this checklist as a guide, the nurse can augment the mother's knowledge while covering points of growth and development with her. This is an excellent teaching opportunity for the nurse to show the mother graphically the physical characteristics present and to predict the changes that will be occurring during the next few months. It is obvious that, concurrent with this assessment, teaching has been taking place.

CHECKLIST FOR NEWBORN ASSESSMENT FOR COMMUNITY HEALTH NURSE

I. Appearance
    Skin: texture
          color
    Eyes: color of sclera
          movement
          drainage
    Hair: amount: head
                 body

II. Posture: sleeping
           waking
           crying
           position of head

III. Physical: shape, size of *head*
             shape, size of fontanelles
             symmetry of facial features
             nose: any nasal flaring?
             buccal cavity, gums: condition
                               color
                               appearance
             ears: presence of cartilage

Neck: shape and size; extra folds at back of neck
Chest: shape: any retraction noted
Respirations: rate and quality; easy? retractions?
Pulse rate: regular? rate?
Breasts: presence of maternal hormones? breast tissue present?
Genitalia: testes descended? pseudo-menstruation?
Temperature: range
Umbilicus: drying? infection? bleeding?
Elimination: voiding — how often?
                          color
                          odor
        stool — how often?
                          color
                          odor
                          consistency
                          flatus?
Buttocks: extra gluteal folds present?
              symmetry of legs and equal length
Legs: symmetrical
      bowlegs?
      clubbed feet?
Reflexes: Moro   swallowing
         grasp   rooting
         sucking   dancing
Cry: sharp, high-pitched
     deep, raspy
     moist
Eating: how often?   satisfied?
        how much?   irritable?

Concomitant with the nursing assessment of the infant's status, an assessment will be made of the mother's specific needs within the family unit.

Nursing Formulation

The nurse in the home formulates plans with the mother to meet the direct needs of mother and infant. This may be the appropriate time to refer the mother to the well baby clinic or private physician for health care. All too often nurses casually tell mothers to keep their clinic appointments. If they questioned mothers in more depth, or listened more closely, nurses might be surprised to learn that some mothers go to clinics because they were told to do so; others just stay away. How much more effective it would be if mothers really understood why they take their babies to clinics for "shots" and checkups!

Most nurses find that if they plan their future visits with the mother before leaving the home a certain amount of support and security is provided the mother. She can save her questions for the nurse and does not feel alone in caring for her infant.

Later the nurse records the visit on the family record. At that time she formulates her nursing diagnosis, nursing goals, and nursing plan to meet these goals. Priorities are delineated for a plan of action. The nurse needs to keep in mind that goals must be tailored for the individual family, and priorities are assigned to the felt needs of the families, not to the needs felt by the nurse to be important.

Implementation

This is the stage at which the nurse takes direct action toward a goal based on her nursing plan. This includes making referrals that are deemed necessary. If the newborn was visited upon request of another agency, then a report is sent back to the referring agency. Referrals are important in the complex structure of community health care. The important aspects of referrals are awareness of their function, appreciation for appropriate timing in executing the referral request, and realization that maximum effectiveness is gained through communication back to the referring agency.

A major task is to bring into action all the resources available to a family. These resources include financial aid, assistance from other agencies (e.g., homemaking services, welfare departments, voluntary infant interest groups, etc.), the help of friends, and many other sources. Supervision or monitoring of these resources after they have been mobilized is urged.

The author had an experience which dramatized the need for supervision of resources mobilized. A student was visiting a family whose mother was a food faddist and had two toddlers in addition to a new baby. The mother believed that the juice from ground grass blades prevented and/or cured all infections. This mother would not listen to anyone from a health agency. The student with her instructor enlisted the aid of a neighbor, formerly a dietitian, who had a good relationship with Mrs. X. The neighbor was to help Mrs. X understand the need for immunizations, health supervision, and a more appropriate diet for the family. At the end of six weeks, the neighbor was drinking and feeding her family the juice from ground grass blades.*

The nurse's next visits would be centered around putting into action the nursing care plan based on the felt needs of the family. This might include formula preparation, teaching, following through on referrals, etc.

Any concern the nurse feels about the physical inspection of the newborn should be immediately reported to the proper health facility.

Evaluation

After each subsequent visit, the nurse needs to look critically at her nursing plans and test their validity. Are they meeting the needs of the family and the nursing goals? If not, why not? Are these plans practical or realistic? Should an alternative plan be used? The overall evaluation of the results obtained from nursing care implementation is a continuous process. Each contact with the family produces data for evaluation and replanning.

*The author will supply the method for the preparation of grass juice upon request.

SUMMARY

In modern nursing practice the newborn infant is brought into the family setting. The nursing emphasis is placed upon his individualized needs within the family grouping. The infant becomes a part of the family and this addition alters the nature and enlarges the scope of nursing care.

The nursing process can and should be utilized in every nursing situation. The majority of the references in nursing literature place the nursing process in the hospital setting, but it is equally effective to provide the best possible nursing care in the community. The major difference is the extensive reaching-out process for mobilizing resources. The health team is enlarged, for it may include friends, relatives, church members, local tradesmen, pharmacists, etc.

By using the nursing process in the community, public health nurses draw closer to the nurses in the hospital setting. By reaching out into the community for continuity of nursing care, the hospital nurses draw closer to public health nurses. With concentrated and united efforts on the part of all nurses, the citizens of a community will receive preventive, continuous, and comprehensive nursing care for the whole family.

REFERENCES

1. Adams, Margaret: Appraisal of a newborn infant. *Am. J. Nursing*, 55:1336–1337, Nov., 1955.
2. McKusick, V. A.: *Human Genetics*. 2nd Ed. Englewood Cliffs, New Jersey, Prentice-Hall, Inc., 1969.
3. Department of Health, Education and Welfare: *Bureau of Handicapped Report, 1967*. Washington, Government Printing Office, 1968.
4. Ohio Department of Education: *Revised Budget, FY 1967*, Board of Education of the Cincinnati School District, Project Number 00130.
5. Rogers, C. R.: The Characteristics of a Helping Relationship. Paper presented at University of Wisconsin, 1962.

41
Adolescents and VD

Mary Agnes Brown

One facet of normal adolescent development is increased sexual awareness. The teenager has many questions and feelings about sex. Family and peer relationships are affected as the adolescent becomes sexually active. For the nurse, this means that the sexual dimension of adolescence must be understood and accepted. Mary Brown discusses one of the problems resulting from sexual activity, venereal disease. Community nurses can be influential in the eradication of venereal disease among teenagers, but first they must deal with their own attitudes toward sexual behavior.

"VD? You've got VD?" says the starting-to-tremble voice of the young girl on the telephone in a recent TV commercial. "Then ... I've probably got it, too...." Thus begins a chain of reactions which may or may not lead to treatment and help for one of 300,000 teenagers reported to have VD each year in this country. The seriousness of the epidemic has meaning for all health care professionals, particularly nurses; it's time to get down to the serious business of helping adolescents prevent and/or receive treatment for venereal disease.

Many young people have no idea of what the symptoms of gonorrhea and syphilis are, or how these diseases are transmitted. Therefore, even though treatment is fairly simple, it is often delayed, either because the teenagers do not recognize the symptoms or because they do not want their families to find out they're having sexual relations. Most adolescents respond to the first symptoms of VD by hoping that they'll go away. When they *do* disappear, as the first symptoms always do, the teenagers gain a false sense of relief. Treatment is delayed, and the disease progresses.

EPIDEMIC PROPORTIONS

Whenever a communicable disease epidemic strikes, usually all available health personnel, including nurses, are mobilized into action. However, because of its insidious nature, the gonorrhea-syphilis epidemic has taken quite a while to surface and be recognized, and to have organized efforts directed toward its eradication.

The rate of cases of gonorrhea has increased to one-and-a-half to two million new (reported) cases a year, and ranks first among reportable diseases.[1,2] Syphilis now occupies third place, and it is estimated that 250,000 cases of all forms of syphilis are diagnosed and treated each year. Although the rate of increase of VD in adolescents is high, recent studies show that the increase in the 40 to 49 age group is greater than those in either the 15 to 19 group, or the 20 to 24 group.[3]

Most cases of VD, however, are never reported. Private physicians treat about 80 percent of the diagnosed gonorrhea and syphilis cases, but they report only one in nine cases of gonorrhea and only one in eight cases of syphilis. This means that over three-quarters of the cases are not reported, and so the disease continues to spread through unidentified contacts.[4,5]

The discovery in the late 1940's of penicillin as an effective cure for both diseases created a false sense of security among professionals and the public alike, and led to a relaxation of vigilance and reduction of funds in the campaign to eradicate venereal diseases. The result was a rise in VD rates, and growing resistance of the VD organisms to penicillin.

Other reasons for the present increase includes changing sexual patterns, lack of education on sex and venereal disease, breakdown in the family unit, increased mobility of the population, changing attitudes and cultural mores regarding sex, and the widespread use of oral contraceptives in place of condoms.[6-9]

ATTITUDE TOWARD TEENAGERS

If we as nurses are to be a therapeutic force in the eradication of teenage VD, we must examine our own attitudes toward sex and our feelings about adolescent sexual activities. How will we as individuals respond to a group of teenagers seeking venereal disease information and guidance or to an infected adolescent's request for help? Will we be shocked? Can the adolescent be considered a child under the circumstances? Should the parents be told? Can the teenager be cared for without the parent's knowledge or consent? From whom was the disease contracted? Should the nurse report the case? In fact, what is the nurse's professional responsibility in such a situation?

Before we can realistically answer these questions, we must work through our concerns about ourselves — particularly as sexual beings. Without this insight it will be impossible to think about and behave objectively in terms of our role with teenagers, parents, physicians, and the community. For some nurses, it will also mean making a conscious effort to understand and accept the nature of adolescent sexual activity.

Teenagers are vulnerable to venereal disease because of many intrinsic and extrinsic factors. They are very casual in their social relationships, and just as casual about sex. It is difficult to prescribe contraceptives and anti-venereal disease methods that are satisfactory to them because their sexual encounters are apt to be sporadic, impromptu, and may take place anywhere, at any hour. Most teenagers respond to their urges immediately; they see no reason why they shouldn't. Therefore, they are unlikely to be prepared to prevent a pregnancy or venereal disease. In addition, they take their cues from adult behavior and attitudes. They know that sexual experimentation has always been considered "normal" for men, and that is now becoming acceptable for women as well.

Teenagers are also under tremendous pressure regarding sex. Their parents tell them not to engage in anything sexual — don't neck, don't pet, don't go to bed with anybody, while the mass media scream at them continually that sex is fun. They have become the target of a carefully researched and calculated advertising campaign to separate them from their nine billion dollars spending money. They are urged through books, newspapers, posters, and magazines to engage in sexual activities and to try every conceivable position and gadget devised to enhance sexual pleasure.

The pressures which adolescents inflict upon each other are even greater. Girls are told, "You owe it to your boyfriend," or "You'll lose him if you don't." Boys are said to be "square," if they don't try to "make" the girl, and they are dared to visit a prostitute at least once. Thus, girls often engage in sex hoping that it will lead to marriage, while boys are doing the same in order to stay out of it.

SEX EDUCATION

To date, sex education has proven inadequate to remedy the situation. Mary Calderone, executive director, Sex Information and Education Council of the United States, has condemned past attempts at sex education for adolescents as "inadequate, hypocritical and completely superficial."[10] Her organization, as well as the American Association of Sex Educators and Counselors continues to develop programs and train educators to meet today's young people on their own level and to speak to them in language they can understand.

Ideally, sex and VD information should come from parents, but most parents shun the whole idea because of their own hang-ups. Some *could* answer their sons' and daughters' questions but don't know how to express themselves; others don't know the answers and are unable to say that they don't know. Too many times children, even teenagers, are told that it is not nice to ask these questions, or that they are too young to know now and will find out later. They surely will — but how, and from whom? In most instances, they will learn from their peers and playmates, often in a traumatic way and by being given distorted information.

Recent studies show that the schools and mass media can offer facts about VD more objectively than either parents or friends can because they are not emotionally or socially involved.[11] In 1966, venereal disease education was begun as a pilot project in six senior and vocational high schools in New York City. By early 1967, there were 40 more, and by fall of that year, all the city high schools offered VD information and counsel.

It seems that the teenage students are often not as hung up and hesitant as are the teachers who offer the sex education program. Gordon reports that many teachers "beat around the bush" and do not give the straight facts or discuss issues of concern to students — homosexuality, masturbation, and venereal disease.[12] But, lack of appropriate sex education is not the only problem; deficiencies exist in treatment services, too.

LACK OF SERVICES

Public health facilities for the treatment of teenagers infected with venereal disease leave much to be desired. The average central city social hygiene clinic is overcrowded and understaffed, and care is impersonal. There are no special teenage sessions, as there are in prenatal and family planning clinics, and the crowded conditions afford little comfort or privacy. Nurse counseling is at a minimum, if available at all.

Nevertheless, young people do attend these clinics and benefit from the examination, treatment, and medication, for which there is no charge. Their requests for confidentiality are respected. Public health-oriented physicians treat and report each case and U.S. Public Health Service investigators, mostly young adults, follow up these reports. Usually, they are able to gain the trust and confidence of the teenagers, and eventually identify and trace sexual contacts.

Many private physicians, sensitive to the specific needs of adolescents are scheduling special office hours with fewer appointments at these times so that they can spend more time with each youngster, counseling and answering his/her questions.

Adolescents in suburban and rural areas may or may not be as fortunate as their urban brothers and sisters. While they lack free clinic facilities, they have more money to spend, and some people think they might benefit from paying their own doctor bills. However, anonymity and confidentiality cannot always be guaranteed. In such communities, social pressures and local politics often affect physicians' practice and their policies with regard to the parents of teenagers. Also, school health services, including nursing care and counseling, may not be available or may differ from one locality to another.

Most states now permit a physician to treat youngsters for venereal disease without parental consent. For example, the New York State law, which became effective May 1, 1970, reads: "A licensed physician may diagnose, treat or prescribe for a case of venereal disease in a person under the age of twenty-one years without the consent or knowledge of the parents or guardian of said person."[13]

Some physicians, however, are only now beginning to come to grips with the issue of confidentiality. In large public clinics there is usually no problem; parents are not sought out and informed. In many cases, the youngsters do not give their right names and addresses, anyway.

The issue of confidentiality does pose a dilemma for many private physicians. One physician has suggested in an article in a British journal that teenage patients, parents, and doctor should come to some understanding about the involvement or noninvolvement of parents in the patient's care, based on the feelings of all of them about the matter.[14]

Another physician, responding to the article, said that the question is not one of moral values for doctors are concerned with health. Adolescents, he thinks, can be shown the effects of behavior — heavy drinking, smoking, use of drugs, promiscuity, and irresponsibility in sexual matters — on their health. It is therefore not a question of going to parents and informing them, but of advising the young people themselves about the consequences of their behavior.[15]

Teenagers would like to be involved in the planning of their own health care and education. At a recent 2-day workshop on "Teenagers and Contraceptive Services," sponsored jointly by two units of the New York City Health Department, some of the young people had an opportunity to make their needs and wishes known. A committee of 18 teenagers worked together with a similar number of adults in planning the program. Among the speakers were teenage high school students who identified their needs and feelings as follows.

Teens *are* sexually active, a fact made apparent by the rise in teenage pregnancies. Teenagers should not be punished for engaging in premarital sex, and family planning services should be made available to them. Requiring consent for treatment from someone other than the patient is a refusal to recognize the patient as a person, and a denial of his/her right to make his/her own decisions. Young people should not be the focus of discussion about teenage family planning; they should be the controlling factor. Any facility that is to serve youth effectively must be youth-oriented.

REMEDIES OFFERED

From the conference, attended by health workers, family planners, and sex educators from all over the country and Puerto Rico, came new ideas and approaches to teen services. Among these were: models for revising existing health care delivery systems; a new awareness of the teen as a human being with specific and legitimate needs; and plans for additions to existing services such as peer counseling groups, teen outreach workers, teenage control over personnel in the form of screening staff about the attitudes, and adolescent advisory boards.

Several new approaches to teenage education are working successfully in New York City. One is the "rap session," in which a small group of teens gather with one or two informed young adults, and together they discuss feelings as well as facts about specific subject matter. As the group members build up a trusting relationship among themselves, barriers to communication are let down, and soon they are sharing experiences and learning from each other, without any of the distrust and inhibition that have blocked attempts to educate them in the past. Feelings are expressed, and reasons for behavior are sought and talked about. Myths are picked apart, and factual information is given where needed and requested. These sessions are for the most part unstructured; the leaders take their cues from the teenagers.

Public Health Service workers are using another approach to teaching about venereal disease. In response to requests from a community, they present a brief film and discussion-type program at school assemblies, teenage dances, and other activities where teens gather. Young people welcome these programs, and are not embarrassed to ask for them, or to participate in them.

NURSES' CONTRIBUTION

These approaches are only beginnings; far more could be accomplished — particularly by nurses — in improving sex education and treatment services for teenagers. For example, in large urban social hygiene clinics, public health nurses could urge special sessions for teenagers and demonstrate that this system will not increase staff workloads but will improve the quality of services.

School nurse-teachers, particularly those in suburban and rural areas, are in strategic positions. Besides casefinding and getting infected youngsters under proper medical care, they have the unique and difficult job of interpreting students' needs, legislative changes, and innovations in health policy to other teachers, parents, school boards, and the community in general. The counseling role of these nurses is of tremendous importance because of the tendency of teenagers to trust and consult their school nurse, sometimes more readily and comfortably than other educators.

The school setting, however, involves problems of confidentiality, since traditionally parents have been notified about a pupil's medical problem. In the case of the teenager with venereal disease, we now have a whole new ball game. How the school nurse-teacher will handle the matter depends not only on his or her professional judgment, but also on the school physician, local school boards, parent-teacher groups, and the policy of the school district.

Nurses working in doctors' offices may have a different set of concerns, depending upon their role-relationships with their employers. If a doctor diagnoses a case of venereal disease, it is that doctor's responsibility to report the case to public health authorities. What if the doctor does not carry out this responsibility? What does the nurse do then? Perhaps she can help the employer understand the seriousness of the consequences, especially in the case of teenagers. Or, perhaps she can volunteer to talk with the teenager about contacts and report the case for the doctor. Perhaps the nurse doesn't feel the need to do anything. It is a matter of commitment and involvement; again, the answers lie within the individual.

Nursing educators, as well as in-service educators are looking at the specific needs of nurses who are involved in teenage programs. They realize that these nurses must develop skills in communication and group leadership to prepare them to work effectively with adolescents. These educators might involve teenagers in planning and conducting classes or refresher courses, as teenagers are experts on adolescent affairs, and many of them aspire to be teachers. Why not foster that interest and at the same time help close the communication gap between two age groups and life styles?

COUNSELING TIPS

Nurses attempting to counsel adolescents on sexual matters ought to be clear about their own sexual attitudes and hang-ups, so as not to allow them to get in the way of professional purpose. It is of no importance to the teenager what your sexual preferences are; but it does matter that you be comfortable enough with yourself to allow that teen to be himself or herself. *This* kind of adult behavior they feel can be trusted.[16]

Knowing something about a young patient that his or her parents do not know can produce anxiety and guilt in a nurse. However, the energy generated can be used in a constructive manner. Adolescents would like very much not to have to sneak behind their parents' backs when they become sexually active. A nurse can explore with the teenager what would happen if the parents did find out from the teen himself. Perhaps the youngster can see where some communication between his parents and himself, however unpleasant, is better than none at all. The nurse can also help the parents to accept the new information from their teenager.

In counseling adolescents in venereal disease prevention, it is wise to relate to their struggle toward adulthood. Further, nurses can help them define what maturity means to them and explore with them their concept of health. Adolescents also need factual information about symptoms and treatment and the importance of *early* diagnosis and treatment for venereal disease. There are several books, some excellent films, pamphlets, and a rash of new little booklets being published by government agencies, drug companies, and college groups that can be used by nurses to supplement their work with adolescents.

Finally, the ability to use self therapeutically is probably the most important tool the nurse has in working with young people, and should be a part of every nurse's professional repertoire. When we can honestly say that we have carried out our responsibility to the young people in our care, nothing is left but *to trust them* to make the wisest decisions about themselves. Trusting is not easy, but it is vital in helping adolescents achieve maturity.

REFERENCES

1. Rosebury, Theodore. *Microbes and Morals: the Strange Story of Venereal Disease.* New York, Viking Press, 1971.
2. Deschin, C. S. *The Teenager and VD: a Social Symptom of Our Times.* New York, Richard Rosens Press, 1969.
3. DeCosta, E. J. Gonorrhea — treatment in the female. *ACOG Technical Bull.* Vol. 16, Feb. 1972.
4. Barton, F. W. Venereal disease (editorial). *JAMA* 216:1472—1473, May 31, 1971.
5. Block, Victor. The growing menace of VD. *Parents Mag.* 45:86—87ff, Nov. 1970.
6. Wilson, C. C., ed. *School Health Services.* 2d ed. Washington, D.C., National Education Association, 1964.
7. Greenblatt, Augusta. *Teenage Medicine.* New York, Cowles Book Co., 1970.
8. U.S. Public Health Service, Disease Prevention and Environmental Control Bureau. *Syphilis: a Synopsis.* (Publication No. 1660) Washington, U.S. Government Printing Office, 1967.
9. Hanlon, J. J. *Principles of Public Health Administration.* 5th ed. St. Louis, C. V. Mosby Co., 1969.
10. Calderone, M. S. Sex and the adolescent. *Clin. Pediatri.* 5:171—174, March 1966.

11. Yacenda, J. A. Survey of VD knowledge among young people. *Health Serv. Rep.* 87:394–398, May 1972.
12. Gordon, Sol. What adolescents want to know. *Am. J. Nurs.* 71:534–535, March 1971.
13. *N.Y. Public Health Law: Section 310* (McKinney, 1971).
14. The doctor and the adolescent (editorial). *Lancet* 1:955–956, May 8, 1971.
15. Ellison, S. E. The doctor and the adolescent. (Letter to the Editor) *Lancet* 1:1068, May 22, 1971.
16. Murray, J. B. Self-knowledge and the nursing interview. *Nurs. Forum* 2(1):69–78, 1963.

42

The Family That Fails to Thrive

Ruth F. Stewart

As community nurses work with families they must assess each family's stage of development. They need to know the normal family tasks appropriate to each stage. On the basis of this information they can plan nursing intervention. Some families, however, are in a state of disorganization and perhaps crisis. They cannot cope with the stress of daily living. These are families that fail to thrive. Ruth Stewart examines the causes of this family condition and suggests ways in which the nurse can deal with it.

The failure to thrive of children without organic disorders is an indictment of society, and yet one that occurs frequently. The maternal deprivation associated with the syndrome is often part of a complex cycle of inadequate mothering breeding a succeeding generation of inadequate mothers. This malady will be perpetuated if professional recognition of a need for help occurs only with a major health crisis. Identification of high-risk families and early therapeutic intervention are critical aspects of health care. Nurses' involvement with the situational and interpersonal factors affecting family wellness puts them in a strategic position to help families who fail to thrive.

THE FAMILY

Reproduction and nurturance of the young are virtually universal responsibilities of the family. Other functions vary somewhat with the culture, but commonly provide economic and psychosocial support, as well as for sexual needs for adult members (Ackerman, 1958, p. 16). The dominant family pattern of Western societies assigns primary responsibility for childrearing to the biological mother. Her charge is to cultivate the societal ideal in the helpless and need-engrossed infant she has borne. It is her duty to satisfy the physical and emotional needs of her child, as well as to provide the training and discipline necessary to his adaptation to society. The mothering process, however, is not an automatic response to parturition, but depends on a variety of individual, as well as cultural, determinants.

Success and satisfaction as a woman are related to motherhood in United States culture. Because of this, there are women not maternally inclined who are nonetheless pressured into the mothering role. Others may succumb to the cultural persuasion despite their inability to meet the demands of an infant (Anthony and Benedek, 1970, p. 102). Motherhood is often embarked upon with far less rational consideration than that given to marriage, although its ramifications are far more pervasive. It results, also with no conscious decision for or commitment to it, through accidental impregnation.

Problematical, too, is that training for motherhood is inadequate in the modern, urban United States. Small families and mobility have altered the traditional pattern of learning the mothering process and practices within the family milieu. Institutional efforts to provide this are limited to high school courses in home economics and family life and to public health nurses' involvement with expectant or new families. Even these opportunities are limited, as policy or mores often restricts participation to families in low-income groups. Society, whose future is assured only through the health and well-being of its young, must give serious consideration to motherhood as a skilled and essential craft.

MATERNAL DEPRIVATION

The need of infants for a mothering relationship was demonstrated in thirteenth century Germany when Frederick II, King and Emperor of the Holy Roman Empire, decreed the separation of infants from their mothers. The infants died. Scientific awareness in the twentieth century brought about study of the relationship of developmental retardation to maternal deprivation. The earliest studies focused on children who were institutionalized, and thus physically separated from their mothers. World War II produced additional studies of children dislocated because of war-related incidents. Later studies have identified the maternal deprivation syndrome in families that are physically together but psychologically distanced. The distancing may be initiated because of the mother's insufficient or distorted relationship with her child, or by the child's inability to respond to the mothering attempts. These dimensions of maternal deprivation, i.e., discontinuity, distortion, and insufficiency, are all encompassed by Ainsworth's definition as "insufficiency of interaction between a child and a mother-figure" (1962, p. 98).

Deprivation Outcomes

The accumulated data leave little question of the adverse effect of maternal deprivation on infant development, despite inadequate understanding of the dynamics involved. The reversibility of developmental damage resulting from this deprivation can be viewed from several theoretical positions, including learning theory, psychoanalytic theory, and "critical periods." Ainsworth (1962, p. 152) believes that these can be compatible, and explains.

Some impairment (is) . . . overcome through learning after deprivation has been relieved, while some impairment resists reversal to a greater or lesser degree . . . while still other impairment may persist because the sensitive phase has passed.

The age at which deprivation occurs and is relieved is undoubtedly a pivotal variable, though little is understood of this (Ainsworth, 1962, p. 153). Studies of children separated from their mothers have indicated that a child is most vulnerable from three months until about five years of age, with the last half of the first year a particularly critical period (Ainsworth, 1962, p. 21; Spitz, 1946, p. 338). At this time a child is normally differentiating himself from his mother, and developing a primitive body image. An impaired relationship with his mother during this period may interfere with this ego differentiation (Ainsworth, 1962, p. 21).

The extent of the deprivation is also related to the permanency of its effects. Any problems brought about by a single and short-term deprivation experience can be reversed almost completely, though a child is more susceptible thereafter to threats of separation. Longer or more severe deprivation, however, increases the possibility of continuing consequences (LaMarre, 1967, p. 584). Genetic differences are possibly a factor in the impact of deprivation on a child, though this is conjectural at present (Ainsworth, 1962, p. 23; Clarke, 1968, p. 1074; Schaffer, 1966, p. 595).

Language and abstraction are particularly vulnerable developmentally in a deprived child, with a resulting effect on intellectual maturation. Personality may be hampered by an inability to control impulses in the interest of long-term goals and from difficulty with interpersonal relationships (Ainsworth, 1962, p. 119).

FAILURE-TO-THRIVE SYNDROME

The failure-to-thrive picture is remarkably similar to the classical description of mourning and melancholia, with silent despair the overriding depression (Spitz, 1946, p. 320). The child's expression may be soberly watchful (Leonard, 1968, p. 468), apprehensive (Spitz, 1946, p. 326), searching, or frozen. Little interest is evidenced in toys or his own body, and he may ignore activity going on around him. Warding off of stimuli occurs through averting his face (Spitz, 1946, pp. 313–314) or covering it with his hands or clothing (Leonard, 1968, p. 468; Barbero and Shaheen, 1967, p. 640). He will often remain immobile, with his body either rigid or flaccid (Barbero and Shaheen, 1967, p. 640). In contrast, though, some children cling tenaciously to any adult, and look woebegone when left behind (Spitz, 1946, p. 326). An obsessional need to stroke soft, silky materials when under stress may be manifested when the need for human warmth has been unsatisfied (Freudenberger and Overby, 1969–1970, p. 302).

Physical development is impaired, with weight more affected than height (Leonard, 1968, p. 469; Barbero and Shaheen, 1967, pp. 639–640). Gross motor development is delayed, as well (Barbero and Shaheen, 1967, p. 640; Leonard, 1968, p. 470; Spitz, 1946, p. 328). Other problems may include anorexia, vomiting, diarrhea (Barbero and Shaheen, 1967, p. 640), and insomnia (Spitz, 1946, p. 313). Deprived children are extremely susceptible to infections, and react more acutely to ordinarily minor ailments than would be expected. In Spitz's foundling home groups, thirty-four of the ninety-one children died within a 2-year period, from such illnesses as respiratory and gastrointestinal infections, measles, and otitis media (Schaffer, 1966, p. 313).

PROGENITORS TO FAILURE TO THRIVE

The ability of the family to meet its responsibilities to its members and to society is precarious at best. Comparing the family to other systems in society, Reuben Hill (1965, pp. 33—34) points out the handicaps imposed by family organization. He notes that the age composition is heavily weighted with dependents, and the weak or incompetent members cannot usually be expelled. Acceptance results from membership, with no additional requirements. It is a puny work grouping and awkward for decision making. Despite burdensome responsibilities, its structure is not organized to withstand stress. Stress, though, is a frequent occurrence in family life, deriving from situational or interactional factors. The disorganization of the family may be minor and transitory, but can quickly become a crisis. Manifestations of family disorganization, minor or major, are varied. Failure to thrive is one expression of this.

Situational Progenitors

Situational factors common to modern family life that are stressful include changes of job or residence, movement upward or downward in social status, illness, and increase of members. Additional strain is imposed by inadequate food supply, poor housing, indebtedness — constants in a life of poverty. An abundance of children multiplies the family expenses and magnifies its deficits. This often necessitates "moonlight" efforts of one or both parents in the attempt to support the family. One-parent families result in the assumption by one individual of most of or all parental functions, ideally shared. Physical or intellectual handicaps of any family member alter the usual role or task performance of all family members. Considerable pressure results when knowledge or skill is inadequate for implementing family or societal roles. Identification of any of these situations in a family suggests a high level of vulnerability to disorganization at that time.

Interactional Progenitors

The family, an "arena of interacting personalities" (Nye and Berardo, 1966, p. 100) can be viewed from an interactional frame of reference when considering its level of organization or disorganization. A child's failure to thrive, when pathology or malnutrition are ruled out, indicates interactional problems between that child and the mothering person. Basic to this, however, are interactional difficulties within the mother's family of orientation and within the current family of procreation.

   The childhood relationships of the mother influence her perceptions of the roles in family life, and her ability to fulfill those roles assigned to her. Gender identity is a major facet of stable personalities and is learned from identification with the parent of the same sex. This identification may result in distorted psychosexual development if there are variances in the parents' sex roles. These may be manifested in overt role reversals, or by an incapacity to adequately fill the expected role. A cold, unyielding mother is particularly detrimental to her daughter's gender identity (Lidz, 1968, pp. 59–60), and this may foment masculinity and humiliation at being female (Anthony and Benedek, 1970, p. 398). On the other hand, a child's perception of insufficient mother-love creates the same results, even when this was not the case. This can occur when rivalry with siblings for maternal attention or love remains unresolved.

The mother-child relationship must also be viewed relative to other current family role reciprocities, such as husband-wife and father-child. The role of wife usually precedes, chronologically and affectionally, that of mother, and the achievement in the first role affects achievement in the other. Dissatisfaction with any of the processes involved in marital life, including sex, influences the mothering. Performance as a mother is related to the performance of the father in his role as well. Values held by the family regarding children, ranging from their number and timing to their sex and coloring, influences the maternal reaction to them (Ainsworth, 1962, p. 18; Rhymes, 1966, p. 1973).

A child's own behavior can be the initiating factor in his subsequent deprivation. He may be an "overactive" or "colicky" baby who creates sufficient stress that resentment and, subsequently, rejection may result. The phlegmatic infant courts deprivation because of this low-response level to maternal overtures, thus depriving his mother of positive reinforcement of her mothering role (Bullard, Glaser, Heagarty, and Pivchik, 1967, p. 688).

PREVENTING FAMILIES WHO FAIL TO THRIVE

"Give me good mothers and I will give you a good society," challenged Huxley. This society, as evidenced above, needs to heed the challenge and systematically promote better mothering. Nursing, whose focus is the individual, his health-related situation, and his perception of it, provides a critical mode for this within the health care system. The nurse has been traditionally accepted as a helping person, with less threat or stigma to the family than often associated with other health team members (Rhymes, 1966, p. 1975). A deliberative nursing process is an appropriate frame of reference for operationalizing the nursing intervention, with the goals falling within one of the three levels of prevention. *Tertiary prevention* (prevention of complication in an irreversible condition) will be instituted when the process begins with identification of a child with the failure-to-thrive syndrome, and where there is no apparent malnutrition or organic pathology. The child may have irreversible developmental damage, so that nursing goals will be focused on promoting sufficient family interaction and mothering that further deterioration may be averted, and infections prevented. [*Mothering* is defined for the purposes of this chapter in accordance with Freudenberger and Overby as "a process that may be performed either by men or by women. By the mothering process we mean a capacity to care for and relate to another in terms of the *other's* needs — especially as this process applies to the care of children by adults" (1969–1970, p. 299).]

Secondary prevention (early diagnosis and treatment) is involved where the inferential nursing diagnosis indicates mild to moderate family disorganization and poor mothering, but where there are no observable symptoms of failure to thrive in a child at the time. The goal in this situation is to promote family inter-action and mothering conducive to the well-being of the progeny (present and potential) and to the prevention of symptoms.

Primary prevention (avoidance of the condition) is the level appropriate to families currently well-organized, with maintenance of this equilibrium and the mothering process as the goal. Child care practices aimed at primary prevention are the ultimate in family health patterns, but are only cursorily noted in this chapter. A primary aim, herein, is to suggest that problem families can be identi-fied and assisted before the child and the family organization suffer irreparable damage.

The early identification of a family who has a potential for failing to thrive requires independent and sophisticated assessment by the nurse, as there is no observable physical pathology. It necessitates collection and analysis of data that encompass the parental attitudes and values related to family life and motherhood, as well as to each other. Collection of pertinent data can be insti-tuted through inclusion in a guide for the nursing history or assessment. Other data may be revealed directly or indirectly through discussion between the nurse and the family members, through family interaction, and from nonverbal behavior. Limited contact with the family necessitates collecting only samplings of family interaction, such as how a woman holds and responds to her baby, how a spouse describes his marriage, or how a decision is made regarding health care. A woman's attitude toward a possible or existing pregnancy may be predictive of her interaction with her child in the future. Should these samplings suggest the need, methods should be instituted for further data collection. If the initiating nurse cannot follow this through, a referral should be made to a community-based nurse.

Nursing Process: Initiating Event
The initiating event for prevention of failure-to-thrive families is the coming together of a nurse with a family, or any of its members, in the early stages of family development. This may be at the stage of betrothal, honeymoon, pre-natality, natality, or early childrearing. The predictability of problems with childrearing in this society should suggest to the nurse the data to be collected in order to assess the family for a possible need for help toward parenthood.

Nursing Process: Data Collection

The data necessary for assessment of a family's potentiality for failure to thrive are determined from the research discussed above. The data should be organized in a way that they can be easily used by all health team members, and specific history or assessment systems (i.e., family sociocultural assessment, individual client assessments) simplify the organization.

Situational variables, the tangible facts of daily life, can be gathered by routine interview. Sociocultural data that are useful include:

Household composition
    Head of household
    Relationship and ages of family members
    Nonfamily members living in household
    Family members not living in household
Educational level(s)
Ethnicity and language(s) spoken
Religion and involvement level
Employment: type(s) and duration
Financial factors
    Income and other resources
    Indebtedness
    Insurance, including health
Housing status
    Utilities available
    Soundness and size
Transportation

Health status is another fact of daily life, and the family's perception of this (realistic or not) is an important facet of the data. These data should reveal the family's view of:

Current health status of members
Past illnesses, health problems, deaths
Expectations regarding size of family
    Contraceptive practices
Health care facilities used, regularly or occasionally

Interaction of members is a crucial index of the organizational strength of the family. The interactional conceptual framework views this through the dynamic relationships relative to needs, behavior patterns, and adjustment processes. If the nurse-family relationship exists over a period of time, the processes to be studied include:

Communication patterns
   Who talks to whom
      how frequently
      conditions involved
      response to
   Who does not talk to whom
      regularly
      occasionally
   Who speaks for family to outsiders
   Nonverbal communication
      touch
      eye contact
      other
   Clarity of communication
      to nurse observer
      to family members
   Handling of anger
      verbally
      nonverbally
      conditions involved
   Decision-making patterns
      egalitarian family
      parent only
      husband only
      wife only
      influence on by extended family
      consistency of perceived to real patterns
   Role relationships
      consistency with societal expectations
      acceptance of assigned roles
      competency in assigned roles
      role conflicts

Other processes of interaction that might be identified relate to family norms, recreation, and child socialization.

Nursing Process: Ordering and Selection of Data

The data need to be organized so that deficiencies or irrelevancies, as well as priorities, are revealed.

Nursing Process: Inferential Nursing Diagnosis

This step of the process involves "the active, conscious, deliberate consideration of the meaning of the data" — forming a hypothesis or hunch (Bregg, 1971, p. 6).

The success of the nursing intervention hinges on the validity of the inferences. The inference necessary here concerns the adequacy of the family organization and the ability of the (current and/or potential) mothering individual to meet the nurturance needs of the (present and/or potential) children.

Nursing Process: Setting Goals

Goals established for nursing intervention necessarily rest on the previous steps of the process. To be operational, the goals cannot be an ideal, or wishful thinking, but must reflect the realities of such family and nurse resources as interest, energy levels, abilities, and time. They may require modification as the family progresses or regresses in its functional adequacy. In order to evaluate any change in the family, the goals need to be stated in behavioral and temporal terms.

Long-term (3 to 6 months) goals and short-term (each contact period, or a series of contacts) goals are necessary to provide direction for and to suggest methods of intervention.

Nursing Process: Intervention

Nurse-Family Relationships. The relationship of the nurse with the family is the pivotal factor in any nursing intervention. The nurse must be viewed as a family nurse, concerned about and working toward maximum wellness for the total family. The interaction will probably be channeled through the wife, because of the traditional role assignment for management of health and childrearing. Because of this, methods of including the husband in the interaction may need to be contrived. There may be occasions when he is present in health care settings or in the home at the time of a nursing visit, and needs only to be specifically invited to participate. Men often feel that they are intruding, or modifying their role, by "sticking around" when health or child care is the issue. Their participation, though, can be legitimated on the basis of family responsibility and decision making. Indirect contact can be maintained through the wife, by soliciting his opinion or his sharing in a decision.

Nursing interaction with a woman who is recognized as inadequate for carrying out the mothering role needs to be cautious and creative. Her feelings of inadequacy or dismay with the mother role are in direct conflict with cultural expectations, increasing even more her anxiety and guilt. Her behavior, because of this, will be suspicious and aloof. A suggestion, however indirect, that she is or will be a poor mother will establish an insurmountable barrier.

The relationship with the woman needs to be established as separate and distinct from the nurse's interest in her child, possibly to the extent of ignoring the child during initial contacts. The mother must feel the nurse's interest in her as an individual, with needs and rights outside her mothering role. She also needs to be recognized for the things she *is* doing well; there are always positive elements to be found in any situation. The nurse must be truthful, however, or he will discredit himself as a trustworthy individual.

Because of the probability that the woman has not resolved her own dependency needs (Anthony and Benedek, 1970, p. 536), a minimal dependency on the nurse during stressful situations in family development can prevent panic. With this support, then, she may be able to accept the dependency of her own child on her. This relationship must be considered as long term, as learning will be slow and family stress will predictably continue.

With the nurse's assistance in discussing her activities and concerns, the woman will very likely identify her own difficulty in dealing with her child, or an anticipated child. Such comments as "Children bother me," "They are too much work," or "I don't want to give up my career," may be admissions of the problem, and can be explored further. A woman who is considering pregnancy, but not yet pregnant may be aided in analyzing her own needs relative to the mother role. If the family postpones pregnancy until she is ready to accept its responsibilities, this family has achieved a higher level of organization and an opportunity for success. At this point the mother has involved the child in the picture, and he can now be introduced into the nursing intervention.

Child Care

With the advent of the child into the discourse of the mother and nurse, care needs to be exercised that the mother does not need to compete with her child for the nurse's attention. The mother's problems with child care can be the focus, rather than the child, with the mother and nurse collaborating on working these out. The self-concept of the mother is not diminished by the nurse assuming an authority role, and she is learning to think through her own problems and assume responsibility for making decisions.

Interaction of the mother with the child can be reinforced by pointing out the child's responses to her, however slight these may be. If the mother indicates interest in a specific activity or goal for her child, this can be used to structure interaction. An example of this is the mother who thinks her child should be walking. Whether or not this is developmentally realistic, the nurse can suggest the mother have a "class" with him for 10 minutes each day. He and the mother can develop a plan that is compatible with the child's motor coordination, but more importantly, includes the mother's handling and talking to him. Reinforcement will be needed for the baby's response to the mothering attempts, with care that the mother's expectations of the child not exceed his potential. Nursing intervention with mothers in other areas of child nurturance have been discussed by Rhymes (1966, pp. 1975–1976).

Family Planning

A family's control over its size is a fundamental factor in maintenance of organizational integrity. There is some evidence that the birth of a first child is provoking, even when the pregnancy is planned (Le Masters, 1965, p. 113), as well as when it is unplanned (Dyer, 1963, p. 199). In another limited study, all the failing-to-thrive children had been unwanted (Eckels, 1968, p. 15).

Nursing intervention is appropriate when the family has indicated they do not plan for family expansion within the next 9 months, but are not using reliable contraceptives. The intervention may be limited to giving information regarding contraceptive methods and resources for obtaining them. Usually, though, there are more complex factors when contraceptives are not used and, these must be considered. Concerns that commonly interfere include cultural or group taboos, fear of loss of sexual potency or satisfaction, concern about partner becoming promiscuous, and cancer phobia.

The usual communication and decision-making patterns of the family will affect any behavior change, and need to be considered in planning the intervention. Attempts to have the wife attend a family planning clinic will come to naught if her spouse makes all the decisions and their communication patterns do not allow for discussion of this topic. In such a case, the nurse may need to talk directly to the man, or to involve others relevant to the family in this direction.

Abortion has recently become an acceptable method for controlling family size once impregnation has occurred, and it is being used by many women. Nursing intervention, if abortion is being considered, may begin with suggesting resources. It is possible that further intervention will be indicated by the woman's fear of the procedure, her guilt reaction to it, or increased family strife resulting from it.

Communication Patterns

Although many nurses are not qualified to function formally as a family therapist, most nurses can assist family members in improving basic communication patterns. Successful communication is gratifying, bringing with it a sense of inclusion and security which is essential to family organization. Intervention consists of assisting family members toward an effective feedback system, appropriate verbal and nonverbal messages, efficiency of terminology, and flexibility (Davis, 1966). Families at any level other than highly organized, can improve family interaction through effective communication.

Crisis Intervention

A crisis results from an event that is perceived by the family as stressful, and for which they lack coping resources. Many events occur throughout a family's existence that might precipitate a crisis, such as birth or death, getting sick or getting well, promotions or demotions. It is the defining of the event as a crisis, and the inadequate resources for coping, that differentiate a crisis from simply an event. In working with families who are vulnerable to stress, the nurse can predict that certain events will trigger a crisis and then be available for assistance. This immediate help, whatever the source, is the critical element in crisis resolution. The results have been found to have far greater impact than a remedy for a given problem, and promote increased skill in dealing with subsequent difficulties. If however, the problem and its concomitant anxiety persist, ability to cope with future situations will be lower than the precrisis level (Hill, 1965), and family disorganization may result (Caplan, 1964, pp. 39—41).

General principles have been identified by Cadden which can be applied to intervention at the time of crisis:

1. Help the troubled to confront the crisis by helping him to verbalize and to comprehend the reality of the situation.
2. Help him to confront the crisis in doses which he can manage, being cautious not to overly dampen the impact. The reality of the situation must be kept in the forefront, although some periods of relief from looking at alarming reality are necessary.
3. Help him to find the facts since these are often less awesome than speculations about the situation. Fantasies can be more frightening than reality, however threatening it may be.
4. Help him by not giving false reassurance. Acknowledge the validity of fears and give reassurance that there is faith in his ability to manage.
5. Do not encourage him to blame others, since blaming is a way of avoiding the truth. Blaming may give momentary relief, but will lessen the likelihood of a healthy adaptation.
6. Help him to seek and accept help because he needs it and because, by seeking it, he is acknowledging that trouble exists.
7. Help him to accept assistance with his everyday tasks, since a crisis disorganizes and disorients energies due to the excessive amount of energy diverted to the task of resolving the problem (Robischon, 1967, p. 32).

Anticipatory guidance in family development and other family health areas can be useful to many families by providing them with a coping resource (understanding of situation) necessary to avert a crisis in the future.

Nursing Process: Evaluation

The effectiveness of the nursing intervention must be routinely evaluated on the basis of the short-term goals. If these goals have not been met, the reasons for this must be identified and the process reconsidered. Modifications may be necessary at any step.

Achievement of these goals reflects progress of the family toward a higher level of wellness, and subsequent goals can continue to guide the nurse and family efforts toward optimal family health.

COMMUNITY ACTION

Huxley's contention that good mothers make a good society might now be reconsidered. Could he have said as well that good societies make good mothers? Many of the situational factors increasing the family's vulnerability to disorganization are a direct outgrowth of social conditions. Poverty is an obvious example, but basic to this is unequal access to education, occupation, and power related to race or sex.

Health care is not available to all families, even for the acutely ill, and few families have access to services promoting wellness. Very few families will have an opportunity for the nursing intervention discussed above.

Changes in health care will result, not just because a need exists, but because the economics or politics of the situation make change attractive. These realities, once accepted, can be utilized by nurses to promote the community changes necessary for family health. The professional responsibilities of nursing necessitate active involvement at the community level. Nursing intervention is most effective when it results in community wellness, with fewer families that fail to thrive.

THE LUNAS: A FAILING-TO-THRIVE FAMILY

A Working Relationship: The Initiating Event

The Lunas (names are fictional) came to my attention through the personnel of the County Outpatient Clinic. Cynthia had been seen in the clinic for diarrhea, and it was noted that at ten months of age she weighed eight pounds (birth weight, five pounds four ounces) and was developmentally slow. A social service conference with Mr. and Mrs. Luna provided additional information, including Mrs. Luna's limited intellectual capacity and her negative feelings about children. A referral was made to the health department, and I arranged with this agency to assume the nursing supervision of the family.

The nursing process began (initiating event) with my acceptance of the family as a client, but an essential corollary was yet to be decided — would the family accept me? Ordering the limited data available, and relating it to study findings, resulted in the initial inference that this acceptance would not be easily won. Mrs. Luna was undoubtedly conscious of her inadequacies as a mother as well as an individual. Having someone visit her as a result of this could increase her own self-doubts and result in a defensive or hostile reaction. I hoped to have an advantage from the prevailing view among the poor that public health nurses are helpful. The Lunas did not have a phone, but even if they had, I would have chosen to make my first contact in person in order to foster positive personal interaction.

The first goal set was to be accepted to the extent of getting inside the house and agreement for a return visit. Intervention, for the initial visit, was planned as presentation of myself as a public health nurse, a caring and helping person. To be perceived this way by Mrs. Luna, I would need to focus the visit on her rather than on the children. To examine or discuss Cynthia would emphasize the inadequacy of her mothering, and probably establish a barrier between us. The children's welfare, in the long run, was dependent on their mother being able to assume a nurturant mothering role. It was she who had to be the primary client in this failing-to-thrive family.

On my first visit to the Luna household I introduced myself as Ruth Stewart, a public health nurse. I explained that the clinic personnel had said that she had told them she was having problems with the children and they thought she might like to have someone to talk to about this. She replied that they had told her a nurse would be coming (which I had not known), but right now she was moving out of the apartment for a week. The electricity and water had been turned off because of overdue bills, and they were moving in with her husband's family until they had a paycheck. After establishing that they expected to return on Friday, I then asked about returning the subsequent Monday. Mrs. Luna agreed to this and we decided on a mutually convenient time. Evaluation of this visit relative to my short term goals indicated satisfactory, though not glowing results. I did not get inside the house, but with an acceptable reason for this. Mrs. Luna received me with minimal suspicion and no hostility, and agreed to a return visit. A nurse-family relationship was begun on the second visit when Mrs. Luna met me at the door and invited me in.

During the next several visits to the Luna home (or rather, homes — they had moved again) I concentrated the nursing process on developing a working relationship with Mrs. Luna. Despite this focus, I learned a great deal about the family through discussion with her and her husband, as well as from observation.

The Family: Data Collection

Alicia and Guadalupe (Lupe) Luna have lived their young lives in this southwestern city noted for its Mexican-American culture and its poverty. The Lunas share in each of these heritages, but hold to the Great American Dream of a home of their own, nicely furnished. Meanwhile, they have moved through a series of small and shabby apartments, with periodic interludes with Mr. Luna's parents, as rent and utility bills got ahead of their pocketbook. They have recently moved to another part of the state in search of a job that might prove more satisfying to Mr. Luna than his night-shift operation of the elevator in a drab mid-town hotel. Perhaps he found use for the bookkeeping he studied cursorily between elevator runs at the hotel.

Mr. Luna was definitely the dominant member of this family, and Mrs. Luna recognized her dependence on him. This husband-father dominance can be expected from study of Mexican-American family patterns but was intensified by personal characteristics in this family. Mr. Luna was slightly built and handsome, and he seemed much younger than his 26 years, possibly because of his boyish gregariousness. He described his high school career as though it was the proving ground for his machismo (the uniquely Latin virility) so that it was not surprising that he did not graduate. His interest in women had not diminished, apparently, as his wife complained about his flirtations with her sister and others. He spent many of his evenings away from home with his male friends, another concern to his wife.

As many of the poor, he considered the daily grind of life rather futile and articulated this dramatically. His hopes for the future, however, belied this apparent anomie. His religion, Catholicism, provided no solace or satisfaction because he "had too much church" when he was a child. His family and his home were a source of pride and he was more actively involved in them than would be expected in Mexican-American, lower-class families. The decor of the apartment was livened by his efforts, one a golden-hued figurehead — a discarded styrofoam wig stand, gilded. He was demonstrably affectionate with both the little girls in the family, one his own child and one a step-child, and helped his wife care for them.

Mrs. Luna was a pretty nineteen-year-old with black eyes and long black hair. She always dressed neatly and attractively, though simply. Her intellectual ability was limited, typified by her being unable to shop without her husband, because she would be short-changed. Communication with her necessitated use of simple, concrete phrases, with continuous evaluation of her understanding. Her husband would take over for her, conversationally, if this was allowed. She accepted her dependence on him as proper. She was an immaculate housekeeper and derived pleasure from this. Her primary sources of enjoyment were shopping trips or movies (particularly horror-type) with her husband. Occasionally, she visited her mother's to watch television because their own set was not working. As her husband, she grew up within the Catholic church, but agreed with his view that she had "too much church" then.

Interaction was limited almost exclusively to the extended family, her own or her husband's. She said she did not have any friends, but that she liked people "who are nice to me." She readily identified her dislike for children and complained about her own making her tired and nervous. Both Mr. and Mrs. Luna wanted to avoid further pregnancies "until we have more money," so she was taking "control pills." Each of her two children had been conceived prior to her marriage, the first occurring when she was sixteen and in the sixth grade. Her mother was "mad" about the pregnancy and insisted that the baby would be placed for adoption. However, when Sally was born she "was so pretty" that her grandmother relented and kept her. Less than a year later, Alicia and Lupe began their courtship, which resulted in her second pregnancy and later, their marriage. Cynthia was born when her mother was eighteen and Sally was twenty months old.

A major theme of any discussion with Mrs. Luna was her reaction to her children. She recognized their dependence on her and used the housework to justify her inattention to them. I never observed her voluntarily initiating verbal or nonverbal interaction with either child. She responded to Sally's active overtures for attention by limited touch or comments, and occasionally would allow Sally to join her in the chair. Cynthia received attention only when she cried, and then primarily through care-taking tasks. Her usual docile inactivity did not provide much stimulus to encourage a response from her mother. During early visits, Mrs. Luna held her stiffly by the arm and at a distance, which reduced body contact between them to a minimum. Mrs. Luna said that her husband would get angry with her because she treated Sally better than she did his baby.

Sally was a bright-eyed, alert 2½ year old, constantly active and demanding attention.

She responded with obvious pleasure when she received attention, and especially when this resulted in her being held or sitting close to others (family members or me). She chattered on in a patter that was seldom understandable, even to her mother. She would, on occasion, slow down sufficiently to talk and play with Cynthia, and sometimes tease her. She liked to play with other children, and would dash outside to find some if not watched carefully. Her mother did not approve of this because she got "too dirty."

Cynthia, at ten months, looked like a forlorn, limp doll and reflected many of the characteristics described for the failing-to-thrive syndrome. Her expression was one of "silent despair" and "soberly watchful" most of the time. She showed no interest in her own body, but would respond to items handed to her. She did not have toys because they "mess up the house." Cynthia watched others around her intently and responded to attention from family members (but not from me) by smiling. Other than her plaintive cry, she did not vocalize. Her mother said that she cried "a lot" at night, though this seldom occurred during my visits.

Her physical development was impaired with her weight more affected than her height. She could not sit without support or roll over. She grasped objects held toward her. She remained flaccidly immobile wherever her mother left her — in the playpen or on the couch. She had never rolled off the couch.

Cynthia's failure-to-thrive is only the most dramatic manifestation of the disorganization in the Luna family. The history of the family provides a classical cycle of the problem situations and relationships that trigger further problems.

The Lunas' decision to organize as a family resulted from the circumstance of an unplanned and undesired pregnancy. Another child, also unplanned, is a member of the family by virtue of her stepfather's acceptance. He provided for her as well as his own child and wife on $60 weekly income. The usual stresses of poverty were routine in the family life, and resulted in frequent change of residence. The educational limitations of both spouses and Mrs. Luna's intellectual limitations created additional hazards to family organization.

Mrs. Luna, in discussing her problems within her family, frequently referred to her childhood. Her father had deserted the family when the children were young and he "has nothing to do with us." Her mother remarried, but nothing was mentioned of her stepfather other than he is no longer living. Mrs. Luna always spoke about her mother with anger and described her as "lazy" and "mean." Mrs. Martinez was said to have "kicked out" both Alicia and her brother because they "wouldn't help." She would not allow the Luna family to move in with her when their finances didn't provide the essentials of life, but "she should." Although Mrs. Luna did not feel welcomed by her mother, she talked about her dependence on her. Data are insufficient for definitive inferences, but they suggest a pattern of unresolved dependency needs.

It is the story of Mrs. Luna's life with her mother that offers a clue as to why Sally thrived while Cynthia failed to thrive. At the time of Sally's birth, it was Grandmother Martinez who responded to her, deciding that she would remain in the family. It is probably that Grandmother also assumed major responsibility for Sally, delegating some to her other daughters, so that Alicia was not burdened with the total dependency of her progeny. Only when Cynthia was born while the Lunas were establishing their own family unit was Alicia expected to bear the full responsibility of motherhood. The family structure could not tolerate this additional — and major — stress, and disorganization resulted.

Goals and Nursing Implementation

Goals, with this family, were established on a long-term basis, with one year chosen as the appropriate interval. Evaluation at the end of the year would indicate the extent to which the goals had been achieved, and provide baseline data for reestablishment of goals and redirection for methods of implementation.

A primary goal, basic to all others, in working with the Lunas was the establishment of trust. In order to evaluate the relationship relative to trust, specific behavioral goals were established. At the end of one year, Mrs. Luna will:

1. continue to agree to nursing visits every two to three weeks;
2. discuss freely the family problems; and

3. talk with the nurse when available about her increased anxiety level rather than cleaning house.

Mr. Luna's perception of my role was critical to achievement of the goals. Important as this is to the nursing relationship with any family, it was doubly so because of Mr. Luna's dominance in his family. His trust of me would be evaluated through his:

1. continued agreement to nursing visits to his family every two to three weeks; and
2. participation in nursing visits when awake.

Implementation geared towards these goals included planning for home visits every two to three weeks with the family's permission and agreement with the timing. Visits were rescheduled, even though previously arranged, when the situation indicated I was not welcome at the time (i.e., when Mrs. Luna was feverishly cleaning house, probably to reduce her increased anxiety or when Mr. Luna awoke early and wanted to take the family shopping). Permission was requested from Mr. Luna to visit his family, initially through Mrs. Luna and later from him directly. Occasionally, visits were arranged at times at which Mr. Luna could participate. When visits were not specifically scheduled ahead, for various reasons, I would write to Mr. and Mrs. Luna suggesting alternative times, including a postal card for their reply.

The paramount goal was that Mrs. Luna would modify her behavior to provide more adequate mothering for her children. Because her own inadequate self-concept and dependency needs were very likely interfering with this, it was here the implementation had to begin, and not with teaching the tasks of motherhood. It was through the tasks, though, that evaluation could take place, so specific goals were established in relation to the children. Mrs. Luna, at the end of one year will:

4. describe a positive behavior of each child and relate this to her interaction with each;
5. provide toys or toy substitutes for children to play with indoors;
6. allow Sally to play outdoors two to three times weekly;
7. hold Sally, when child initiates this;
8. hold Cynthia three times daily, ten minutes each time; and
9. talk with Cynthia three times daily.

Mrs. Luna's dependency needs were met to a limited extent by my being available on a periodic basis for her discussion of her problems, and for assistance in handling those relative to her children. A positive self-concept was fostered through focus on her and her problems, rather than the children, as well as by avoidance of comments or behaviors that might be interpreted as critical. I also legitimated for Mrs. Luna the reality of the problems of motherhood and housekeeping, and the needs of women beyond these roles. I identified and reinforced the attributes and behaviors that contributed positively to the limited family organization. There was always something positive I could pick up on within the situation and the bounds of truth. An incidental, but important consideration, was my inquiring of Mrs. Luna what she wanted me to call her . . . and her reply was Mrs. Luna.

Data collection was a continuing process, partly because of situational changes, but also because the family's increasing trust in me allowed them to disclose more about themselves and their history. Other data resulted from very specific collection methods [see Client Assessment] that I employed once we were well into a working relationship.

I implemented the client assessment by suggesting to Mrs. Luna that getting more information from her about her own health and the problems she had been discussing would be helpful in our working together to decrease the problems. I explained that I would use a form that nurses used on everybody with whom they work, thus establishing it as a routine procedure, not differentiating her or her problems. She agreed to this readily and a time was arranged for this. Despite the assessment focus on Mrs. Luna, many of the answers involved concern for and problems related to her children. This, then, was used as an approach to suggest doing assessments on the children as well. The same assessment guide was used, in this case, for the children.

The information from the assessments was useful in validating inferences made previously on the basis of limited data and findings from the literature for comparable situations. It was most useful in that it brought the problems Mrs. Luna faced in mothering her young daughters to an operational level. In responding to questions on the guide, Mrs. Luna identified several specific problem areas in the tasks of child rearing. Because of this, additional goals were established as a basis for working together in such areas as controlling Sally and feeding Cynthia. It was Mrs. Luna, though, who initiated the discussion of the problems. At this point, Mrs. Luna and I began working toward her increased interaction with Sally and Cynthia. Unfortunately, it was about this time that Mr. Luna decided to move to an area that appeared more promising economically.

Evaluation

The goals established for the Luna family could not be validly evaluated because the nursing process was interrupted before the evaluation term was completed. However, nursing methodology could be assessed informally relative to family responses.

Contact with the family was maintained until they left the community, with their agreement on the frequency and timing of visits. There were some occasions when they were not home, however, at the time agreed on. Mrs. Luna would later explain, voluntarily, that Lupe had awakened and wanted to go shopping or to visit. Because this was typical of his behavior, it was very probably the reason. My encouragement of Mrs. Luna to do things she enjoyed, as well as maintaining her household roles, may also have contributed to this. I did consider the possibility of avoidance, but the data did not support this.

Mrs. Luna said several times that she liked to have me visit her and contrasted this to the "other nurse" that told her to "feed the kids more."

Correspondence to Mr. and Mrs. Luna suggesting possible visit times was always answered on the enclosed postal card by Mr. Luna. A couple of times he explained that they were to be out of town, but told when they would return. He volunteered that they liked getting these letters.

As the nurse-family relationship continued, Mrs. Luna articulated more specifically and clearly her interpersonal problems, not only with her children but also with her husband and her mother.

After several months, Mrs. Luna identified that she was not as tired as she used to be, and was sleeping better. She attributed this to Cynthia's "getting older." Since, in these few months, Cynthia's needs and behavior had not changed, it suggested a change in her mother's acceptance of her.

Mrs. Luna's mothering behavior modified somewhat during this time. Although she did not hold Cynthia very often, she did begin holding her close to her and in a more relaxed manner. She volunteered that she was "doing more" for the children, although I had never suggested this to her.

The few changes highlighting the eight-month nursing intervention with the Lunas seem woefully insufficient when looking at those problems that remain. Modification to any extent, however, increases the family's capability for coping with the remaining problems, and increases their potential for wellness.

Client Assessment

Head of Household: Guadalupe Luna
Address: 321 Culebra
Name: Luna, Alicia Sanchez
Name prefers staff to use: Mrs. Luna
Birth Date: 3/24/52
Religion: Catholic (not practicing)
Medical Dx: None
Nursing Dx: Inadequate and insecure mother

Interviewee: Alicia Luna
Interviewer: Ruth Stewart, R.N.
Date: 5/17/71
A. Significant biopsychosocial data related to activities of daily living
    1. Rest and sleep
        Often wakened by children during night and wakes up tired. Likes to sleep late in morning. Does not nap.
    2. Elimination
        O.K.
    3. Eating
        Very good appetite, eats three to four times daily if food available (financial problems with this). Likes meat particularly.
    4. Breathing
        O.K.
    5. Skin
        O.K.
    6. Senses
        O.K.
    7. Mobility
        O.K.
    8. Recreation
        Shopping with husband, favorite recreation. Likes movies, particularly horror. Can only do this if sister will babysit. Goes to mother's home occasionally to watch T.V. (None in own home.) Does not attend church (too much when a child).
    9. Communication
        Limited because of problems of understanding. Need to use very simple concrete statements with her. Husband will take over communication for her if he's around. She enjoys talking with nurse when alone.
    10. Interpersonal relations
        Interaction only with family. No friends. Likes people "who are nice to me."
    11. Temperament
        Placid and accepting. Admits nervousness with children, but can't get adequate Hx (see A. 9.).
    12. Dependence/Independence
        Identifies dependence (extreme) on husband, mother.
    13. Education
        6th grade (at 16 years).
    14. Work
        Maintains household. Immaculate housekeeper. Does laundry in bathtub.

15. What is important to person
      To remain nonpregnant.
      To have a house and furniture.
B. Sociocultural
      See family sociocultural assessment.
C. Data related to person's health needs
      1. Patient's and/or family's understanding of condition
            Attributes problems in family to having the children. She does not
            like children. They make her tired and nervous. Doesn't "have time
            for them" because of house work.
      2. Patient's and/or family's understanding of condition and events leading
            up to it
            Expects problems (C. 1.) to be reduced because Cynthia is getting
            older (Sally not mentioned) and if she does not get pregnant.
      3. How condition is managed in home
            Children have been cared for physically, but given little attention or
            affection by mother. Mr. Luna does assist her with care of children.
            Generally, situation is just "muddled through."
      4. Previous health care and reaction to this
            Emergency care and prenatal care.
            Now on contraceptive pills – taking O.K.
Nursing Goals: At the end of one year Mrs. Luna will:
      1. Continue to agree to nursing visits every two to three weeks.
      2. Discuss freely the family problems.
      3. Talk with the nurse, when available, about her increased anxiety level,
            rather than housecleaning.
      4. Describe a positive behavior of each child and relate this to her inter-
            reaction with each.
      5. Provide toys or toy substitutes for children to play with indoors.
      6. Allow Sally to play outdoors two to three times weekly.
      7. Hold Sally, when child initiates this.
      8. Hold Cynthia three times daily, ten minutes each time.
      9. Talk with Cynthia three times daily.

BIBLIOGRAPHY

Ackerman, N. W.: *The Psychodynamics of Family Life,* New York: Basic Books, Inc., 1958.
Ainsworth, M.: *The Effects of Maternal Deprivation,* Public Health Paper 14, Geneva: World
      Health Organization, 1962.
Anthony, E. J., and T. Benedek (eds.): *Parenthood,* Boston: Little, Brown and Company,
      1970.
Barbero, G. J., and E. Shaheen: "Environmental Failure to Thrive: A Clinical View," *The
      Journal of Pediatrics,* 71(5):639–644, 1967.
Bowlby, J.: *Maternal Care and Mental Health,* 2d ed., Monograph Series #2, Geneva: World
      Health Organization, 1952.

Bregg, E. A.: "Curriculum Conceptual Framework," The University of Texas Clinical Nursing School (System-Wide), October 1971. Mimeographed paper.

Bullard, D. M., H. H. Glaser, M. C. Heagarty, and E. C. Pivchik: "Failure to Thrive in the 'Neglected' Child," *American Journal of Orthopsychiatry*, 37:660–690, 1967.

Caplan, G.: *Principles of Preventive Psychiatry*, New York: Basic Books, Inc., 1964.

Clarke, A. D. B.: "Learning and Human Development," *British Journal of Psychiatry*, 114:1061–1077, 1968.

Davis, A. J.: "The Skills of Communication, " in D. Mereness (ed.), *Psychiatric Nursing*, Dubuque, Iowa: W. C. Brown Company Publishers, 1966, pp. 44–48.

Dyer, E. D.: "Parenthood and Crisis: A Re-Study," *Marriage and Family Living*, 25(5): 196–201, 1963.

Eckels, J. A.: "Home Follow-up of Mothers and Their Failure-to-Thrive Children Using Planned Nursing Intervention," *American Nurses Association Clinical Sessions*, New York: Appleton-Century-Crofts, 1968, pp. 12–19.

Freudenberger, H. J., and A. Overby: "Patients from an Emotionally Deprived Environment," *Psychoanalytic Review*, 56:299–312, 1969–70.

Hill, R.: "Generic Features of Family under Stress," in H. J. Parad (ed.), *Crisis Intervention*, New York: Family Service Association of America, 1965, pp. 32–54.

LaMarre, C. J.: "Psychological Aspects of the Development of the Young Child," *Medical Services Journal*, 23:580–586, 1967.

Leaverton, D. R.: "The Pediatrician's Role in Maternal Deprivation," *Clinical Pediatrics*, 7(6):340–343, 1968.

Legeay, C.: "A Failure to Thrive: A Nursing Problem," *Nursing Forum*, 4(1):56–71, 1965.

LeMasters, E. E.: "Parenthood as Crisis," in H. J. Parad (ed.), *Crisis Intervention*, New York: Family Service Association of America, 1965, pp. 111–117.

Leonard, M. F.: "The Impact of Maternal Deprivation on Infant Development," *Connecticut Medicine*, 32(6):466–472, 1968.

Lidz, T.: *The Person*, New York: Basic Books, Inc., 1968.

Lo, W. H.: "Aetiological Factors in Childhood Neurosis," *British Journal of Psychiatry*, 115:889–894, 1969.

Nye, F. I., and F. M. Berardo: *Emerging Conceptual Frameworks in Family Analysis*, New York: The Macmillan Company, 1966.

Parad, H. J., and G. Caplan: "A Framework for Studying Families in Crisis," in H. J. Parad (ed.), *Crisis Intervention*, New York: Family Service Association of America, 1965, pp. 53–71.

Rapoport, L.: "Working with Families in Crisis," in H. J. Parad (ed.), *Crisis Intervention*, New York: Family Service Association of America, 1965, pp. 129–139.

Rhymes, J. P.: "Working with Mothers and Babies Who Fail to Thrive," *American Journal of Nursing*, 9:1972–1976, 1966.

Robischon, P.: "The Challenge of Crisis Therapy for Nursing," *Nursing Outlook*, 15(7): 28–32, 1967.

Schaffer, H. R.: "Activity Level as a Constitutional Determinant of Infantile Reaction to Deprivation," *Child Development*, 37:595–602, 1966.

Spitz, R. A.: "Anaclitic Depression," *Psychoanalytic Study of the Child*, 7:313–341, 1946.

Taylor, A.: "Deprived Infants: Potential for Affective Adjustment," *American Journal of Orthopsychiatry*, 38:835–845, 1968.

Wiedenbach, E.: *Clinical Nursing: A Helping Art*, New York: Springer Publishing Co., 1964.

43

Working with Abusive Parents

Anne B. Savino
R. Wyman Sanders

*Suspecting that a child has been neglected or abused by its parents is one thing.
What to do about this is another. Although the nurse is concerned for the
child's well-being, in most situations the parents also need assistance. Understanding, patience and skill are all needed by the community nurse in assisting
these parents. The following chapter is an account of a successful group-therapy
and home-visit program for abusive parents.*

Today, there is less thought of placing abused children in foster homes and
more of helping parents so they can provide an adequate home. This shift has
come with the growing realization that the parental problems that are responsible
for the child's injuries may be amenable to treatment, and so more treatment
programs have begun. Interest in the whole area of abused children has increased
in the past 10 years.[1]

One such program for parents is conducted at the UCLA Neuropsychiatric
Institute. The Institute provides an outpatient therapy group for parents who
have been charged in court with either "child abuse" or "maintaining an unfit
home."

The self-help approach was adopted for several reasons. The literature indicates
conventional individual and group psychotherapy has been unsuccessful.[2,3] Also,
these parents are immature, impulsive people who need assistance in learning to
set limits. They are depressed and self-deprecating and are desperately looking for
a "good" mother surrogate. They are acutely aware of their problem situation
and, therefore, are looking for someone who can help them without being judgmental or critical.

Since we at the Neuropsychiatric Institute believe that both parents are involved in the child abuse phenomenon, a criterion for joining the group is that
both parents must attend. The only exception has been in cases where only one
parent was living in the Los Angeles area. The group meets one evening a week
for an hour and a half. The number present for each session has varied from
none to eight. When parents do not attend, we call them and encourage them to
return the next week.

GROUP PROCESS

The therapists are a child psychiatrist and a public health nurse. Thus, the group
members have both a "father" and a "mother" model. When parents first enter

the group, they usually show strong feelings of rage toward society for "causing" them to be in this predicament.[4] They usually direct this anger at the pediatrician who made the initial diagnosis and the social worker who worked with them during the court proceedings. Many look at the social worker as someone who has control over their future; it is she who must ultimately write a report recommending continued placement or return of the child to the home.

After a few sessions, the couples become less angry and the group process moves in two directions. One aspect is dealing with the resistance the parents feel toward discussing the problems which ultimately led to the abusive act; the other deals with being a parent.

The parents who benefit most are those who finally become comfortable enough to talk about the abusive acts. The types of difficulties these parents have demonstrated are long-standing isolation, poor peer interactions, severe marital conflict, and life-long patterns of inadequate family interaction.

All the families display marked deficiency in their knowledge about being parents, so the second focus in the treatment group or program is on child care. For example, during one session all parents agreed that a nine-month-old baby should be able to stop crying when told to do so. The instruction includes normal physical and emotional developmental patterns — feeding, toilet training, discipline, sibling rivalry, and the like.

HOME VISITS

The public health nurse makes home visits whenever a group member requests it. Care can be individualized more when the public health nurse works directly with the mother and her child in their natural environment.

Since these parents are filled with rage toward authority figures (particularly due to their relationship with their own parents and partially due to the way society has "rebrutalized" them), it is of utmost importance that a positive relationship be established between them and the nurse before teaching can be done.[4–6] Abusing parents are sensitive to domination and control.[2,7] On the other hand, these parents do need "mothering," and so the first few meetings with the family may include just sitting and listening with undivided attention.

At first, only minimum attention must be placed on the child. The situation has brought the parents in contact with persons who were concerned about the welfare of the child, and now for the first time someone is focusing attention on them. One of the dynamics behind the child abuse phenomenon is that the mother or father feels that the child is getting more attention than she or he and, therefore, focusing on the child may be perceived by the parents as another act of rejection. Although the goal is to make the home a safe one for the child, the parents are the only persons who can actually change the environment. The nurse's responsibility is to help them accomplish this.

When the nurse enters the picture, many authority figures (family, physician, protective services, and perhaps even the court) have already told these parents either verbally or nonverbally that they are not doing an adequate job. It is important that the nurse therapist not fit into this same mold. In an attempt to cover up her own discomfort in dealing with these families, however, she can easily approach them in an intrusive way by coming on too strongly with direct interviews and excessive instructions, thus communicating rejection. If this happens, the parents may become even more negative and distrustful. They may be polite, but they may also feel too threatened to express their own honest feelings and, instead, will give only lip service to what the nurse is saying.

The nurse's best assessment tool is observation. If she takes the time to sit and listen or chat, slowly building a positive relationship, she is more likely to obtain important information. Later, the nurse can acquire more material by questioning in a nonthreatening manner.

Since marital conflict plays a big part in most of these families, arranging some of the home visits when both the mother and father are present is important. The nurse can then take that opportunity to foster better communication between the parents.

SUPPORTING A MOTHER

The nurse can also point out normal child behavior in a noncontrolling and nonthreatening way. Mrs. A., during a home visit, became irate when her two-year-old daughter responded to one of her requests with a loud and hostile "no." The nurse then said:

Most mothers feel that this particular age is a very difficult one, because it is a time when children are testing their own control and independence. It is a trying and difficult time; and I can see that it is this way for you.

Here the nurse is telling Mrs. A. that what her child is doing is normal and opens the door for this mother to express her strong feelings of frustration over the child's behavior.

Unintrusive modeling is another tool, once trust has been established. If the nurse is unsure of rapport with the parent or if she has the vaguest feeling that the child will be punished for receiving attention, she does best to focus her attention on the mother. A child who places her head in the nurse's lap is difficult to ignore. Allowing the child to do this without pushing her away, while continuing to talk with the mother, keeps the focus on the mother's problems and, at the same time, initiates modeling. In some cases, the nurse can show affection for the child if she feels certain that the mother will not feel rejected. The rewarding feeling of then watching the mother imitate this action is indescribable.

Interpretation is another tool. Once during a visit a mother gave a younger, favored child a security blanket to comfort him. The older, abused sibling then attempted to place her head on the blanket. Her mother immediately reprimanded her. The nurse then commented, "It looks as though Mary wants a blanket, too." The mother looked surprised and commented that perhaps she did and immediately got a second blanket, stating, "Here, Mary, here is your blanket." The child appeared pleased, and the mother continued her conversation with the nurse.

If a nurse witnesses child abuse, she is required by California law to report it. However, to gain the mother's trust and establish good rapport, the nurse must learn to tolerate all other types of discipline. These are impulsive, acting-out parents. At times, the nurse may witness discipline which seems excessive or unnecessary. In these cases, it is important not to interfere or the child's position may be jeopardized; and after the nurse leaves, he may receive even more punishment. Many of these parents view punishment as the only way of controlling a child's behavior. The nurse must evaluate carefully whether she is witnessing discipline or clear child abuse. This may not be easy, as the dividing line between maximal discipline and minimal abuse is fine.

CHILD MANAGEMENT CLASS

The nurse can also suggest alternative means of handling a child's undesirable behavior. One such approach used here is a Child Management Parents Class, which the nursing staff of the UCLA Neuropsychiatric Institute of Child Outpatient Clinic established. This class stresses behavior modification techniques, using Patterson and Gullian's *Living with Children*.[8] This is an excellent help in modifying maladaptive behavior. Much information gathered from this class is used individually with these abusive parents.

The nurses teach parents the principles of reinforcement and extinction. When parents complain about a child's behavior and describe their handling of it, they are asked if they would like to try another method which has proved successful. The nurse describes a simple intervention, the principle being an immediate reward for the desired behavior, thus strengthening it. The parents are further instructed to pair nonsocial with social rewards. For example, a hug and praise are given simultaneously with a star on a chart or a piece of candy. The nurse recommends that such undesirable behaviors as tantrums be ignored, which will lead to their extinction. The parents are told beforehand that when a behavior is ignored, they should expect that the behavior will first increase before it drops off.

If the public health nurse approaches families with self-assurance and understanding and keeps some basic principles in mind, the door is open for a worthwhile experience for all involved.

REFERENCES

1. Kempe, C. H. Battered child and the hospital. *Hosp. Practice* 4:44ff, Oct. 1969.
2. Helfer, R. E., and Kempe, C. H., eds. *Battered Child.* Chicago, University of Chicago Press, 1968.
3. Paulson, M. J., and Blake, P. R. The abused, battered, and maltreated child: a review. *J. Trauma* 9:1−136, Dec. 1967.
4. Terr, L. C., and Watson, A. S. Battered child rebrutalized: ten cases of medical-legal confusion. *Am. J. Psychiatry* 124:1432−1439, April 1968.
5. Golub, S. The battered child: what the nurse can do. *RN* 31:42−45, Dec. 1968.
6. Morse, C. W., and others. Three-year follow-up study of abused and neglected children. *Am. J. Disabled Child* 120:439−446, Nov. 1970.
7. Elmer, E. Child abuse: the family's cry for help. *J. Psychiatr. Nurs. Serv.* 5:332−341, July−Aug. 1967.
8. Patterson, G. R., and Gullian, M. E. *Living with Children.* Champaign, Ill., Research Press, 1971.

44

Maximizing Health Care to Families

Leonard T. Maholick
Josephine Graham

Many families experience mental health problems but the ways each copes with these problems vary in effectiveness. When unsuccessful, a crisis occurs. But psychiatric help is often not available or too expensive. The authors of this chapter propose that good psychological care can be given to a large number of families by a small number of health personnel. In the following three-act drama, an actual situation is described in which the public health nurse is the primary therapist with the psychiatrist as consultant. It is a part of her family counseling role.

PROLOGUE

There are, perhaps, millions of people living unhappy, frustrated, meaningless lives, burdened with a host of unsolved personal problems. They can be found in Anytown, U.S.A. However, professional problem solvers are a relatively rare and scarce commodity. Long will be the day before the supply of such help exceeds the demand for it.[1]

Using the principle of parsimony, "the best care for the most with the least by the fewest," we believe it is possible to deliver a broad spectrum of helping services to troubled people without the full-time presence of the traditional mental health team.[2]

The essentials are (1) the public health nurse in her familiar role of family counselor, (2) the strategically limited use of psychiatric consultation, and (3) a painstakingly designed program of therapy (see Figure 1).

This drama of real-life problem solving takes place in a rural community, 100 miles from any psychiatric resources.

ACT I: A CRY IN THE COMMUNITY

Scene I: The Emergency Room

In the Emergency Room of a 50-bed general hospital, a general practitioner faces a dilemma. Mrs. John Doe, a 28-year-old beautician, has impulsively climaxed three months of despair by swallowing thirty Triavil tablets. The policy of the general hospital is not to admit psychiatric cases. The family's income eliminates private hospitalization. The husband opposes commitment to a state institution. A compromise is reached: home care and a trial of counseling at the personal problem center of the local health department. The doctor arranges an appoint-

From "Parsimony Applied," *American Journal of Public Health,* Vol. 60, No. 1, pp. 51–55, 1970. Reprinted by permission of the publisher and the authors.

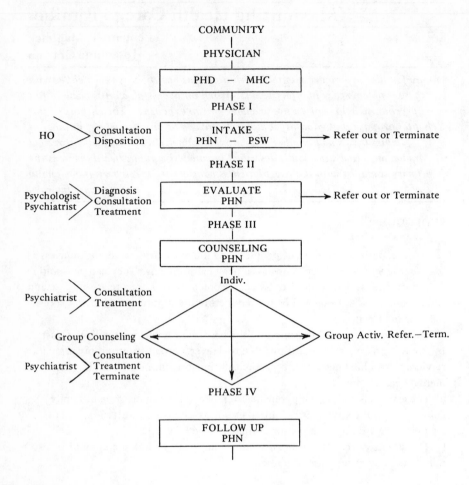

COMMUNITY

PHYSICIAN

PHD   —   MHC

PHASE I

HO   >   Consultation
Disposition

INTAKE
PHN   —   PSW
→ Refer out or Terminate

PHASE II

Psychologist
Psychiatrist   >   Diagnosis
Consultation
Treatment

EVALUATE
PHN
→ Refer out or Terminate

PHASE III

COUNSELING
PHN

Indiv.

Psychiatrist   >   Consultation
Treatment

Group Counseling   <   →   >   Group Activ. Refer.—Term.

Psychiatrist   >   Consultation
Treatment
Terminate

PHASE IV

FOLLOW UP
PHN

Figure 1. Service Operational Flow

ment by telephone and completes a brief written referral on a form supplied by the agency.

Scene II: The Personal Problem Center

Mrs. C, the public health nurse, and the patient meet. Mrs. Doe stares at the floor and answers questions in scarcely audible monosyllables. Mrs. C patiently explores her feelings about the referral and extracts largely factual information relative to the admission. The young woman remains guarded and aloof but does finally say, with some tears, "I just made things worse by what I did last night. I need help."

Then, the nurse explains the contents of a Personal Data Kit in which the patient is to write about herself and her situation as she sees it, using a structured biographical review as a guideline. She is also to complete a specially designed companion Problem Check List and return all the completed material within two days.

Mr. Doe expresses bewilderment as to the cause of the depression and listens intently as the nurse reviews suicidal precautions with him. Daily 30-minute nursing contacts are set until Mrs. Doe can be seen by the psychiatrist at the next clinic, five days hence. The general practitioner is notified of the plans and agrees to retain the ongoing medical responsibility for the patient.

During the initial exploratory interviews, Mrs. C encourages the patient to express her feelings of inadequacy and futility. The patient cautiously reveals how unpleasant her in-laws have been to her, how unfairly she believes her own child has been punished by her husband, and how forgiving and understanding she has tried to be. Throughout the budding relationship, Mrs. Doe expresses much relief during the solely supportive and nonconfrontive sessions.

ACT II: ENTER THE PERSON

Scene I: Consultation and a Helping Plan

Before the patient is seen directly, the nursing counselor, Mrs. C, using information from the Personal Data Kit, presents her written summary to the consulting psychiatrist on a specially developed Summary and Planning Guide. It is to be noted that the nursing counselor has been fully trained in the use of these specific tools.[3]

The picture as developed by the nurse is one of a 28-year-old beautician with a chief problem of "nerves — there is no reason to go on living." Overdose of Triavil and gastric lavage done at general hospital. For three months Mrs. Doe has had loss of energy, lack of interest, no appetite; is moody with weeping spells, wants to stay in bed and be left alone. Husband is a truck driver, 30 years old. Second marriage for each. He has a daughter, ten; she, a son, seven, and they have one daughter, four. Both have high school education and she trained as a hairdresser; has one-chair shop in her home. Combined income of about $7,000 a year; many debts, car, home, doctor bills, and so on. The Problem Check List is peppered with indications of much internal distress and a host of personal problems, most of which relate to economic conditions and personality deficiencies. So far has talked of feeling she is to be blamed for the ten-year-old's failure in school last term and her present floundering; she suffers from the excessive criticism of her mother-in-law, fear of losing her husband's love, and terror that somehow her child will get a fatal disease and die as did a friend's child. First marriage in teens failed; both "too young"; husband was abusive. Present husband is perfect; "too good for me." Parents living; father laborer, mother does housework; neither understood her as child. Little contact with them at present.

The nurse considers Mrs. Doe's major assets to be (1) youth, (2) education, (3) motivation for help, and (4) interest of husband. Liabilities could be the (1) censure by in-laws, (2) inability to continue communicating with husband, (3) possible reluctance to forgive self, (4) relative social isolation, (5) high level of inner discomfort and, (6) preoccupation with and history of suicide attempt.

After having made a preliminary estimate of the patient's inner distress, personal problems, and her strengths and weaknesses, she is seen jointly by the nurse and psychiatrist. Afterwards they discuss the case: there are the classical symptoms of depression (rated moderately severe) with anxiety. Identifiable stresses are: rejection by her relatives, guilt over sexual indiscretion, the school failure of her stepdaughter. The patient's present coping mechanisms are massive withdrawal and isolation, denial, repression, and acting out in suicide attempt. Therapeutic plans call for the establishment of a continuing professional relationship in which the patient can ventilate and abreact. Medication is prescribed for symptomatic relief. Search for other current stresses is indicated, especially marital and familial. Aim for modification of current methods of coping. After symptomatic relief, stabilization of emotional control, and good individual therapeutic contact have been achieved, place in group counseling and group activity program and press for resocialization. The patient agrees to return for continuing help.

Scene II: The Individual Counseling Interviews

Mrs. Doe makes good use of her scheduled hours. Her defensive facade is relinquished even when she fearfully introduces hints of her flirtation with a male neighbor. Later she revealed a previous sexual affair about which she felt intense guilt. The nurse accepts this confession with the same composure maintained during previous revelations. Rapport seems completed at this point. The relationship is firmly established and Mrs. Doe comes to her appointments with increasing eagerness and is much more expressive.

Scene III: Family Involvement

The nurse investigates the ten-year-old's school performance. The teacher has some suspicion that the child is disturbed by the unspoken conflict between the parents. A psychological evaluation done at the clinic verifies the girl's above-average mental ability. Mrs. C interprets the findings to the school and the parents and explains the recommendations in the report. Mr. D is astonished to learn how his wife felt about this and encourages her to tell him of her other concerns. For the first time in months they begin to communicate meaningfully.

Scene IV: Group Counseling

Following the six individual counseling interviews, Mrs. C introduces Mrs. Doe to four other women who meet one hour weekly for discussions of their personal problems. Mrs. Doe is uncomfortable and silent but pays close attention to what is being said. During the second session, she asks a few questions and reveals a little of the unhappiness she has been experiencing. She expresses surprise that others have felt much the same as she has: "I thought I was the only one with a problem just like mine." By the third week she is speaking freely and frequently, trying not only to elicit encouragement from others but, in her own way, attempting to offer reassurance to the group members.

Scene V: Group Activities

Mrs. Doe and two others move from group counseling into socializing activities planned weekly for 90-minute periods. Although Mrs. Doe is timid at first, she is coaxed to help prepare the refreshments by one of the older members. Her efforts are praised and she slowly gains confidence in planning and working with others. At the third meeting, when the other patients ask her to show how she does a hair style, she seems to be very comfortable throughout the demonstration.

ACT III: EXIT THE PERSON

Scene I: Termination Planned

At this point Mrs. Doe has had the intake interview, four 30-minute interviews with the nurse, one hour with the psychiatrist for evaluation, six individual counseling sessions with the nurse, a second psychiatrist appointment of 30 minutes, six hours of group counseling weekly, a 20-minute appointment with the psychiatrist, six hours of group activities weekly, and now a 30-minute interview with the psychiatrist for possible termination and aftercare. (Total time: 21 hours with the nurse, 9 hours individually, 12 hours in groups, and a total of 120 minutes with the consultant psychiatrist; all this over a period of 14 weeks.) At this appointment the results are evident. From a rather bedraggled morose young woman with averted eyes, Mrs. Doe makes her appearance smartly groomed, neatly made-up, and smiling pleasantly. Her tensions have vanished, the depression is relieved, life is worthwhile, the marital climate is more favorable ·than ever, the stepchild's school performance has improved to a passing standard. She has learned that she can disagree with others without losing their love and respect, a crucial lesson for her. She is scheduling her former patrons in the beauty shop; beginning with one a day, she increased her work load rapidly. The family makes plans for church and inexpensive outings to the country on Sundays.

There are still momentary lapses of regret for her past behavior but she does not dwell on them. She feels that now she can manage all right if she can talk occasionally with the nurse when she needs to.

Scene II: The Follow-up Clinic

Nine months after the suicide attempt, Mrs. Doe is at the clinic for a ten-minute contact with the public health nurse. The level of improvement is being maintained without medication. The nurse schedules a ten-minute appointment with the psychiatrist for reevaluation. His decision and recommendation are: discharge to care of general practitioner, condition improved, further care not indicated.

EPILOGUE

This individual solved her problems — at home, relatively quickly, efficiently, with minimal disruption of family and work activities, and at low cost — through the use of an on-the-scene nurse-counselor and the judicious use of an outside consultant. This real-life drama need not be a singular nor a unique experience. It is fully repeatable by others.

A small band of six public health nurses have been doing this regularly and systematically since 1964. In 1967, devoting 25 percent of their time to mental health work, they conducted 7,800 counseling interviews with patients and their families plus 1,000 patient contacts in 175 group counseling sessions. This same small group saw 245 new and reopened cases in 1967 and maintained an average monthly caseload of 303 patients. Less than $24 per patient was spent for the most costly services of the consulting psychiatrists (three days per month) and psychologist (two days per month).

Using the nurse as the provider of local mental health services and the primary therapeutic agent within the context of a small public health department is surely an outstanding example of Parsimony Applied.

Note: The training materials found in the Personal Data Kit, The Biographical Questionnaire, The Problem Check List, and The Summary and Planning Guide are available upon request.

REFERENCES

1. Maholick, Leonard T., and Graham, Josephine L. Problem Solving for Troubled People — One Approach at the Local Level. *Alabama Ment. Health,* Vol. 18, No. 13 (Mar.), 1967.
2. Hollister, William G. The Principles of Parsimony in Mental Health Center Planning. Ibid. Vol. 19, No. 1 (Jan.), 1968.
3. Shapiro, David S., Maholick, Leonard T., et al. *The Mental Health Counselor in the Community. Training of Physicians and Ministers.* Springfield, Ill.: Thomas, 1968.

45

The Family with an Elderly Member

Lucille Gress

*The aging process creates difficulties for many people. It requires adjustments
for both the aging individual and the members of his family. As the elderly
person's dependency needs increase, community nursing assistance is often
needed. When aged individuals remain at home, they need counsel, physical
care and assistance in the use of community resources. Later the nurse may
assist the family in selection of a nursing home. In this chapter the author uses
a case example to describe the nurse's role with the elderly person and his family.*

While professional nursing has long been concerned with the expanding nuclear
family, there has been little attention focused upon the contracting nuclear family
and the problems that arise as the remaining aged family members approach the
end of the life cycle. Undoubtedly, the disruption that occurs when the aged
individual must change to a new environment has as much potential for becoming
a crisis episode as that occurring with the birth of a child. In either case, there is
a psychological reaction that creates a state of disequilibrium until the family
learns ways of coping with the change and adapts to such change. Usually assistance is sought from extrafamilial health professionals during these periods of
disequilibrium. When the professional nurse becomes involved, nursing intervention must be predicated upon those principles related to psychosocial needs
as well as those related to physical needs if the intervention is to be appropriate
and effective.

In order to provide some basis for appreciation of the role of the nurse, a
general definition of nursing and a definition of gerontological nursing will be
given. In a basic definition of nursing, Henderson (1966, p. 15) states:

The unique function of the nurse is to assist the individual, sick or well, in the performance
of those activities contributing to health or its recovery (or to a peaceful death) that he
would perform unaided if he had the necessary strength, will or knowledge. And to do this
in such a way as to help him gain independence as rapidly as possible.

Referring more specifically to care of the elderly, Stone (1971, p. 1a) writes:

Gerontological nursing is the nursing care of the elderly based on scientific knowledge from
the fields of gerontology and nursing. It encompasses preventive care, maintenance and
rehabilitative aspects of health care. It requires an understanding of the process of aging
and its relationship to nursing intervention.

These definitions give direction to the nurse practitioner and describe the locus
of practice.

In addition to direction from the definitions of nursing, the professional nurse may benefit from developing and using a conceptual framework appropriate to the chosen field of practice. Such a framework may be eclectic in nature, leaving some freedom for creativity in the development of a plan for nursing intervention.

Using a developmental conceptual framework, the family may be viewed as a social system experiencing developmental stages just as individual family members do. The family may be defined as a nuclear unit including husband, wife, and children. The nuclear family ends with the death of the last spouse. This family unit functions as a dynamic social system in an interdependent relationship with extrafamilial social systems. These social systems engage in a reciprocal give and take relationship with certain shared expectations that often are not formally stated.

An example of the interdependent relationship of the social systems may occur as the aged family member approaches the end of his life cycle. Because of the increasing dependency needs of the aged family member, assistance may be sought from an extrafamilial system. The nurse often becomes involved at this point. The family expects help with one of its traditional functions, i.e., care of its aged family member. The nurse, in turn, as he interacts with the family and assumes some responsibility for care of the aged individual, expects certain behaviors of the other family members. For example, if the aged individual is being institutionalized, provision of clothing, cosmetics, and visits from the family are expected. If the nurse chooses to conceptualize the family seeking assitance as a "patient" with certain needs, rather than to limit concern to the aged family member, he may function in a role that can be supportive of the continuing developmental process of the entire family and of individual family members.

The following case study of Mrs. Rowe (fictitious name) will provide the basis for consideration of the ways in which the professional nurse might function with the aged individual and his family. The fact that a professional nurse was not formally involved with the Rowe family does not necessarily negate the need for, or possibility of, a nursing role at that point in time. Part of the problem in terms of the nursing role, is related, no doubt, to the nurse's perception of his role in continuity of care. The nurse in the emergency room functioning within the framework of family nursing might have interpreted continuity of care and needs of the family as being part of his responsibility. His role might have become increasingly visible by means of a referral made to a community nurse who could, in turn, have worked with the family. The community nurse could have perhaps been effective in listening to the expression of feelings about the change in Mrs. Rowe's condition and the need for other arrangements for her care. Pointing out available community resources and being supportive during the institutionalization process might have enabled him to alleviate some of the feelings of anxiety of the Rowe family. Not only would this kind of nursing intervention make visible the role of the nurse in a family-centered nursing approach, it would also give visibility to the nursing role of meeting needs of the aged individual and his family, as the older person experienced the last stage of his life cycle.

CASE STUDY

Mrs. Rowe, a 67-year-old widow of Catholic faith, continued to live in her own home following the death of her husband 10 years ago. There were 13 children, the youngest died at the age of one month. The ages of the living children ranged from 28 years to 49 years. These children, 4 daughters and 8 sons, lived nearby. Of these children, one son, 28 years old, was single; two sons, aged 35 and 37 years, also single, were mentally retarded and institutionalized; the rest have children of their own and were living with spouses except for the 44-year-old son who was recently widowed. He and his sons continued to maintain their own home.

Busy with her family during the years, Mrs. Rowe had not developed hobbies. She had a sixth grade education and regretted not having more. She tended to be moody and to cry frequently with little provocation. Although finances were limited, especially following the death of her husband, Mrs. Rowe managed to meet her own needs and, on occasion, extended financial help to some of her married children. The children visited at intervals as circumstances permitted, but did not assume responsibility for their mother's care, or for making decisions regarding her care, with the exception of Mrs. Green [fictitious name], the oldest daughter. Mrs. Green had been the mainstay of the entire family.

In recent months, Mrs. Rowe had been hospitalized several times because of illness related to arteriosclerotic heart disease. Mrs. Green, in seeing her mother's changing health status and recognizing her mother's increasing need for supportive care, invited her to live in her home. Other family members accepted this arrangement and continued to visit their mother as usual.

Soon after going to live in her daughter's home, Mrs. Rowe began making numerous telephone calls to various family members, often calling the same individual at frequent intervals during the day. The family attempted to set limits by asking Mrs. Rowe to make only one call to each family member daily. One son obtained an unlisted number as a means of controlling the incoming calls because his wife, under treatment for emotional problems, was disturbed by the calls.

Mrs. Rowe's sleep pattern began to change. She was up frequently at night and usually went to the refrigerator to get something to eat. One night Mrs. Green, awakened by her mother's "prowling," found Mrs. Rowe sitting on the edge of her bed eating chocolates. Melting chocolate was running down her face and dripping on her gown. Mrs. Green commented that her mother looked like a child sitting there. She did not scold her mother "because there was no use." Instead, she cleaned her up and helped her back to bed.

Mrs. Green, relating her feelings about her mother's condition, said her mother looked to her more than to the others because she was more sensitive and responsive to her mother's feelings and needs. If the rest of the family were unable to help Mrs. Rowe, she always tried to help. Mrs. Green said she loved her mother and wanted to do whatever she could to make her happy. Sometimes she was concerned with the seeming lack of attention given her mother by her brothers and sisters. She acknowledged the fact, however, that they had other family responsibilities and were concerned with financial problems.

Another change in Mrs. Rowe's behavior became obvious. Several times in the absence of Mrs. Green (beautician), Mrs. Rowe called the police and an ambulance to take her to the nearby medical center. In spite of the fact that these trips were unnecessary for medical reasons, the cost was the same as for a true emergency (four times in one week totalled $120 that was paid by Mr. and Mrs. Green). At this time, Mrs. Green began to realize that her mother could no longer be left alone.

Mr. and Mrs. Green, both nearing retirement, needed to keep on working to prepare for their own future, as well as to contribute toward the support of Mrs. Green's mentally retarded brothers and their own children. It was decided, therefore, to hire Mrs. Rowe's sister to stay with her during the day. However, this arrangement soon proved unsatisfactory. Mrs. Rowe continued to insist on making frequent telephone calls and became very agitated when attempts were made to dissuade her. On one occasion, she managed to cross the street to a neighbor's home and reported that her daughter was withholding her medication and poisoning her.

In the meantime, Mrs. Green acknowledging the fact that she could no longer cope with her mother's unpredictable behavior, began looking for a suitable nursing home. She reported feelings of ambivalence as she made the search. Taking her mother outside the family for care was in opposition to the family value system and to her mother's expressed aversion to going into a nursing home. Some of the family members expressed rejection to the idea of institutionalization for their mother, but offered no alternatives. Mr. Green, anxious about his wife's mental well-being, was supportive of the plan.

Mrs. Rowe quietly accepted going to the nursing home the day of admission. Mrs. Green, on the other hand, felt more uncomfortable than ever. Lack of the "common courtesy of a greeting" from the staff necessitated inquiry as to where to leave her mother and added to the feeling of "coldness" she experienced. Overhearing an aide "threatening an elderly man with a cold shower if he became incontinent," did little to relieve her anxiety and concern for her mother's welfare. "I almost gathered my Mom up and brought her back with me," she said in recounting the experience.

Since the staff, composed of a registered nurse, licensed practical nurses and nurse aides, did not ask for any information, Mrs. Green was uncertain if they had a telephone number in case of emergency. She decided to visit her mother after work to see how things were going. In the meantime, because of her anxiety and concern, she called the social worker on the case to determine whether or not the admission procedure in this situation was the usual approach.

During the early postadmission period, Mrs. Rowe began to have crying spells. The staff was puzzled about the reason for the episodes but assured Mrs. Green that her mother was receiving good care.

Mrs. Green said that although she felt the right decision was made regarding institutionalizing her mother, she was saddened by the thought that she could not take care of her mother during her time of dependency as her mother did for her when she was a baby.

Although the role of the professional nurse is hardly visible in the case of Mrs. Rowe, functions of a nurse in the role will be explored in the analysis of the case.

THE ROLE OF THE NURSE

Perhaps a look at the role of the nurse as it developed historically is a useful way to point out why the role of the nurse is being considered. According to Virginia Stone (1970, p. 106):

In the past nursing care of older people was delegated to the good natured, kind, ill prepared people with kind feelings toward old people.

However, because more people are living longer and are being cared for in institutional settings and because consideration is beginning to be given to a quality of life that is more satisfying, the need for nurses prepared to function in a different way is essential. Having lived longer, with the likelihood of becoming more differentiated, aged individuals have some needs that are unique in addition to those needs held in common with their fellow human beings. Rights of the aged are being recognized with societal expectation tending toward respect of those rights in terms of health care. Equal status recently given by organized nursing to geriatric nursing with other specialities, such as medical-surgical nursing, has been cited by Stone (1970, p. 108) as reflecting this trend and is indicative of the need for reexamining the role of the professional nurse.

No longer is it acceptable for nursing practice to be based upon intuition or to have those nurses who think of care of the aged as being out of the "mainstream" of nursing responsibilities, be responsible for care of the elderly. Rather, the professional nurse should be prepared to work with the elderly and their families wherever they are developmentally, or on the wellness-illness continuum. In this role, the nurse is changing from functioning as a custodian of aged individuals to functioning as a "counselor, teacher, researcher, consultant, and patient-side practitioner" (Davis, 1968b, p. 1106).

An analogue of the development of the role of the nurse might be made to the development of the aged individual. The nursing role, developing over a long period of time, is also becoming more differentiated. While there are areas contributing toward the development of specialities in nursing practice, i.e., pediatric nursing, coronary care nursing, geriatric or gerontological nursing, there are components of nursing shared with practitioners in any locus of practice. The differential in gerontological nursing arises out of the physical and psychosocial needs of the aged individual and his family, according to their individual and collective developmental levels and where they are on the wellness-illness continuum. Just as the aged individual should be viewed as a member of his family rather than a separate entity, the role of the gerontological nurse should be viewed within the context of the "whole" of nursing. In order for the nurse to function effectively with the aged individual and his family, knowledge of the developmental levels of the individual and his family and the aging process is essential.

ASSESSMENT

Regardless of whether the nurse's initial contact with the family occurs during a relatively quiescent period of development, or during a time of disruption and crisis as in the case of Mrs. Rowe, an assessment of the family and its needs should be started.

Assessment, in this case, may be defined as the process of collecting data as a means of learning about the family and acquiring information that will provide the basis for nursing intervention. Setting of priorities should be determined by the present needs of the family. Since the family is assumed to be in a continuing state of development, the need for a continuing process of assessment is implied.

Assessment in the case of Mrs. Rowe will be made within a modified developmental conceptual framework of the family. Concepts from the crisis theory will be incorporated into the framework to allow for a more comprehensive assessment. While the modified developmental conceptual framework of the family will be used here, it is well to acknowledge that other conceptual frameworks might be equally useful. The crucial factor hinges upon use of a more formalized, systematic, and deliberative approach to nursing intervention. Assessment can be an important part of formalizing the nursing process.

The focus of the assessment in this situation will be upon the psychosocial parameters. This is not to deny the need for assessment of physical parameters, but is in cognizance of the impact of institutionalization and the importance of preventing depersonalization. Usually, attention is given to the more obvious physical needs almost to the exclusion of attention to the psychosocial needs. In an institution providing long-term care for the aged, it is important to help the aged individual to retain his personal identity and his identity within the family group. This task is facilitated by assessment of the family dynamics.

In beginning assessment of the family, the nurse should observe the interaction of family members as a means of learning about the dynamics of their relationship. The level of anxiety of family members should be assessed during the process of institutionalization. Although Mrs. Rowe and her daughter were the only family members present initially, the composition of the family as a whole and where they lived could have been a part of the data obtained. Additional information about the strengths and weaknesses of the family might also have been elicited. During such an assessment process, the nurse would have an opportunity to convey understanding and empathy to the family. This interchange should be helpful in decreasing the level of anxiety and in building a trusting relationship that would enable the family to feel more comfortable in expressing their concerns verbally.

The impact of institutionalization should have been explored with Mrs. Rowe and her daughter. Institutionalization constitutes a crisis episode for many aged individuals and their families. According to crisis theory, the family should be more open to therapeutic intervention during periods of disequilibrium, therefore, the nurse-family interaction at this point may markedly influence the outcome of the crisis episode. Providing opportunity for these family members to express their feelings and offering support while they do so, should be helpful in relieving some of their anxiety and contributing toward initiation of the coping process.

It is important for the nurse to have an understanding of some of the factors contributing to the impact of institutionalization. The Rowe family, after exhausting its own resources, sought help from an extrafamilial institution. Separation anxiety occurring in the anticipated loss of privacy for family intimacy and realization of the ultimate separation by death, probably influenced the reaction of the family. Families often experience guilt feelings about institutionalizing their aged family member while the aged individual often experiences feelings of rejection and abandonment. This reaction is not unusual in spite of the fact that institutionalization seems to be the only viable alternative to care of the older person. Taking these factors into account and having knowledge of the increased mortality rate that occurs in the immediate postadmission period, the nurse should carefully examine ways in which he can interact responsibly with the aged individual and his family.

A more detailed assessment of the aged individual than of the family as a whole is necessary. Although the primary emphasis in this situation is on the psychosocial parameters, the physical parameters cannot be completely ignored. These parameters are so closely related that it is difficult to separate them for the purpose of analysis. Focus on the psychosocial dimension, in this case, is to point out the tendency to overlook psychosocial factors that also influence the well-being of aged individuals. The impact of institutionalization and the potential for depersonalization are documented in research findings. Since reaction to institutionalization occurs over time, there is need for a continuing assessment of the aged individual, including his way of coping with the major change in environment.

In most cases, a physical examination is a part of the admission requirement and provides some useful information. However, the nurse should also make some physical assessment of the older person. For example, Mrs. Rowe was quiet at the time of admission to the nursing home. Did she give any indication of hearing impairment, i.e., lip reading, inappropriate responses to questions? Sensory loss may be the result of impacted cerumen and temporary or permanent pathological change in the eighth cranial nerve. On the other hand, was Mrs. Rowe's quiet manner a reflection of feelings about institutionalization and the marked change in environment? The nurse should make an assessment with interpretation of the data and exercise judgment in determining the appropriate nursing intervention.

Physical assessment should be useful in determining capacity to perform activities of daily living such as ambulation, dressing, eating, toileting, and bathing. Such assessment of functional ability should also include attention to any help that might be necessary, or to aids needed to support ability for self-care, such as a hearing aid, a walker, or special eating utensils. Eliciting this kind of information conveys interest in the individual and is useful in helping the person make an easier transition into the nursing home setting. Observation of the individual's normal pacing of activities should be made to facilitate planning that would avoid rushing the person beyond his capacity. Hurrying the individual sometimes leads to confusion and does not give the individual time to do what he could do for himself.

Mental status should be assessed in an effort to learn the person's ability to initiate and carry on usual activities. Orientation to time, person, and place is a part of this assessment. The amount of freedom allowed, or supervision required, is partially determined by this assessment.

Since Mrs. Rowe was a new admission, she and her daughter had a right to be oriented to the nursing home environment. During the orientation further assessment of Mrs. Rowe's mental status could have been made. Learning how she interacted with other residents would have given some idea of her ability to socialize. Simple testing of her ability to recall the location of her assigned room, and certain other areas, might have been helpful in evaluating mental ability. Additional observation of the interaction between Mrs. Rowe and her daughter could have been made during the tour of the nursing home. Other information about Mrs. Rowe's care and previous life style might have been elicited at this time.

Assessment of emotional status may be a means of picking up information regarding behavior patterns and predictability of behavior. Mrs. Rowe's history of frequent crying episodes shows a tendency toward a labile emotional status. Given this information, the nurse should explore further to try to determine what triggers this behavior and how to effectively support Mrs. Rowe. If change occurs in emotional status that may be the result of pathological processes, the family may need help in learning how to cope with the change. Effort should be made to prevent the family from becoming unduly emotional, thus diminishing its coping ability. In any case, an attempt should be made to identify any correctable problems that might be disturbing to the emotionally labile aged individuals and to learn ways of dealing appropriately with the disturbed individual and his family.

Additional information about other family members to determine their reactions to the institutionalization of Mrs. Rowe might be helpful in assessing their possible need for counseling. Some family members find it hard to visit the individual in the nursing home. In some situations this may be because of problems with transportation. In others, it may be that the psychological reaction to the institutionalization is an inhibiting factor. Working within the conceptual developmental framework of the family makes it imperative to identify the problems if the nurse is to discharge responsibility for preventive care, maintenance, and rehabilitative aspects of health care of the aged individual and his family. The nurse must seek to determine ways of helping the family to learn how to use its capacities to continue development of potential for meaningful family relationships.

To assess the role of the nurse in the Rowe case necessitates calling attention to the basic developmental task of the nurse/family in the nursing home situation. This task is that of developing a trusting relationship. The fact that the role of the nurse is unclear in this case does not rule out the need for a nurse who will define and clarify the role in the interaction with the aged person and his family. If the nurse is unable to meet with the family, he should have a staff that is prepared and expected to extend a warm greeting to the family experiencing the crisis of institutionalization. This is important in establishing a trusting relationship.

One of the major nursing goals in the Rowe case, and other similar situations, should be to prevent depersonalization. This goal should pervade the total of the nurse/family interaction. Health for the older person and his family in the nursing home experience depends, to a great extent, on the continuing interaction of individual family members in a supportive and affectional relationship. The knowledgeable nurse functioning in an effective role will be sensitive to the human needs of these people. He will be seeking to promote continuing growth and development of potential for a more satisfying experience for all concerned.

The professional nurse role can be further developed in the nurse/family interchange during the crisis episode related to institutionalization of the aged family member by use of available knowledge and skills in a responsible way. To formalize and systematize a deliberative nursing approach is to take nursing out of the realm of intuition through application of principles of the behavioral, social, and physical sciences. Assessment is an important part of the deliberative nursing process. The outcome of the nursing intervention under such conditions should be the enrichment of the living experience of the aged individual and his family wherever they are in the life cycle. This process should also bring fulfillment to the nurse experiencing the nursing role in dynamic interchange with the family.

To paraphrase Schwartz (1969, p. 79), the unique function of nursing centers upon care of families seeking health care in situations in which they lack the ability or knowledge to care for themselves. If the professional nurse is to accept the challenge and act responsibly, he will need to use his knowledge and apply skills important to the humaness of the aged person and his family as well as skills important to physical well-being.

BIBLIOGRAPHY

Ackerman, W.: *The Psychodynamics of Family Life,* New York: Basic Books, Inc., Publishers, 1958.

Benjamin, F.: "The Role of the Geriatric Nurse in Health Maintenance," *Geriatrics, 22:*58–64, 1967.

Brody, E. M., and G. M. Spark: "Institutionalization of the Aged: A Family Crisis," *Family Process,* 5:76–90, 1966.

Brown, M. M.: "Personalization of the Institutionalized Older Patient," *ANA Clinical Sessions,* American Nurses' Association, 1969, New York: Appleton-Century-Crofts, Inc., 1969, pp. 118–124.

Davis, B. A.: "ANA and the Geriatric Nurse," *Nursing Clinics of North America,* 3:741–748, 1968a.

———: "Coming of Age: A Challenge for Geriatric Nursing," *Journal of the American Geriatrics Society,* 16:1100–1106, 1968b.

Deutsch, S., and B. Krasner: "Meeting the Needs of the Patient through Comprehensive Planning," *Journal of Geriatric Psychiatry,* 3:107–120, 1969.

Henderson, V.: *The Nature of Nursing,* New York: The Macmillan Company, 1966.

Kalis, B. L.: "Crisis Theory: Its Relevance for Community Psychology and Directions for Development," in D. Adelson and B. L. Kalis (eds.), *Community Psychology and Mental Health,* Pennsylvania: Chandler Publishing Company, 1970, pp. 69–88.

Kent, E. A.: "Role of Admission Stress in Adaptation of Older Persons in Institutions," *Geriatrics,* 18:133–138, 1963.

Knoll Pharmaceutical Company: "Psychodynamics in Extended Care of the Aged: Illness, Loss of Function: A Special Kind of Stress," *Geriatric Focus,* 6:1, 56, 1967.

Knowles, L. N.: "Nursing Care to Increase Older Patient's Potential in Potentialities for Later Living: A Report on the 17th Annual Southern Conference on Gerontology, University of Florida, February 4–6, 1968," Gainesville, Fla.: University of Florida Press, 1968, pp. 53–62.

Lawton, M. P.: "The Functional Assessment of Elderly People," *Journal of the American Geriatrics Society,* 19:465–481, 1971.

Leiberman, A.: "Institutionalization of the Aged: Effects on Behavior," *Journal of Gerontology,* 24:330–340, 1969.

Parad, H. J. (ed.): *Crisis Intervention: Selected Readings,* New York: Family Service Association of America, 1965.

Robischon, P.: "The Challenge of Crisis Theory for Nursing," *Nursing Outlook,* 15:28–32, 1967.

Schwartz, E.: "Aging and the Field of Nursing," in M. W. Riley (ed.), *Aging and Society: Aging and the Professions,* New York: The Russell Sage Foundation, 1969, p. 79.

Shaughnessy, E.: "Emotional Problems of Patients in Nursing Homes," *Journal of Geriatric Psychiatry,* 1:159–166, 1968.

Spark, M., and E. M. Brody: "The Aged Are Family Members," *Family Process,* 9:195–210, 1970.

Stone, V.: *Gerontological Nursing,* Student Syllabus, Evanston, Ill.: Video Nursing Inc.,
    1971, p. 1*a.*
———: "Nursing Services to Meet the Needs of the Aged," in M. Field (ed.), *Depth and
    Extent of the Geriatric Problem,* Springfield, Ill.: Charles C Thomas, Publisher, 1970,
    pp. 106—116.

46

Family Nursing during Death and Dying

Marilee Woehning
Ida M. Martinson

Much of the literature dealing with death and dying is focused on the individual. Thus, most nurses seek to assist the individual through the stages of dying and the family members through the grieving process. An additional emphasis needs to be placed on the effect of this crisis on the family as a unit. What changes take place in family roles and tasks? How can the family be assisted during the necessary adjustments? In this chapter the authors address this issue with a discussion of the tasks that families must undertake in their adjustment to death. They offer helpful insights for the community nurse working with the family during dying, death and readjustment.

The nurse was making a home visit late one afternoon to a family caring for a middle-aged man with lung cancer. He was alert, although his lungs sounded more congested when the community nurse listened to his chest. While standing at the bedside, his condition suddenly changed. His breathing became labored, his skin turned grey and diaphoretic, his eyes rolled back. For half an hour his wife, two sons and daughters-in-law and the nurse stood at his bedside holding his hand, praying and crying, waiting for death, which they knew was inevitable. The presence of the nurse gently giving directions and suggestions reassured this family that they were doing all that could be done for their husband and father and that there was no need to rush him back to the hospital. "How long can he breathe like that?" and "Is he dead yet?" were asked as they stood at his bedside. As a family they needed to stay together at his bedside — an experience unknown to many families.

Currently, most deaths in this country take place in hospitals with nurses as the principal care-givers. Nurses can also be the principal care-givers outside these institutions. We would suggest that the home is a viable alternative for the dying patient and his family, with the support and leadership of the community nurse.

When the dying process and the death occur in the home, the community nurse must deal with many more aspects of death and dying than when death occurs in the hospital. The nurse, when present, is usually the only health care professional in the home, and, therefore, will be responsible for interacting with the family and assisting them. Death requires a multitude of adjustments and tasks, not merely for the person who is dying but also for the members of his family. Dr. Kubler-Ross has described denial, anger, bargaining, depression and acceptance as five phases the dying person may experience.[1] Recognition of these five phases can be helpful to the nurse and family. The nurse in the

This chapter was written especially for this book and has never been published before.

community must be prepared to assist the family in adjusting to the loss from the time they first anticipate a member's death until there is evidence of readjustment following death. In this chapter we shall examine some of the tasks faced by such families and ways in which the nurse can be of assistance during this time.

Lindeman has suggested three stages that must occur during the course of grief. The stages are "emancipation from the bondage to the deceased, readjustment to the environment in which the deceased is missing, and the formation of new relationships."[2] To these we shall add the anticipation stage, and in each one we will look at the major tasks with which the family must deal. Every family member has certain tasks that must be done. These tasks are the assumed or assigned duties and responsibilities each individual member carries out within the family unit. Impending death and death itself create changes and additional family responsibilities and tasks.

STAGE OF ANTICIPATION

The anticipatory period occurs from the time the family suspects death or knows of its certainty until death occurs. This period of time can be as short as a few hours or as long as several years. We have identified two major family tasks that must be dealt with during this stage.

Task 1: Caring for the Dying Member

The difficulties that families experience in caring for a dying member at home will vary. In a family where the husband had lung and bone cancer, the wife debated whether her husband should be admitted to the nursing home or whether she should attempt to care for him at home. Following several discussions with the nurse and a visit to the nursing home, she decided to take her husband home: "I can care for him at home as well as they can at the nursing home." Once the decision was made, the supportive services of the family and a community nurse were initiated. Weekly visits by the nurse gave the family opportunities to ask questions and evaluate their ability to provide care at home. The wife was also taught to use a suction machine that alleviated her fear that her husband would choke to death because he could not cough up the lung secretions.

In another home, Peter,* who was dying of leukemia, was being cared for by his family and the community nurse. Each evening his father carried him downstairs to join the family for dinner. However, the father noticed large bruises appearing on Peter's body as a result of being carried. The father began to question whether he should be carrying Peter downstairs. It bothered him to see bruises developing where his hands had held Peter. He felt responsible for the bruises. The choice between the boy's desire to be downstairs for dinner and the prevention of the bruises was not difficult to make. Peter's desire to be part of the daily life of the family was by far more important.

*The names have been changed to protect the identity of the family.

Some of the fears and difficulties experienced by families can be alleviated by the community nurse's support of approaches to care that are common or innovative. One woman dying at home was too weak to walk more than a few steps. To be carried to the car and taken out for a rootbeer was the highlight of her week. Although it would have been easier to bring the rootbeer home to her, her family supported her desire to change the surroundings and to go to a drive-in, an example of previous normal behavior. She was also able to be carried to the living room from her bedroom for short periods of time to visit with family and friends in familiar surroundings.

Another young man cared for at home spent his last weeks in a recliner chair in the living room so that he could see outside and be central to the family activity. One night Mark's mother, who was tired, told her son that if he kept calling her he would need to be readmitted to the hospital. The next morning Mark shared with her his idea of using a trapeze so that he could stay at home and could manage the bedpan and some movement without calling her so much. His mother shared this incident with the nurse when she came to visit. The community nurse supported the mother's desire to overcome the difficulties and to try keep Mark at home because being at home was so important to him.

Approval by the nurse of the family's preparation of a person's special foods as well as of their imaginative approaches is important throughout the time of care. Mr. Heinz was at home, becoming weaker every day. His ability to swallow became impaired due to cancer infiltrating the central nervous system. Throughout his life, fresh beets from the garden had been a treat. The family had gotten fresh beets for him and, although he was unable to swallow, Mr. Heinz enjoyed chewing the fresh cooked beets his wife prepared. He spit out the beets after the flavor was gone.

The families who care for a dying member at home do not feel the restriction of institutional rules or detailed procedures for making requests. The difficulties they do experience can be reduced by the community nurse's support and encouragement of their approaches to patient care.

Task 2: Dealing with the Life-Death Paradox

The struggle to preserve life and prevent death is commonly experienced. However, when death is inevitable following a critical change in a person's condition there seems to be less desire to forestall death. It has been noted that both the family and the nurse may sense impatience during this time. In addition, the length of time waiting for death appears to correspond to the degree of impatience felt by those waiting. Following months of struggling to preserve life in one situation, the family and nurse found themselves in the last hour before death impatiently waiting for the woman's final breath. The paradox becomes apparent as the struggle for life gives way to the impatience. This impatience is frequently experienced when death is imminent but the patient lingers. Recognition that impatience may be a reaction to part of the dying process enables families and nurses to endure this time of waiting with less stress.

When there is no waiting following an unexpected change in a dying person's condition there is less chance for the family members or nurse to develop impatience. Mrs. Bond, the nurse, was a member of the family who awakened to give the pain medication to her father-in-law who was dying of cancer. She noticed the absence of restlessness and there seemed to be no need for pain medication. His feet were cool, evidence of circulatory failure, and his eyes, which had been glossy for the last day, were no longer glossy. She awakened the wife and the rest of the family members in the cabin. As they came to the bedside, she notified the sister and brother-in-law who were in the summer house next door. They rushed to the bedside, and there was a period of five minutes where each minute was very precious as he looked at each person there. He attempted to smile and to the question "Do you see Jesus?" answered "Yes." His breathing stopped. This family did not experience impatience, possibly because death was not prolonged.

The community nurse's awareness and understanding of these tasks can be of assistance to the nurse as well as to the family while involved in the care of the dying person and his family.

STAGE OF EMANCIPATION

The emancipation stage that Lindemann writes of may be considered as a stage of separation. The death has occurred and the finality of the event is making an impact on the family. In working with families during this period the nurse must recognize two essential tasks in which the families will need to be involved.

Task 3: Expressing Grief

Expression of grief will vary in families. However, freedom of expression should be encouraged by the nurse. Sobbing, screaming out in anger, the need to be alone, the need for an arm around the shoulder and few words are only some examples of the many possible expressions of grief. Cultural influences may affect the expression of grief. For example, in the traditional confucian Chinese mourning rites, the expression of grief is established along the kinship relationships. When the father dies the eldest son would be involved in a three-year period of mourning.[3] Not only is a longer period of mourning encouraged but one finds a more demonstrative expression of grief in the Chinese family than in northern European families, which tend to have a more stoic public expression of grief. In caring for families with a dying member the nurse must anticipate a variety of possible expressions and individualize responses to best meet their needs.

Task 4: Relinquishing the Person

Relinquishing the dying person is another task that the family must face during the stage of emancipation. Some families are not able to consider the separation until the death has occurred. However, most families have begun the process of relinquishment before death. The family may not be aware of beginning this process until after the person has died. This was evident in one family where Brian cared for his wife at home until she died. In reflecting following her death, he said it was easier for him to accept Mary's death after seeing her in continuous pain day and night. Mary had always put on a good front while in the hospital so her husband and family were not aware of the constant pain until she was at home.

In another family, a young mother of four children had a short time to live. She wanted to be at home. After two days at home she realized that it was too difficult for her husband to care for her and she could not bear having him or her children watching her so closely. For that reason she chose to return to the hospital where she died three days later. This decision helped her husband realize and face the impending death and separation.

Other individuals have expressed varied degrees of beginning to face separation after death. One woman, immediately following her husband's death, wanted to continue holding his hand and did not want to leave his bedside. Even after a half hour at his bedside it was difficult for her to leave. Another man after his wife died said, "She's finally at peace." Only one more look before leaving the room was a daughter's request after her mother's death.

It is important for the nurse to realize that the process of relinquishing a person varies from individual to individual and realization of separation following death takes time. However, the nurse can facilitate the process and realization of separation if she is willing to take time to listen to the family.

STAGE OF READJUSTMENT TO THE SOCIAL ENVIRONMENT

Following death comes the realization that the person is gone but that the surrounding environment remains, even though the situation has changed. It is important to remember the seriousness of unresolved grief. There has been increasing evidence in the literature suggesting that unresolved grief may cause illness and even death.[4] The environment of the family may appear the same but a great deal of readjustment must be made. At least two tasks are involved in the transition and readjustment following death.

Task 5: Dealing with the Vacant Role

In all families roles are assumed by each member. When death occurs roles are disrupted and reorganization is necessary. Following Mrs. Turner's death, her husband had to assume the role of both mother and father for the three young children. Because he was not able to find a housekeeper, he relied on his parents and neighbors to assist in caring for the children. In addition to his previous responsibilities he took over preparing meals, washing clothes and helping the children with their homework. Gradually, Mr. Turner was able to delegate some of the work load to the children. Although he began to involve the children in the family responsibilities, he missed having someone with whom to share decision making and planning for the future. It was not possible to replace the part his wife contributed in sharing and planning for the family.

In another situation, the husband had taken care of all business and financial matters. The wife had not been involved in payment of bills nor did she have any understanding of the overall financial situation. The role of financial manager became a new and difficult assignment after the husband's death. It became essential for her to keep track of the bank balance to maintain solvency. In this situation a son was able to give guidance. The nurse in the community may become involved in helping or finding help for persons undertaking new responsibilities.

Task 6: Adjusting to External Institutions

Occasionally the nurse may need to suggest alternatives to the family regarding changes in living arrangements or work situations. For example, grown children might encourage their mother to leave the family home and move to an apartment. Perhaps another arrangement would have been to bring in a companion or student renter so that the mother could stay in her own home.

Shortly after the death of Joan's mother, the daughter wondered if she would be able to go to the Girl Scout mother-daughter banquet. The community nurse suggested that the grandmother attend the dinner with her.

The community nurse might also be in a position to suggest that a previously planned early retirement be postponed for a year or two to promote socialization and thereby assist in the process of readjustment. The time of readjustment to the social environment varies, but some period of readjustment is essential to all families following death.

STAGE OF FORMATION OF NEW RELATIONSHIPS

Following death, the family is dealing with and adjusting to many altered relationships. However, it is also important at this time for the nurse to recognize and encourage the task of the development of new relationships.

Goldberg's article brings to focus the need to remember the total family constellation.[5] There will be a need for new family relationships as well as new relationships for individual members of the unit. Joining and participating in new groups is one means. For example, one young father joined a single parents group following his wife's death. He enjoyed the social gatherings as well as the stimulation and support of other adults similarly adjusting to a loss. Another means of forming new relationships is to take part in volunteer services, which may open up a very satisfying outlet for energies. This stage of formation of new relationships is an ongoing process throughout life, but following death it is important for total family readjustment.

CONCLUSION

The community nurse must constantly remember these stages of adjustment to death and dying and the resultant tasks when involved with families caring for a dying member. The nurse in the community is frequently the person called on to assist the family before and following the death, in its readjustment to the environment and the formation of new relationships.

REFERENCES

1. Kubler-Ross, Elisabeth. *On Death and Dying.* New York, Macmillan, 1969.
2. Lindemann, Erich. "Symptomatology and Management in Acute Grief," *American Journal of Psychiatry* 101 (1944), pp. 141−148.
3. Yu-Lan, Fung. *History of Chinese Philosophy.* Princeton University Press, 1952.
4. Parkes, Colin Murray. *Bereavement: Studies of Grief in Adult Life.* International Universities Press, 1972.
5. Goldberg, Stanley B. "Family Tasks and Reactions in the Crisis of Death," *Social Casework* (July 1973), pp. 398−405.

VIII

Community Assessment and Health Planning

*Community nursing means more than working in the community.
This point has been emphasized throughout the preceding chapters. It is service to the community. Community nursing is concerned with community health. Consequently, in addition to understanding patients and families, the community nurse must grasp
the nature of communities. How are they organized? What are
their characteristics? What are their needs? Also, the nurse must
know how to plan for community health services. What factors
should be considered in this planning? What persons and groups
should be involved? These are some of the questions answered
in Part VIII.*

*Every community is a system of parts, each influencing the others.
The political structure determines many decisions affecting the
community. A conservative faction may keep the community from
developing an innovative health program. Schools, churches and
clubs influence the thinking and behavior of the people. Geography
can influence the community's economy. Location on a river may
encourage certain types of industry and provide jobs for many area
residents. A community located in the center of a farming area may
bring in migrant farm workers with their special needs and concerns.
The health care system of a community is not isolated from these
other features of community life. It must be seen as one part of a
complex system. Only then will service to the community be effective.*

*One reason community nurses must understand the community
is to carry out effectively their services to families. They must
know what services are available and how to put people in touch
with them. They need to understand the influence of various
community characteristics on the families and individuals they
are serving. But this is only one aspect of community nursing. Its
broader goals must also be considered. Nurses are members of
the health care team and also members of the community. Therefore they have a dual responsibility for understanding and involvement in larger community concerns. Their charge is to serve
the community.*

*Community nursing is future-oriented, seeking to increase the
level of health in the community. Its aim is distributive care,*

particularly emphasizing prevention, which requires effective long-range planning. The conceptual framework for understanding the community and planning within it as well as specific examples of nurses working to raise the level of health care are examined in Part VIII.

47

Assessing Community Characteristics

Donald C. Klein

Because everyone belongs to a community, it is easy to take for granted that everyone understands communities. In this chapter, Donald Klein challenges that view. He maintains that as people get involved in some health care program or agency they often lose an objective and comprehensive understanding of the community. Although this chapter was originally directed to those who work in community mental health, it has wide application for all areas of community health, including community nursing. It provides an overview of the various aspects of a community such as its self-image, physical environment and social organization. In addition to providing a conceptual framework for under-standing the community, the author relates this framework to the goals of community health workers.

The clinical worker new to community work and his citizen collaborators in the community may question the need for a special conceptual view of community to guide them in their work. As life-long participants in multiple communities, they justifiably may lay claim to knowledge based on firsthand experience. To suggest that they do not have, on the basis of their experiences, sufficient under-standing of the communities in which they work may seem strange to some. The suggestion is analogous to that of dynamic psychology when it questions the adequacy of the average person's common sense view of himself. This paper is based on the assumptions: (a) that it is important for professional mental health workers to maintain an objective and comprehensive view of community processes; and (b) that it is often difficult to do so, especially when the worker is confronted by community issues and events which are personally involving or which appear to threaten the very program to which he is committed.

The image of community which is developed in this paper is intended to serve as a rough territorial map which may help the mental health worker maintain some bearings as he functions within the complexities of the community. It is an attempt at a dynamic synthesis of a clinical point of view, with research and theory drawn from the social sciences, and empirical observations made within an ongoing community mental health program at the Human Relations Service of Wellesley, Inc.

It is believed that any comprehensive view of a community for mental health purposes should take into account (a) the physical and topographical character-istics of the setting, (b) the community's "self-image," that is, the view of the community held by its inhabitants, (c) the nature of community groups and their characteristic interaction patterns, and (d) the dynamic interplay of dominant

From Donald C. Klein "The Community and Mental Health: An Attempt at a Conceptual Framework," *Community Mental Health Journal*, Vol. 1, No. 4, pp. 301–308. Copyright © 1965 by Behavioral Publications, 72 Fifth Ave., New York, N.Y. Reprinted with permission.

community forces. In the discussion of each area which follows, there is no attempt to be categorically comprehensive. Rather, the effort is made to indicate the scope of the phenomena and their implications for the development of mental health programs.

PHYSICAL CHARACTERISTICS OF THE COMMUNITY

Where is the community located geographically and with respect to such things as: (a) natural resources, (b) trade and travel routes, and (c) other communities? It should be apparent to the casual observer that the natural resources available to any community dictate to a large extent the character of its economy. The suitable natural resources of some communities are organized around tourists and the tourist trade. Other communities find themselves engaged in mining and the extracting and processing of these natural resources. Other communities are manufacturing centers, and so on.

Trade and travel routes determine the extent to which residents of the community may be in contact with other areas and surrounding regions. Is this the kind of community which is accessible to the outer world? Is this a remote and isolated community into which strangers or "furriners" rarely come? Finally, is the community larger, smaller, or the same size as the surrounding communities? Is it a "satellite community," adjacent to a county seat, or a larger city or town in which are located most of the educational, trade, and cultural resources of its region? Perhaps it is one of the many burgeoning suburban towns growing up around our metropolitan areas from which wage earners emerge in the morning and to which they return at night, the so-called "bedroom" communities of modern America.

Physical Size

Size of a community can be expressed in population density and in trends of population growth or shrinkage, as well as in sheer physical dimensions. Most communities have grown since World War II, sometimes markedly so. Therefore, in most cases it is appropriate to consider what resources, what agencies, and what people in the community are paying attention to population trends? Is there any integrated plan with respect to this? What are some of the effects of this community's growth? What happens to the new people? Are these conflicts between newcomers and the old timers?

Population Density

The factor of population density is just beginning to be studied from the standpoint of mental health. Plant and animal biologists have some notion about the importance of this factor. When two kinds of distribution of the same number of items in the population exist, the conditions under which these trees and other plant and animal life live are very different. A striking and often used example involves two groves of redwood trees, each consisting of one hundred trees. In one grove the trees are much closer together while in the other they are spread out over a considerable area. The sun penetrates one grove and not the other. Certain kinds of fauna and flora will flourish in one environment and not in the other. There have been some studies of urban communities which suggest that different kinds of behavior and emotional difficulties occur in the center of congested community areas than occur in outer rings of a community. Outer rings are usually less densely inhabited, and inhabited by different kinds of individuals.

Location and Resources

Another significant physical characteristic is the location in the community of the various services, agencies, and institutions: schools and hospitals, the main shopping areas, the main arteries within the town, and connecting roads that link one section of a community to another. The consideration of location is obviously important when thinking about the placement of a mental health center, since experience indicates that different clientele are attracted to a clinic depending upon its physical locus within the community. In some places, both the disadvantaged and elite groups in the population often reside in sections which are isolated from the main body of the community and which have few roads connecting them to the rest of the town. Such isolation may well affect the extent of use to which a mental health center or other community resource may be put by either group.

Topography

Common sense recognizes the influence of topography upon community life. In literature it is common for authors to think of regional differences in terms of topographical features, i.e., the frequent reference to the *"rock-ribbed,* reserved New Englander."* Whether or not topography influences character formation, it does affect real estate values and population distributions. In many communities, for example, the more economically favored sections of the population are more apt to live in the geographically more elevated sections of town.

THE COMMUNITY'S VIEW OF ITSELF

Attention should be directed to the "phenomenology" of the community, that is, the ways in which residents view their community (Sanders, 1953). Such perceptions constitute a kind of community self-image, usually based on history and traditions handed down from the past. How are such self-images organized? Each community seems to be able to say about itself, "We are such and such kind of folks." Some communities think of themselves as friendly places; others consist of people who "mind our own business"; a few communities have been studied where the residents accept a self-appraisal which essentially states "we are a bunch of no-goods"; another community may consist of "hustlers and go-getters"; and still another may be inhabited by "rugged individualists." It seems reasonable to expect that such differing community self-images would lead to quite varied responses to the introduction of mental health programs.

Guiding Values

There are the values upheld in the community which guide and direct action: "We hold these truths to be self-evident" in *our* community. Some causes are readily mobilized around certain dominant values and still other causes will not flourish because they seem to be inconsistent or opposed to them.

Several often divergent and even conflicting values may coexist in a single community. Often separate values are upheld by different segments of the population but sometimes the same individuals may appear to subscribe to apparently conflicting value orientations. How does this affect the mental health field? As an example, one might think that the acceptable value of the need "to care for our own" would facilitate the organization of a local mental hygiene clinic to treat adults and children. On the other hand, such an enterprise might seem to conflict with a different value orientation espousing free enterprise because the mental health center becomes viewed as an expression of socialized medicine. Conflicting values in the same individual as well as in the same community are integrated in a variety of ways. But such integrations of dissonance are only beginning to be understood by students of personality, let alone observers of the modern community.

A value conflict frequently observed in such institutions as mental hospitals and in prisons is the conflict between the "soft," treatment-oriented, remedial values as opposed to the sterner, more "hard-headed," punitive and judgmental values. Both coexist and are strongly upheld in American society. Usually, mental health centers seem to have relatively little difficulty in entering into contact with the educational segments of the community, but have much more difficulty in establishing cooperative relationships with the law enforcement segments. It may be speculated that communities do not encourage a close cooperation between the "soft" values of the mental health center and the "hard" values upheld by the more punitive agents. Mental health enterprises in some communities may be allowed to flourish just because they do not unduly affect the conflicting values as often expressed and fulfilled by the law enforcement people, among others.

Community Style

Each community seems to say in one way or another, "we have our own ways of doing things." It is useful to look at how decisions are made in a community and how new ideas may be proposed and implemented in the population. In one community, luncheon meetings seem to be favored; in another, letters to the editor have greater impact; and another may launch a new idea with great public fanfare in a central auditorium accompanied by considerable community-wide publicity.

In the organization of mental health associations and mental health centers, it would seem important to: (a) pay attention to the community's view of itself, (b) determine what kind of folks the inhabitants of this town feel they are, (c) ascertain which truths are upheld as self-evident when applied to human nature and community life, and (d) note the acceptable ways in which new ideas are proposed and decisions are made.

STRUCTURAL CHARACTERISTICS OF COMMUNITY GROUPING

The social-psychological structure of the community can be viewed from the standpoints of the socioeconomic characteristics of the population, and patterns of interaction between groups, agencies, and institutions. Looking first at socio-economic characteristics, the observer would do well to note the nationality groups represented, the religious institutions present, the educational levels of the population, the occupations pursued, and the age distribution. Such factors would appear to influence the way in which the mental health resources as well as other community services are used. On the other hand, these factors also affect the nature of the problems to be found in the population. There is a grow-ing body of evidence to suggest that mental illnesses are distributed differentially in the population according to socioeconomic characteristics. The studies by Hollingshead and Redlich (1958) indicate that, in New Haven at least, there is a far greater prevalence of diagnosed cases of schizophrenia among working class segments of the population than among middle and upper class groups. Even the nature of treatment provided by professionally trained people in the hospital setting differs according to the socioeconomic background of the patients.

It is useful for the observer of the community to attempt to map or diagram the patterns of interaction between groups, agencies, and institutions. What are some of the social-psychological features which can be noted from a structural point of view?

Authority

First, there are those segments of the community occupying positions of authority *vis-a-vis* other segments. Authority in this sense is being used to designate the formal responsibilities given to governmental and other bodies. Authority may or may not be accompanied by an equally high level of prestige. Such authority is often accompanied by power, but is by no means synonymous with it.

Power

Power is the ability to influence decisions and actions of other people. Viewed in another sense, it is the extent of the individual's or group's ability to block or facilitate the gratification of the needs of other people. Power over all mankind would be secured almost immediately by the individual or group who learned how to control the supply of air which people breathe. Obviously, power viewed in this way can be seen to vary according to the area of need in question. For example, the county commissioners may have great influence and power over the mental health center where finances are involved but it may be counterbalanced by the commissioners' recognition of the professional skills which can be provided by the staff. Such a reciprocal or interdependent situation is perhaps the optimal one for the development of close working relationships and shared problem solving between the governmental body and the mental health center, a sharing based on recognition of mutual needs.

Power patterns in communities differ according to the degree to which they are stable and fixed, or unstable and fluctuating. Expanding population areas, for example, often seem to be typified by highly unstable power structures. They are often marked by sharp cleavages between the newcomers and the old timers. As a result, social planning for health, education, and social welfare enterprises may become inadvertently enmeshed in the already existing struggles for power on the part of different factions. A mental health center thus may become a political issue, although it would hardly appear that one political party would in actuality tend to be more mental health oriented than another. Such cleavages may run through all aspects of community life and may set up barriers to planning in the area of mental health until the reasonable issues regarding the mental health needs of the community are clearly separated from the less reasonable ones grounded in such factors as unstable power distribution.

The well-known studies by Hunter (1953), Freeman, et al. (1960, 1962), and others indicate that recognized top power-figures or decision-makers in most communities are drawn from the following groups: those controlling natural resources, those controlling financial reserves, those in charge of means of production, as well as certain prestige-figures and certain professionals, with an occasional political leader thrown in for good measure. Hunter maintained that such top power-figures do not usually operate visibly in the community or through official channels. Later students of the subject have not confirmed his thesis, however.

A significant power group in the typical modern American community consists of those realtors who act as so-called "gatekeepers," occupying a role which may impinge upon the mental health of newcomers and others. To a greater or lesser extent, they determine into which communities people will move and into which neighborhoods they will settle. Often the realtors feel that economic security and success is bound up with their skill in assigning suitable newcomers to various sections of town. The criteria the realtor uses in his gatekeeper role and the consequences of the sorting process for mental health is not yet sufficiently understood.

Prestige

Most community agencies seek to attract to their boards or other sponsoring bodies prestigious figures in the community. Prestige is usually based on social position, family background, and inherited wealth. It may also reside in individuals whose deep devotion and good sense is recognized when it comes to matters affecting the entire community. Hunter stresses that prestige-figures often may have a latent power position in their communities which they choose to use only on certain occasions.

COMMUNICATION

The communication network of a community represents an extremely important feature which often is dimly perceived and ill understood. Who talks to whom, about what and under what circumstances? Not only do people of similar socio-economic characteristics sometimes reside close to one another, they also frequently interact with and communicate with one another more readily than with other groups in other sections.

Certain individuals or places in the community serve as communication centers. For example, in one New England community the largest supermarket was found to be the gossip center. Any item of information discussed in the supermarket would spread through the community. In other towns the barber shop, the beauty parlor, the local bar, and even the town dump may serve as gossip or communication centers.

In considering communication, it is customary to distinguish between formal and informal communication. The community observer would do well to note which open formal communication channels exist between various groups. Some groups have well-established intercommunications; between others there are no such channels. When formal communication channels do not exist, informal contacts between single individuals often are relied upon. Very often one group believes it has "communicated" with another group through an informal contact of this nature when in actuality no transmission of information has occurred on an intergroup basis. As a result, under some conditions, the first group may reject the second group and may fail to note possible points of alliance because it has misinterpreted inadequate communication to be rejection. Hunter's (1953) study of a southern city provides a case in point. He found that the top power-figures in the white community rarely knew and therefore could not communicate with their counterparts in the Negro community. Conversely the Negro power-figures were not in touch with the white leaders. Both top power-groups instead were in contact with "second echelon" power-figures in the other communities. Under such circumstances, it was very difficult indeed for these two subcommunities to come together to identify mutual needs and to solve mutual problems. It is clear that the board of a mental health agency cannot assume that effective communication with a group exists simply because a member of that group is "represented" on the board.

THE DYNAMIC INTERPLAY OF COMMUNITY FORCES

Because community structure and dynamics are closely interrelated, some issues of the dynamics of the community have been touched on in the foregoing discussions of power and communication. In order to consider this topic more systematically, it is useful to consider the community as an integrated field of forces. This assumption leads one to attempt to identify the instrumentalities whereby the various community values, interests, and groups become coordinated. Some communities have truly coordinative community councils or health bodies. In other communities, apparently coordinative groups in actuality represent restricted segments of the population. One may well raise the question of the extent to which the board of a mental health service should seek to serve the community in a coordinative way. To what extent can such a board attempt to assess and interpret community needs in the area of mental health? Is such a coordinative function possible when the agency must, at the same time, represent one of the value areas of the community and, in so doing, compete in the market place with other values and interests?

One of the most significant integrative dynamics of a community from a mental health standpoint concerns the processes whereby help is made available and sought by those in need. More simply stated, what kinds of problems are brought to which resources in the community? Some observers have suggested that in the lower socioeconomic groups as much as 80 percent of the complaints brought to the general practitioners and health clinics have no organic basis but are instead an expression of social and emotional malfunction. Problems which arise from bereavement are obviously more apt to come to the clergyman. In recent years family agencies in many communities noted that they tended to serve lower socio-economic groups and, in some cases, have attempted to alter this state of affairs. On the other hand, it appears that mental hygiene clinics are turned to most readily by middle class segments of the population. The community observer or planner may wish to ask himself and the community whether such patterns of helping should be altered or whether they should be reinforced and strengthened? The board and staff of a new mental health center may wish to consider what will happen to help-seeking and help-giving patterns as the center becomes established in a community. Should the mental health center take over responsibilities for certain psychiatric problems from the caretaking groups already dealing with them in one way or another? Or should the mental health center be in the position of strengthening these caretaking groups in their mental health operations?

The community is a dynamic system; each segment is related to each other segment. Moreover, the community is what Kurt Lewin (1951) called a "unified field." By this he meant that a change in one region would affect all other regions. Since the community is a dynamic system and a unified field, it follows that the entry of a mental health team will induce effects of one sort or another through-out the community. These reactions probably will be quite varied depending upon the ways in which the agency is perceived and experienced. One segment of the community may rush forward to collaborate with the mental health effort, and to make use of the resource. Another segment may attack the agency and perhaps even attempt to have it ejected as something alien or dangerous. Still another segment might simply seek to establish as much social psychological distance as possible between it and the agency. Whatever the pattern of response, the notion of the dynamic community would compel the assumption that these responses, in toto, represent an over-all pattern rather than haphazard reactions or reactions based primarily on idiosyncrasies of individual citizens or community leaders.

In the community there are groups which are highly receptive to certain influences from the outside, whereas other segments of the community are correspondingly hostile to or avoidant of outside influences. Which groups are receptive and which hostile depends on such factors as the nature of the community and of the outside influence itself. With respect to mental health issues, the pattern of response in various places throughout the country has appeared to be that of relatively greater receptivity on the part of the educational and certain religious systems, antagonism and attack on the part of exponents of law and order, and avoidance on the part of those people and groups most concerned with the maintenance of such cherished community values as neighborhood integrity, real estate land values, and the like.

As a dynamic system, a community exists in some kind of equilibrium or balance of its forces, which, while not static in nature, do act to maintain some form of homeostasis. In some communities, however, the regulatory mechanisms seem relatively poor and there are extremes of oscillation back and forth as, for example, in political power between radical and reactionary groups, or in the commonly observed alternation of government by reform movements and entrenched political bosses. In such communities, a mental health enterprise may enter as part of one phase in the oscillation and later may find itself under severe attack as the system moves back to the other extreme. Moreover, the entry of a mental health center may itself induce oscillation as opposing and restraining forces are mobilized. If not reckoned with, such oscillation might ultimately lead to unforeseen limitations on or even ejection of the center. It is wise for the board and staff of a mental health center to maintain continuing assessment of forces and factors opposing movement towards mental health values with the goal of understanding and, conceivably, altering and reducing rather than overriding them.

A social scientist may view the mental health movement with some skepticism. There are some who go so far as to postulate that the equilibrium of communities depends upon the existence of social pathology, delinquency, mental illness, and other deviant behaviors. This postulate suggests that the stable segment of the society in some way "needs" the unstable. Another way of putting this thesis is to ask, "How can we understand and practice virtue if we cannot observe and know about sin?" Those upholding this position assert that, even when causes of certain kinds of social pathology are well understood, communities seem remarkably unable to mobilize to deal effectively with them. They note, as further corroboration, the ready tendency of social groups to establish scapegoats and marginal members of one sort or another.

The writer's own observations indicate that in virtually every neighborhood area studied residents can and do identify individuals or families disliked by their neighbors. Those disliked are viewed as marginal or deviant in that they cause trouble, seem peculiar, are emotionally upset, or simply are "not like us." Neighborhoods appear to respond in a variety of ways to behaviors which are considered to be deviant, objectionable, or "sick." Under some conditions certain neighborhoods seem to be able to integrate marginal people and to deal effectively with certain problems. Under other circumstances some neighborhoods appear to reinforce and enhance the marginality through a hostile system of isolation and "quarantine." Such community processes are at present little understood. It seems clear, however, that neighborhood patterns and expectations may have considerable influence on the social learning of children, the quality of coping behavior, and the emotional well-being of individuals and families. The child who is having difficulties in relationships with parents, and is expressing these difficulties via destructive and aggressive behavior in the neighborhood, may find that neighborhood a force for health, or an additional force for emotional maladjustment, depending on how neighborhood forces are mobilized.

The foregoing cognitive map of community is necessarily limited. In addition to omissions arising from the author's inadequacies, there are inherent limitations common to most maps. The function of a map is to assist the user to accomplish certain specific purposes. Thus a map of transportation facilities may not include the elevations and other details needed for a topographical map. The objective of this paper has not been to provide specific guidance for the mental health worker in the community. Rather, it has been to stimulate his interest in the community and underscore patterned interactions having to do with certain fundamental functions for which communities exist. Clinically trained psychiatrists, psychologists, and social workers develop an ingrained feeling for the dynamics of personality as they are expressed in the behavior of their patients. It is hoped that, for some, these remarks will point the way towards the development of a similar "sense of community" as manifested by the behaviors of clients, consultees, board members, and the many other citizens with whom they work.

REFERENCES

Freeman, L. C. et al. *Local community leadership.* Syracuse: University College, 1960.
Freeman, L. C. et al. *Metropolitan decision making.* Syracuse: University College, 1962.
Hollingshead, A., and Redlich, F. *Social class and mental illness: A community study.* New York: John Wiley & Sons, 1958.
Hunter, F. *Community power structure: A study of decision makers.* Chapel Hill: University of North Carolina Press, 1953.
Lewin, K. *Field theory in social science.* New York: Harper & Brothers, 1951.
Sanders, I. *Making good communities better.* Lexington: University of Kentucky Press, 1953.
Sanders, I. *The community: An introduction to a social system.* New York: Ronald Press, 1958.

48

What Is Health Planning?

Tasker K. Robinette

Community nursing is more than service in the community; it is service to the community. Therefore it is important to understand the nature of the community and how to design ways that health services can be improved. The community nurse is in a strategic position to contribute significantly to planning for the health needs of a community, but that requires insight into the nature of planning itself. In this article, Tasker Robinette examines the fundamental features of planning in a wide variety of settings, showing how they can be applied to planning in the health care system.

The dictionary definition of "planning" is "the mental formulation of a proposed method of doing or making something or of achieving a given end." Mannheim describes it as the third evolutionary state of rational thought, after first, discovery, and then inventive thinking. Finally, planned thinking he defines as the deliberate regulation and intelligent mastery of the relationship between single objects or institutions — but for a purpose, not as an activity important in and of itself.[1] In Mannheim's definition, the purpose is rational control of society toward intelligently preselected ends. These definitions illustrate the range of classical use of the term "planning." In its most casual application, it simply means to think out what we want to do before we start to do it.

At a more complex level, as in architecture, engineering, and organization planning, we have developed the idea into a complex and sophisticated technology, the tangible results of which are the familiar — blueprints, specifications, organization charts, policy and procedure manuals. The classical steps in this methodology are:

1. *Form the philosophy* — Who are we, what do we believe in, what are we planning.
2. *Forecast the future without our intervention* — What will the world that concerns us to be like in the foreseeable future unless we do something to change it?
3. *Establish goals* — What do we want to be different as a result of our intervention in the future? What are we working toward?
4. *Gather data* — What is the difference between the world today, and the way we want it to be? What is the extent of our task?
5. *Formulate objectives* — What will we do, in what order (priorities), in what periods of time (given our opportunities, restraints, and resources)?
6. *Analyze alternatives* — What ways are open to us to accomplish our objectives, and what are the advantages and disadvantages of each of these, such as, costs versus benefits?

7. *Select a strategy* — Which alternatives will we select?
8. *Program* — What tasks are required in what order, to pursue our strategy? Who will do these tasks, under what conditions.
9. *Schedule* — How much time is needed for each task, in what sequence?
10. *Budget* — How much, of what kind of resources, is required to support our program?
11. *Management control* — What kind of a system will we establish to keep our program on its predetermined tracks?
12. *Evaluation and feedback* — How will we measure our progress, check our assumptions, and provide a mechanism to feed in new information indicating the need to change any previously listed element of our program?

The creation of buildings, cities, large organizations, and complex machinery (airplanes, missiles, and computers) requires advanced planning technology that is really nothing more than an extension and refinement of the same process used in planning a dinner party. Galbraith, in *The New Industrial State,* however, suggests that our whole society rests on an implicit agreement between government, our largest corporations, and our major institutions to permit and enable this kind of planning.[2] It is this agreement that President Eisenhower warned of when he spoke of the "military-industrial complex."

That this kind of planning is difficult is shown by the problem faced by the manager of the Bölkow Company, a German helicopter manufacturer, who undertook, in 1951, to plan an aircraft that would be up to date, cost effective, and salable 19 years after the start of the project.[3] Development alone was to take seven years, and the helicopter's original design had to incorporate component parts into the final version which were predictable but unknown at the start of the project. That helicopter is now flying, which indicates that, while difficult, the undertaking was possible. We would not have modern automobiles, jet aircraft, or space probes if it was not possible to plan with precision.

ANOTHER DIMENSION

That kind of planning relates to a corporate or product unity, in which some authority has some control over the task to be performed. Social planning, as described by Mannheim and Galbraith, and described by Eisenhower, adds a geometric dimension to the problem. Somebody must apply the classical method to interacting divergent and largely autonomous unities, toward a common goal which is dimly perceived, and with less than enough power and authority to assure adherence to the plan. Other countries have tried it over the past 50 years with mixed results. Now we are beginning to try it, too, but without their willingness to use coercive power. This kind of planning must deal with tangibles, values, and human motivations. Yet the only planning techniques we have mastered are those borrowed from industry. We are in the difficult process of formulating new methods more appropriate to this new, more difficult task. We must do it by borrowing some elements of the classical planning process and modifying them to fit our democratic values, our knowledge of political realities, and our new knowledge from behavioral science.

Americans know the benefits of industrial planning, and it should be no surprise, therefore, that in reaction to rapidly increasing costs, coupled with an increasing sense of social conscience, our representatives would legislate "planning" for the health care fields.

ACTIVITY, NOT PLANNING

Health professionals and concerned nonprofessional citizens picked up the challenge of the 89th Congress (at least in some places) with a zeal which matched their lack of planning knowledge and experience. As a result (at least in some places) there has been much activity, involvement, interaction, frustration, and conflict. There have been many meetings but little "planning" and very little improvement in our health service delivery system as a result of this activity. This is partly caused by: (1) the belief of some that, somehow, it is the activity itself which is important; (2) our lack of familiarity with proven industrial planning technology coupled with our failure to create a carefully thought out newer version more applicable to our situation; (3) our unfamiliarity with the nature, purpose, and need for planning; and (4) unreasonable expectations.

Each of us has different understandings about what planning is, what it does, what it takes, and who does it. I am not sure we are likely to achieve what the legislators had in mind by just *any* kind of new activity, so it concerns me that I have heard the phrase "health planning" used in so many contexts lately, and without any qualifying modifiers.

The phrase, health planning, is being used to signify the opposite of action, as in a "planning" as opposed to an "action" committee. It is used to describe general discussions, as in a "planning conference," and "a planning grant." The Comprehensive Health Planning (CHP) agencies often speak of problem identification as "planning," and the voluntary areawide hospital planning agencies often refer to their attempts to coordinate the plans of individual institutions as "planning." Comprehensive health planning is often used to denote the avoidance of duplication of services and facilities, but is also being used to describe data gathering, involvement, forecasting, regulatory activity, and public information activities. Planning for comprehensive health services is entirely different from comprehensive health planning and is often called "program" planning but then program planning can refer to any health service activity, whether comprehensive or not. It is easy to see why planning is so popular — everybody can do his own thing and say he is fulfilling the legislative mandate. I am not surprised, however, that so little results have come from so much diverse activity, which is all given the label of "health planning."

I have seen the opposite of the classical idea of planning labeled as planning. I have heard of "evolutionary planning," "incremental planning," "developmental planning," "pragmatic evolution," or "stage planning." While some of these terms may have legitimate use in other fields, in health planning I have heard them used mostly to describe a situation in which we evaluate our past experience and correct our past errors after all the evidence is accumulated by others and proved reliable — by others. In other words, we substitute *evaluation* or *problem analysis* for planning.

The confusion in terms is a byproduct of our attempts to modify previous ideas for applicability in health care or more likely, I believe, to try to reduce the ideological opposition to social planning for health services and the controversy and conflict which that opposition causes. The confusion places us in danger, however, of losing our direction. If we lose our direction, we will not achieve the end results we are supposed to be pursuing, and we will not have created an applicable health planning technology.

FUNDAMENTAL CHARACTERISTICS

Returning our attention to the fundamental aspects of planning, which are clearly called for in the new federal health planning laws, let me explain what I think "planning" means.

Planning is always a method — a technology, a tool, a means — for doing something useful. It is a method of predetermining a course of action. It involves a logical thought process, which requires the planner to imagine an end result (the goal) of activity, and presumes the power and intent to control future activity in an environment which is presumed to be at least partially predictable. Let's go back for a moment and pick up some key words and ideas.

1. Planning is always a *means* to an end, not an end in itself. Those who maintain that CHP, for example, has as its end result the establishment of the "planning process," need to explain the value in a planning apparatus with no purpose other than to continue to exist.
2. Planning always relates to the future. Problem solving is management of the *present*. Planning is management of the *future*. When we concentrate on solving present problems, we exclude attention to situations that might become problems in the future.
3. Since planning is a means to a future end, the end result must be visionary, or imagined, since it is in the future. Planning cannot proceed until the end result has been decided upon. The solution of the end result (goal) is always a subjective, judgmental process. Planning, therefore, is a thoughtful process, and thought is an important kind of action.
4. Planning is a *management* technology. It presumes the power and intent to control. Planning activity, separated from the power or intent to control, is

commonly described as research, data or information gathering, reporting, or recommending. Our present attempts to achieve involvement and participation are really attempts to gather power which can later be used to manage or control (influence action), after plans have been prepared.

5. It is the nature and intent of planning to limit future possibilities of action, in order to concentrate available resources on those action probabilities which seem most likely to achieve the desired end results. The tendency to place limitations on freedom of individual action is, therefore, inherent in the idea of planning.

6. It is the purpose of planning to cause or initiate controlled change. Thus, one does not engage in planning unless one wishes to cause change, or unless one anticipates change and intends to bring that change under rational control.

I will be perfectly comfortable with anyone who places a qualifying modifier such as "comprehensive," "program," "institutional," "manpower," "facilities," or "health" before the word planning, as long as the activity he is describing essentially fits the description above. Involvement, participation of consumers, data gathering, organizing a staff, and discussion meetings may well be required in order for plans to be implemented successfully, but they are not in and of themselves planning. They are, no matter how necessary and important, program management, rather than planning activities.

ITS CONTROVERSIAL NATURE

Planning in health care has been accompanied by major controversy and serious conflict. I have implied some of the reasons, but they can be more directly stated.

1. Planning is new in American health care administration. It dates from about 1930, with major emphasis only since 1966; it is new in our larger society as well. As late as 1934, Margaret Mead asserted that no nation on the face of the earth had ever attempted to "program its new normalities" into the next generation, and that is precisely what we are trying to do. All things which are new are controversial in some measure.

2. Planning is an initiatory process, and in the health care field our posture of "responsiveness" to patient needs is a tradition lost in antiquity. (Planning is like preventive medicine as compared to curative medicine.)

3. Planning is a thoughtful process, and those of us who are health professionals have always been strongly "action" oriented. To be caught "thinking" is embarrassing for us; we feel comfortable only when we are "doing" something.

4. Many of us believe that so many important factors are unpredictable that it is impossible to create a reasonable plan. Every existing building and most successful programs disprove this myth, as does the fact that we have not had a major depression in 35 years. If we could not see into the future, our wind-

shields would be firmly implanted in the floor of our automobiles. Even so, our unfamiliarity with planning in health breeds skepticism.

5. Planning is a method of control, and most people resist control in the present, let alone the future. Planning is rightly perceived by them as a means of limiting their individual liberties.

6. CHP, and all new "planning" programs are clearly intended to reduce some people's power while increasing the power of others — to reduce, for example, the power of one hospital's board of trustees to act unilaterally, while increasing the power of consumers participating in a planning council. No one gives up power easily. Rapid, intentional power shifts sometimes become revolutions.

7. Planning proceeds from an agreed-upon philosophy, goals, and objectives. Clearly all participants in the planning process cannot agree on philosophy, goals, and objectives except at the highest level of abstraction. More accurately, different people hold different values, and even when they share values with others they place different weights on the same values. Thus conflict is inevitable. In our society the mechanism we use to resolve conflicts, peacefully, is called politics.

8. The achievement of a political consensus on philosophy, goals, and objectives requires effective communication among participants. We live in many separate worlds, and communication is very difficult. We have no common language, and building one is torturous and time-consuming. Since we are largely unaware of how little shared experience there is among us, we tend to attribute dark motives to those whose disagreement with us is based on perception from a different perspective. Communication requires shared experience.

CREATE THE PATTERN

At the risk of appearing to try to freeze a dynamic language into historical word usages, I have tried to describe a way of doing things which I believe we have been asked to apply to the improvement of our health care services delivery system. Something different than this method may be needed and, if it is, we'll have to create it. Some people say it will evolve, but I think evolution is a word future generations will use to describe what we do, rather than a word we should use to describe our own attempts. There should be method and purpose in our actions. We must create the pattern that those who follow us will say emerged.

I have called for precision in the use of the phrase health planning in order to direct our attention toward a method of developing the best available health care services, for all our people, wherever they are located and whatever their economic or social status — a method which I believe we have been given the chance to test by the legislative representatives of the American people. We cannot test the method, however, unless we know it, understand it, and try it, while always keeping in the back of our minds the fact that it is only a method.

Some different method may be required, but we will not know that until we test our present technology. Too many of us try to avoid the controversy that I believe is an inevitable corollary of all true planning by applying the phrase "health planning" to a lot of related and peripheral (even if necessary and desirable) activity which is not planning, and even by applying it to some activity which is the antithesis of planning.

The Congress stated our philosophy and general goal in the preamble to the Comprehensive Health Planning Act. They asked us to consider alternatives to a fragmented health care system, to historic professional jurisdictional boundaries, and to hospitalization for diagnosis and convalescence. And they suggested a method — planning.

I appeal for a review of the meaning of the term "planning" as it is applied to health in order to remind us of the true nature of the task in which we are engaged. I believe we need to apply all the technology we already have, while all of us together engage in the formidable task of creating a new and more appropriate methodology. A car without a windshield doesn't need a steering wheel; the driver of a car without a windshield and a steering wheel would more appropriately be called an operator. I would rather be a driver than an operator.

REFERENCES

1. Mannheim, Karl. *Man and Society in an Age of Reconstruction.* New York, Harcourt, Brace and World, 1941, pp. 140—155, 163.
2. Galbraith, J. K., and Randhawa, M. S. *New Industrial State.* Boston, Mass., Houghton Mifflin Co., 1967.
3. Schwartz, Walter. Bölkow's rigid rotor. *Rotor and Wing Magazine* 2:18—21, 43—45, Dec. 1968.

49

How to Become Involved
in Community Planning

Helen Jo McNeil

The two preceding chapters presented conceptual frameworks for understanding the community and for planning to meet the long-range health needs of the community. But how does the nurse use these principles in specific situations? This chapter describes one nurse's involvement in community planning. It shows how community nurses can specifically apply the more abstract principles of health care planning.

Do you believe that *you* can help plan the future of our community? The question jumped out at me from the front page of our local newspaper, and I reacted positively to its appeal for citizen participation. As a nurse and consumer, I knew the lack of coordinated health planning in our community, and I was aware from previous studies of the community that health and social services received little attention. I strongly believed then, as I do now, that health is a community responsibility and decided to attend the announced public meeting.

Our community, a suburb of Seattle, is composed of 17,959 families, most of which have moved here within the past ten years. The average household head is somewhere between thirty-five and fifty-four years old, a college graduate, and a professional man. He owns his own home, plans to stay in the community, and works in the city ten miles away. But I knew that the apparent affluence of our community did not preclude health problems or the need for health planning.

The local chamber of commerce had initiated the planning project, I learned from the paper, and had requested assistance from the Bureau of Community Development at the University of Washington, a resource that offers community educational services upon request without charge. A consultant from the bureau had been assigned to assist in the project.

At the meeting attended by 300 concerned citizens, I filled out a card indicating my interest as health and social services and volunteered to serve on the steering committee for the community program. A preliminary survey had identified some of the other areas of concern as traffic congestion, lack of recreational facilities, and problems resulting from the rapidly increasing population in the area.

The steering committee was made up of representatives from each of the community's 17 neighborhoods, plus a few individuals who had special interest and knowledge of the area. One such was the assistant superintendent of the school district, who had served his district for many years and who proved to be an outstanding resource person in education matters. The committee met twice a month.

From the beginning, it was evident that the committee members needed to know more about the community — its resources and needs. So authorities on such subjects as police, highway, and health were invited to discuss their specialties before the group. Community involvement was an important part of the plan and required finding out how people perceived their needs.

QUESTIONNAIRE

To discover people's opinions about their needs, a questionnaire was developed by the subcommittee studying transportation, education, parks and recreation, public services, land use and appearance, health and social services, and government. Each subcommittee contributed questions that would lead to useable knowledge for planning for the future. Steering committee members served as chairmen of the subcommittee and I volunteered to serve on the health and social services one.

This subcommittee defined its goals as: (1) determining the health and social service needs of the community as perceived by its members; (2) identifying health and social areas deficient in service; (3) finding out the community's attitudes to specific known health problems; and (4) providing stimulation for health education by calling attention to specific health problems.

Professional leaders in health were asked to evaluate the questions related to their field as developed by the subcommittee. Included were the hospital administrator, the chief of the hospital medical staff, the local public health officer, the chairman of the dental society, and the director of the mental health center. They gave suggestions and, at the same time, were made aware of the survey. Involving these key leaders, it was hoped, would serve to implement any changes that the survey results might suggest as being needed.

Preparing the questions and organizing the survey took seven months. Captains were selected to head the survey teams and received a 2-hour training session from the steering committee member who headed the survey, aided by the consultant. Each captain selected two lieutenants who, in turn, chose nine interviewers and all members received a training session. Addresses, not names, were obtained from an advertising firm and every seventh address was put on the survey roll.

The teams then went into action. Approximately 400 interviewers surveyed 2,443 of the 17,959 households in a week. Each interview lasted 30 to 60 minutes. Often additional time was needed to locate an address.

The total cost of the survey was $220, which was raised by means of a $3 self-assessment by the steering committee, with a few local business organizations making up the balance. Such a survey, conducted by professionals, would have cost about $50,000, our consultant told us.

The questions we asked our respondents were designed to explore the community's attitude about some of its critical, unsolved problems. The cost of health and social services was not emphasized. One such problem was the increasing number of unwed parents in school grades seven through twelve. The respondents were asked whether they believed more help or information in certain areas should be provided. (See results tabulated below.)

In another instance, citizens twice had voted against addition of fluoride to the drinking water, even though there were a number of young children in the area. We wondered if their attitude had changed since the last vote had been taken, and asked them whether they now favored fluoridated water in the water system.

Another objective of the committee was to pinpoint gaps in health and social services from the consumer's point of view. We hoped the answers to our question would indicate what the consumer saw as his needs, rather than what the professionals thought them to be. Therefore, the needs that the consumer had but did not recognize were eliminated from the study. It was important, also, to learn if the individual knew how to locate the service he sought. Perhaps a needed resource was available in the community but unknown to the individual in need of it — signifying a gap, at least in education. For example, one couple interviewed were caring for an elderly parent who needed professional nursing care at home. Neither the doctor nor the family was aware that this visiting nursing service was available.

RESULTS OF QUESTIONNAIRE

Responses to the health and social service questions was overwhelmingly positive. Often, as professional workers, we hear only negative opinions from the community. The survey brought out more accurate opinions. For example, in response to the question of whether more help or information should be provided in sex education and related topics, the percentages of respondents answering "yes," "no," or "don't know" to each topic were:

Topic	Yes	No	Don't know
Sex education	48	21	31
Venereal disease education	56	13	31
Help for unwed parents	52	12	36
Child adoption	50	14	36
Planned parenthood	51	16	33
Mental health	62	10	28

The consumers' attitude on fluoridation was surprising: 75 percent favored adding fluoride to the water system; 16 percent disapproved; and only 9 percent had no opinion about the matter.

To find out more accurately whether the consumer's need for certain health and social services — many of a confidential nature — were met by existing resources in the past two years, areas of need were listed on a separate sheet of paper. Respondents were asked to fill out the form privately, and then the sheet was sealed in an envelope. (For results see accompanying chart [below].)

Gaps in Community Health and Social Services Identified by Area of Need. Number of People Requiring Service Within Two Years, and Number Who Received Service

Area of need	Required service		Received service	
	Yes	No	Yes	No
Doctor's care	1907	290	1714	24
Dental care	1747	393	1574	23
Hospital care	1005	1065	906	20
Emergency room service at a hospital	698	1293	603	27
Nursing home care	70	1860	47	9
Home nursing care	52	1860	37	10
Psychiatric care	134	1804	93	31
Counseling for marital or child behavioral problems	150	1804	82	50
Emotional problems of adults	107	1819	57	35
Emotional problems of child	141	1807	94	33
Drinking problem	31	1885	21	8
Drug usage	25	1893	17	3
Problems of physically handicapped or mentally retarded	66	1850	46	13
Homemaker service in emergency	112	1810	60	42
Day care for children of working parents	137	1789	74	49
Retirement homes	36	1870	15	14

Responses to this question were not answered uniformly. Of those who did respond, a small percentage requiring medical, dental, hospital, or emergency room service were unable to obtain it. A somewhat higher percentage could not secure nursing home, home nursing, or psychiatric care. About a third of those who recognized a need for counseling on marital and child behavioral problems, and help for emotional problems, did not locate any source of assistance. One-fourth of those seeking help for children with emotional problems did not find it.

Eight of the 31 persons who admitted a drinking problem were unable to find assistance. Three of the 25 individuals desiring help for drug usage did not locate it. Of those needing homemaker service, 38 percent did not obtain it; while 36 percent of those needing day care for children were unable to find it. Retirement homes were not discovered in 39 percent of the cases. The gap in services for the physically handicapped and mentally retarded was noted in about one-fifth of the cases.

While the community's needs identified by the survey are obviously not a complete inventory of all those needed for future planning, the process of planning and conducting the survey did stimulate interested involvement on the part of the consumers. The report of the National Commission on Community Health Services confirms that consumer participation is a primary requirement in improving community health services.[1] At the first public meeting, one year prior to the survey, the response to the need for citizen participation on the health and social service committee was rather limited. At that time the committee consisted of an engineer, a minister, a housewife, an inactive nurse, and a public health nurse. Other citizens interested enough to participate in the project seemed much more aware of needs in land development, recreation, and transportation, than those in health and social services.

The second public meeting was held to report the findings of the survey, and it completed the first phase of the community planning project. A second steering committee then was elected to lead phase two: an analysis of the survey results to seek solutions to the problems identified. An effort was made to involve citizens other than those on the first steering committee, and volunteers were requested. I volunteered for the health and social service committee.

During the next six months, the health and social service committee developed from one of the weakest to the strongest committees on the community council. There are now 50 members, equally divided between consumers and professionals, but the latter are increasing more rapidly than the former. Subcommittees were formed so that the skills of this large committee might be better used in the many areas of identified need. These subcommittees are the youth activity council, the community resource publication, the drop-in center for drug users, family counseling, and the juvenile court conference. This increased interest in health and social services might be attributed to citizens' involvement in the survey, publicity, and, to some extent, competition within the health and social service field.

WHY GET INVOLVED?

The public health nurse-citizen is especially qualified to assist in community health planning. On her daily home visits, she sees the total needs of patients and their families and by assessing the total picture can give the planners a composite picture of health needs of the entire community. Because she is knowledgeable about the available resources, she can make these known to planners, as she does to patients. The nurse's very presence in the community is often a reminder to consumers of their health problems. Seldom does a day pass without someone saying, "You're a nurse; you ought to be able to help me with this problem...." It might be, "My elderly mother is having great difficulty managing to live alone; how can we provide her with a safer, more comfortable situation?" or "Is this chest pain serious enough to bother the doctor about?" The nurse assesses the problem and assists the inquirer by referring him to the appropriate resource.

Since she is skilled in planning for the health needs of a family, she can expand this skill to the community.

Another advantage of the nurse is that she is a salaried worker, one not influenced by profits and losses inherent in the system of health care. She is free to concentrate on the needs of the consumer and be an objective health planner. In her responsibility to promote health, prevent disease, and improve health care, she thereby helps reduce the cost of health care.

As a consumer of health services, herself, the nurse can evaluate those that she uses and see where the services are weak or not available. In the past, the consumer had a voice only in the use he made of the available services. Now it is possible for him to plan for services that previously did not exist.

How does a nurse become involved in community planning? First, she must learn about the community by reading the local papers and by listening and talking to local leaders and agencies' representatives. Once she has found out what needs to be done she should assess her own skills and offer to do the task she is best prepared for. For example, a public health nurse possesses skills in interviewing that are helpful in surveying community opinion. Combining this skill with her experience in group teaching, she can assist in training interviewers.

What does the nurse do in community planning? As a consumer, the nurse might function in many ways, but, as a professional, she has the responsibility to insist upon the development of goals and measures to evaluate the effectiveness of health care. She can help consumers articulate the goals of health service to serve as effective guidelines for health professionals. Because she is acquainted with consumers from many representative groups or has the resources to locate appropriate representatives, she can stimulate their involvement in health planning. Once these consumers are involved, they often need continuous support, which she can and should give. She also knows professionals in the health field and can help involve them and keep them informed of the committee's progress.

Familiarity with current health legislation is essential for the nurse on the community planning council. Sharing knowledge of the legislative action with appropriate members of the council at the proper time is one of her important responsibilities.

One of the main pitfalls is doing *for* and not *with* lay committee members. Many times it would seem more expedient to do the job oneself rather than help others to do it. Nevertheless, guiding rather than doing has proved the more effective method, so that consumers can learn through doing and then help teach others.

Another is restricting one's thinking and efforts to nursing or health services. Nurses must broaden their approach to include all health services and community areas under study. The health and social service committee needs the support of other community committees and, at the same time, must support other committees if changes are to be effective. Finally, there is the danger of professionals outnumbering consumers. Consumers may assume, incorrectly, that they have less to offer than the professionals and may drop out of the council. Their participation and contribution must be fostered and appreciated.

SATISFACTIONS GAINED

Satisfactions are difficult to evaluate, but I believe they outweigh the time and effort one expends in community planning. One is getting to know community leaders and becoming better acquainted with their work and how the various particular jobs are interrelated. Another is seeing the consumer speak out on health and observing his interest and subsequent impact on the community. Sharing in directing the future of the community and helping achieve continuity of care for all is especially satisfying to a nurse. For example, the hospital now makes contact with those giving home care in order to provide continuity of patient care. And finally, it is most rewarding to see communication taking place between voluntary and public agencies and consumers. After committee meetings, members frequently get together and discuss problems informally, with the focus most often on the patient, the client, the parishioner, or the student in need of help, rather than on the agency. As the goals of the professionals and consumers become closer, the more likely they will be achieved.

Smolensky says that health is a social responsibility in and of the community.[2] As nurses, we are in the community as professionals and of the community as consumers; therefore, health planning is in part our responsibility.

REFERENCES

1. National Commission on Community Health Services. *Health is a Community Affair.* Report of ... Cambridge, Mass., Harvard University Press, 1966, p. 160.
2. Smolensky, Jack, and Haar, F. B. *Principles of Community Health.* Philadelphia, Pa., W. B. Saunders Co., 1967, p. 38.

50

A Cultural Approach to the Nurse's Role in Health-Care Planning

Molly C. Dougherty

It is one thing for health professionals to formulate goals for community health, but quite another to translate goals and plans into terms that are meaningful to the community members. When nurses work in a culturally homogeneous setting, the problem of communication is simplified. But most communities have numerous subcultures. Each group may interpret the goals and plans of health professionals differently. Furthermore, innovations must be designed to fit with existing cultural patterns. This chapter provides an essential link between planning and patient acceptance.

Health-care planning, with emphasis on community needs, is an important function in the delivery of health-care services. To nurses involved in delivering these services, the goals of program planning become part of nursing care, for it is often nurses who initiate health-care innovations and translate planning into action.

To bring the planning phase into perspective and assist the nurse in achieving goals with individual patients and families, it is first necessary to understand the development of — and changes in — health-care planning, since the aims and purposes of planning are often altered by time and changing social conditions. Throughout United States history, medicine has been a force in bringing about change; but, as part of the culture, medicine itself has been shaped by the dominant values of our changing society. Before 1960 few physicians expected the consumer to initiate action on health-care problems, either at the community level or through state and federal legislation. However, the influence of consumer concerns *is* being felt and *is* leading to the development of planning programs in the private sector, public agencies, and the federal government.[1] Currently, the prevailing thought is that an effective health-care program should fit the cultural patterns for which it is planned and should incorporate mechanisms for feedback from health-care consumers.[2]

Most existing health-planning programs, however, are developed within complex organizational hierarchies. These hierarchies, which are in effect subcultural groups, are composed of individuals organized into a social structure marked by specialization of work, graded statuses, various levels of command and role expectations, and are identified by a set of values including definite plans toward goals, and mechanisms and motivations for the achievement of those goals.[3]

It is axiomatic that when a plan involves few individuals or systems, goals tend to be specific, but they become generalized as the complexity of the planning

From *Nursing Forum*, Vol. 11, No. 3, 1972, pp. 311–322. Reprinted with permission from Nursing Publications, Inc., 194-B Kinderkamack Road, Park Ridge, New Jersey 07656.

increases.[4] Nurses are more concerned with specific goals, since they are usually involved with individual patient problems that are limited in scope. On the other hand, professionals who create broad health-care programs have concern for a total patient population and formulate goals on this basis. However, nurses involved with a small segment of the population — a segment that represents a subculture for whom the broad program may not be specifically suited — often need to understand not only the objectives of the broad health-care program, but also the perceptions and values of those affected by the program before they can take the responsibility for translating or modifying health-care goals. Since the nurse is a product of the subcultural group that generates health-care planning, understanding the general goals is, in many ways, easier than understanding and ultimately changing the habits, values, and beliefs of patients within another subculture. Still, if a nurse is to bring about change, each patient must not only consent to health-care counseling and intervention, but must frequently alter personal habits and ways of living.[5]

Individuals evaluate advice according to their own matrix of culturally conditioned understanding. There is no simple formula to follow in understanding the culturally conditioned gestalt of another individual; however, studies of change resulting from intercultural health programs have revealed valuable information. It has been found, for example, that many persons fear and suspect the new and novel. The mere fact that the best available method or practice is new may mean that a patient's initial reaction will be unfavorable. Also, individuals or groups may resist change because they think there is little that one person can do to change the course of his life. Or they may fear and suspect any program supported by the government. For some people, religion, too, may present a barrier to their acceptance of a medical program.

Studies have also been made that demonstrate medical personnel are often unable to translate medical descriptions into instructions that are meaningful for the patient. This failure in communication may be due to the patient's apprehension or inability to concentrate, to the professional's use of words not in the patient's vocabulary, or to other language problems.

Divergent perceptions — by medical personnel and by patients — of the significance of a specific health problem can account for many failures. Similarly, health expectations often differ between the population affected and the medical personnel involved.[6]

In this country, "the public-health movement has been conceived and implemented primarily by middle-class people, and directed primarily at lower-class people."[7] Groups described as lower class have certain defining characteristics, such as income or occupation, which set them apart from the population as a whole. While some values and beliefs of such groups are similar to those of the medical subculture and of the dominant social class, others are different. The mixture can be confusing to the health worker, who sees some of his own values and behaviors in another subculture, but also sees many that contrast negatively with his own.

Health care innovations are accepted or rejected depending on their fit or conflict with the patient's existing cultural patterns. If new material is interpreted
in ways that do not violate established patterns, it is more likely to be accepted.
Ideas and methods which least affect the patient's habits, beliefs, and values meet
less resistance than those that attempt to alter existing behavior patterns and
values. For example, the chlorination of water supplies, an innovation effective
in reducing disease, met with minimal public resistance. Apparently it did not
alter behavior patterns or conflict with existing values. On the other hand, voluntary programs of annual physical examinations — however successful in reducing
disease — have not been well accepted. Evidently, the idea of seeing a physician
when one is well is not valued by most people in this culture.

ADAPTING HEALTH-CARE GOALS

To illustrate how a broad health-care goal can be adapted to a specific subcultural
patient, a study involving family planning will be described below, and the nurse's
unique contribution, as an essential link between planning and patient acceptance,
will be analyzed.

Family-spacing programs can be seen as one kind of health-care service having
close ties to the behavior patterns and values of most people. These programs are
now considered high priority by the medical subculture and are founded on
recently formulated techniques, values, and goals. In the subcultural groups to
whom these programs are directed, the techniques are for the most part alien; the
discussion of sexual behavior in medical vernacular is unfamiliar; and the value
placed on family limitation by the medical team may conflict with existing values
and beliefs. A part of health-care planning for only a decade, family-spacing programs undoubtedly represent unfamiliar values and methods to most people and
to many health personnel.

Because family-planning programs are relatively recent and have met with
mixed success, the presentation of contraceptive information provides an excellent example of the nurse's role in innovation. The major change suggested in
the following study is the introduction of the diaphragm; novel since the patient
had not previously used it, and difficult since she expressed some fear about it.
However, behavior changes can be made and made more easily if they are presented in a systematic way that is consistent with established patterns, beliefs,
and values. Certainly, there are alternatives open to the nurse in the presentation
of material. The following illustrates one way a goal may be accomplished with
a particular person.

The nurse who participated in the study has knowledge about family spacing.
She understands the long-range goals of population limitation and the risks involved in too frequent and too numerous pregnancies. She values and shares
with other personnel the goal of providing every woman with the most effective,
acceptable family-spacing technique the woman is capable of using. She has
certain data about the potential patient (her name, age, parity, marital status,

and income) and, most importantly, she knows the woman has indicated a desire to use family-spacing services.

There is, however, a considerable amount the nurse does not know, but which may be important in introducing new useful information. She can collect the needed personal data and present the new information in a number of ways. If the exchange of information is to be of use, however, the patient must believe that the nurse has knowledge of value to her, and it must be presented in a manner that does not threaten the patient's existing beliefs about her physiology and function. To increase the likelihood of success, the nurse must modify the form of the health message so it makes sense to the particular person for whom it is intended.[8]

The nurse is faced with the problem of ascertaining which segments of knowledge will best fit into the patient's system of values, beliefs, and behavior. The novel element (in this situation, family-spacing technique) must be made sufficiently congruent with the patient's understanding. If, in the process of assimilating new information, the patient's framework of understanding is transformed slightly, certain behavioral change may be expected to follow.

Understanding how the patient organizes her ideas and beliefs about herself may be an important aspect of nursing in a situation such as this. Because the nurse is a member of a different subculture, her conceptual organization cannot be assumed to be the same as her patient's.

The patient's perception of reality will usually not emerge if she is bombarded with a series of questions. It is better that the nurse listen closely and direct the discussion gently to encourage the patient to report experiences as *she* perceives them (which may not be the way a professional person would describe them, and which may not represent reality in a medical sense).

The following interviews illustrate what information may be elicited and used by the nurse. The data were obtained during three recorded sessions totaling three hours and fifteen minutes of non-directed discussion about pregnancy. To give an indication of the kind of information revealed with continuing contact, the information is presented in the sequence in which it was obtained.

ELICITING KNOWLEDGE AND BELIEFS

Lisa, who is seven months pregnant, is a 16-year-old, Southern Negro, para 1-0-0-1. She has a seventh grade education. Married to a 30-year-old laborer, Lisa lives with her husband, her brother-in-law, and his wife who is childless. Lisa's first child, 19-month-old Jill, was born before Lisa met her husband. Lisa had Jill by Caesarian section because of a cephlo-pelvic disproportion and will have a Caesarian section with this baby.

During her first pregnancy Lisa went to a local physician who referred her to a medical center. Describing her feelings about her first pregnancy, Lisa said,

Well, I think before I were (pregnant) I want me a little girl so I say it's all right.

During her pregnancy she lived as a dependent in her parents' home; her boyfriend did not help her financially. She was sectioned after an attempted induction. Her reaction to learning that she would be "cut" revealed a somewhat philosophical attitude, and reasonable faith in the medical team.

Well, I didn't like it at first. So I say, well, just go ahead and I say maybe the thing will turn out all right. I say if it don't, it just don't.

When she returned to the hospital four weeks post-partum, birth control pills were prescribed.

I took the pills and the pills mess me up. I had terrible headaches all the time and I just felt bad all the time, just stayed sick. I took the pills for six months and then just didn't have any period. . . . I went to the doctor and he gave me four pills to take and it started it but it never did come back right and I have never seen it since.

Did she think she would use birth control pills again?

No, if I have a Caesarian this time I can't have but one more and they automatically stop me. . . . Well, I couldn't have no more than three cause . . . it would be too dangerous. See, I can have difficulty with this operation and then they have to stop me then. I just wondering what they going to do. . . . I know that if I don't decide to take the foam or the jelly, or the diaphragm, they might tie them.

In a later interview she further described her feelings about pregnancy and children.

When I gets mad with him (her husband) sometimes and I say, "Oh, I don't want the baby," and I just, well, it's the way I be feeling sometime. I don't want it, I just want Jill. . . . I just say I don't want no more children, so after this one I really don't want any more. . . . I figure it, I say, I'm having my kids while I'm young so when I get grown my kids'll be grown. . . . It's all right, kids is nice to have, you know, but I just don't want any more. . . . I say two or three is enough for anybody.

A third interview focused more closely on child-spacing techniques. In her discussion Lisa referred frequently to information she had obtained from other women, reflecting the importance of non-medical communication in selecting and adjusting to a particular device.

Well, this lady, this nurse, came by the house today and she said she knowed three young ladies they had loops and they got pregnant with them. . . . She showed me the loop. . . . So she say that after this one they tell me something about the loop, but I don't want one because they have too much problem with my stomach anyway and so it probably make it worse.

Lisa was asked if anybody in the clinic had been talking to her about what she was going to do after she had this baby, so she would not have another one soon.

Well, no, not yet . . . I don't know . . . I was going to get a diaphragm, but after this lady said this girl she had a diaphragm and it gave her cancer, so I don't know, 'cause, see, you have to have a cancer smear every six months, so . . . you can get cancer between now and six months before you go back, see? . . . I might, you know, get the jelly or the foam, one of the two.

In this discussion Lisa indicated she had eliminated for herself three methods and was considering either foam or jelly. The nurse thought this interesting because in a discussion with Lisa's mother about six months earlier, the mother had given a graphic description of the use of Vaseline as a contraceptive, and reasons for its effectiveness. Lisa's preference for a similar method provoked the question, "Have you ever heard of using Vaseline?" After a positive response she was asked, "What do you think of it?" She answered, "Oh well, it's all right, but I don't think it's too safe." Further conversation revealed that she was using Vaseline when she became pregnant with her first child. She stated that she had heard about it from her mother. Her mother, however, did not tell her how to use it. "She just said pack it, she didn't say how much."

The use of Vaseline, however imperfectly communicated from mother to daughter, bears a strong resemblance to the two methods Lisa was now considering. Her confidence in these methods was strengthened by one other experience.

I knew a girl, now she said she was on the foam, she said she used it for three years . . . so I imagine it done her pretty good, you know.

She mentioned first hearing of foam while in the hospital with Jill. She was questioned about her knowledge of this method.

They just told me how to use the foam, cause see you get an injection with the foam, see, but they haven't told me anything about the jelly or the cream or the diaphragm, or how to use it or anything like that.

Later she was asked about her earlier statements regarding child spacing. How long did she think she should wait until she had another baby after this one?

Well, it's best to wait . . . if you have babies every year it's not good on you, see, your health'll go down real quick. And it's best to have them two or three years apart and you can, you know, do more with them at that age instead of have two small ones right there together.

DEVELOPING APPROPRIATE ALTERNATIVES

Further discussion with Lisa may produce other worthwhile information, but at this point she has expressed enough about herself to suggest what innovations may be adapted to her understanding. She has already eliminated those choices that do not fit into her established cultural patterns, but she isn't sure what other alternatives she might use. She had expressed interest in knowing more about foam, jelly, and, with some reservation, the diaphragm. Foam and jelly have an almost perfect fit with Vaseline, which she has used. She has already incorporated the possibility of this substitution and is apparently ready to change her behavior in this direction, demonstrating the principle that behavior can and will change when a more useful alternative is available, but it will most probably change within loosely defined limits.

At this juncture, the nurse could introduce Lisa to various spermicidal products, explain their use and the reasons for their effectiveness, assure her that a supply of such products is available, and go no further. In doing this she would have supplied Lisa with information for which she has expressed a desire. However, she may also try to promote the process of behavioral change by discussing further the one novel element, the diaphragm. By doing this, she would be moving closer to her own goal — to provide each woman with the *most effective* child-spacing technique the patient is capable and desirous of using.

But will Lisa see the diaphragm as an acceptable solution? The nurse may wish to explore whether Lisa's fear of cancer would prevent her from using a diaphragm. If Lisa's beliefs about the connection between cancer and the use of a diaphragm are too strong, pursuing this method may not be advisable for the time being. If it should turn out that Lisa does want to know more about the diaphragm, the nurse now has the opportunity to show her a diaphragm, and explain how it is applied, the advantages of this technique over others, and why a woman must be fitted for a particular size.

If Lisa can understand how the diaphragm is used, enough to accept it, she might then be given information about the use of a spermicidal jelly with the diaphragm. Either the diaphragm or jelly is a satisfactory method of child spacing, but combined they are more effective. Therefore, the nurse, taking into account what Lisa has already expressed about herself, might suggest the combination as the most effective method and one that might be acceptable to Lisa. This point may be difficult to get across, however, because Lisa doesn't think in terms of reported percentages of women who became pregnant while using a particular method. She draws from her own experiences and from those of women she has known. But if the diaphragm is to be introduced at all, the combination with spermicidal jelly is important and should not be overlooked.

CONCLUSION

Many kinds of patient situations make up a nurse's experiences within a particular subculture. Through experience, however, the nurse begins to see cultural patterns and becomes better able to predict how persons in a particular subculture will express their ideas and beliefs about themselves. With such information the nurse is better equipped to introduce innovations consistent with cultural patterns, and achieve the goals of health-care programs. Also, she can communicate her experiences to other members of the local health team. And with increased understanding of the local subculture the local team can alter its approach to make it more acceptable to the population. Moreover, the nurse can add new information to the body of knowledge about a particular population, thereby helping those responsible for health-care planning to develop programs more acceptable to the consumer. Thus, through direct involvement with communities and segments of communities, the nurse can implement and modify health planning in a unique way.

REFERENCES

1. Mahoney, Margaret E., "Momentum for Change," *American Journal of Nursing,* 69: 2446–2454, 1969.
2. Sigmond, Richard M., "Health Planning," *The Milbank Memorial Fund Quarterly,* 46: 91–117, 1968.
3. Foster, George M., *Problems in Intercultural Health Programs,* New York: Park Avenue, 1958, p. 230.
4. Sigmond, *op. cit.*
5. Simmons, Ozzie G., "Implications of Social Class for Public Health," *Human Organization,* 16:7–10, 1957.
6. Foster, *op. cit.*
7. Simmons, *op. cit.*
8. Paul, Benjamin, and Walter B. Miller, *Health, Culture and Community Case Studies of Public Reactions to Health Programs,* New York: Russell Sage Foundation, 1955, p. iii.

51
The Core Committee: A Model for Decision-Making within Public Health Units
Olga Roman Smiley

Many times health planning for the community will begin within some health care agency. Furthermore, what goes on within such an agency will eventually have an impact on the community. But how should health professionals organize to effectively plan, implement and evaluate improvements in their own work? This chapter stresses the importance of input from every level of a health care organization. Olga Smiley describes the formation of a "core committee" in one public health agency and shows how it worked to plan for that agency's role in delivering health care to the community.

The utilization of a "core committee" to plan, implement, and evaluate nursing programs in a public health unit is the wave of the future. At this time it is new, untested, and perhaps represents "future shock." This article will describe the development of core concepts and a core committee, and the functioning of the core committee, in a health unit in Ontario, Canada.

BACKGROUND

In the summer of 1972 I received an invitation from a health unit to act as a consultant to nursing services. The unit is an official public health agency providing service to 45 communities with a total population of 115,000. It has a central office and six sub-offices. There is a nursing staff of 40. The unit is funded by the Province of Ontario. However, it operates as an independent agency controlled by a local board of directors.

As a consultant, as well as public health nurse, my initial concern was twofold:

1. How can the attachment of a new individual, the consultant, to a health agency evolve?
2. How does the consultant effectively evaluate the needs of the agency and help to bring about change?

I felt the heart of these two concerns was linked to the way the staff nurses view, diagnose, and attempt to solve problems. The understanding and identification of these areas would help to equip the nurses with the methodology and skills necessary to draw on their own resources and solve their own problems. Nursing involvement in the consultation process would contribute to a team approach for the study and resolution of difficulties.

From *Nursing Clinics of North America*, Vol. 8, No. 2, pp. 355–359, 1973. Reprinted by permission of the publisher and the author.

The staff nurse in a public health agency is on the firing line of any community health program. She bears the burden of providing service for individuals and families and for the needs of the community. Her knowledge, skills, and sensitivity are considered crucial to the successful implementation of any program. It is therefore essential to include and involve her in program planning. To accomplish this I decided to try to initiate a core committee.

SETTING UP A CORE GROUP

I recommended to the total nursing staff and the medical officer of health that a representative group from nursing be selected.* The following reasons were given for selecting this group.

1. To broaden the base for decision-making in planning for nursing services.
2. To broaden the base for communication within nursing services and the health unit.
3. To broaden the base for initiating and evaluating change within the nursing programs.

The nursing staff and the medical officer of health accepted this plan. It was then suggested that the total nursing staff assume the responsibility for the selection of core members. Guidelines for the selection process were provided. Membership to the core committee would be selected from:

1. Various educational levels: registered nurses, registered nursing assistants,[†] nurses with a Certificate of Public Health, and nurses with bachelor's degrees.
2. Various sub-offices: there were seven sub-offices in the health unit.
3. Various seniority levels: these ranged from practitioners with less than one year's experience to nurses with over twenty years' experience.

Within two weeks the nursing staff selected seven nurses to represent them as the initial core committee. The members were rotated gradually to insure maximum staff participation.

From within the core committee a liaison nurse was selected. This liaison member represented the core group. She was given the full support of the core committee, and the authority to act on their behalf. She was given the responsibility for making interpretations of core activities to the medical officer of health as well as bringing requests back to the core committee.

The activities of the core group were documented in the form of minutes of their meetings. The minutes were duplicated and a copy was kept on file in each

---

*There was no nursing director or supervisor in the health unit at this time.
†Approximately equivalent to the licensed practical nurse in the United States.

sub-office. The medical officer of health was also given a copy. Core members held meetings in their respective sub-offices at frequent intervals to interpret core committee decisions and to invite discussions of core activities.

Meetings of the core committee were initially set at regular intervals varying from once a week to twice a month. These meetings were rotated among the various sub-offices. The medical officer of health and members of the board of health were invited. The agenda for the core meetings was planned well in advance. The agenda items were organized by identifying nursing priorities through the core representatives.

THE RESULTS

This has been a brief description of a process of staff organization and planning through representation. However, the progress of the work undertaken was affected by the dynamics of the core committee. A positive feeling and pattern of interaction developed through the participation of the core members in the experience of mutual enquiry and decision-making.

We worked very hard at setting a climate conducive to this, I felt the most important aspects of this climate were the attitudes and expectations of the consultant and the staff nurses. My attitude was that of a helper, not a director or a teacher in the traditional sense. I perceived the staff nurses of core as coming for help to discover better ways to perform their nursing functions. I tried to resist placing them into a single staff nurse mold. They were perceived as bringing a variety of experiences, training, and points of view concerning their communities and families. I in turn brought my point of view, training, and experiences. My attitude was to share my experience and training rather than to impose them. This set of attitudes on my part set up the basic requirements regarding the core group attitudes. If a climate of mutual enquiry was to be developed it was essential that the core members come to the meetings with attitudes of enquiry and openness rather than of dependence and passivity.

During the core meetings I presented my ideas with enthusiasm and conviction, but not with the attitude that I had the only answers. I did this in the hope that the staff members in the core group would use my ideas as a basic model to compare and test against their own ideas. My frame of reference was one of initiating and sharing ideas and feelings. I was extremely careful not to be directive or authoritarian.

I encouraged the core group to develop an attitude of gentle doubting. This attitude was helpful to me. I could be less inhibited about forcefully expressing my ideas, assumptions, and convictions if I could rely on the core to doubt, question, and test. Their development of the ability to test new ideas against their experiences and build on them with creativity was invaluable. This creativity eventually contributed to meeting many specific nursing needs in the community.

The core committee made decisions involving several nursing programs and procedures. The decisions concerning current programs related to communicable disease, school health, and maternal and child care. The decisions concerning new programs related to physician attachment, liaison positions, and educational contributions.

The core committee decision-making process revolved around the preparation for and discussions of the current competences and programs. It also included the identification of desired competencies. This required five steps:

1. The development of models of required competences and programs.
2. The assessment of the present performance levels of the nursing staff.
3. The evaluation of the effectiveness of the nursing programs.
4. The assessment of the gaps between the desired models and the present performances.
5. The implementation and evaluation of actions to meet these gaps.

Public health nurses are steeped in the belief that mutual planning for patient care is invaluable. However, the idea that staff nurses can become intimately involved in, and assume responsibility for, planning with nursing administration is in the pioneering stages of development. Consequently what we know about planning with individuals and families we do not apply to the administrative aspects of nursing and community health programs. So, for adventurous nurses and health units, with a high tolerance level for questioning and speculation, a core committee can be exciting and productive.

CONCLUSIONS

It is hoped that this account of a core committee in action may serve as a guide for future planning. It may also serve as a model for problem-solving within a public health unit or other nursing service setting. It is an exciting method of insuring maximum participation of the staff nurses and of the consumers of health care programs. In this way we may come closer to developing health care patterns and programs that are tailored to community needs. This was my challenge, and I hope it will become yours.

52
Planning for Social Change: Dilemmas for Health Planning

John G. Bruhn

Social and cultural change occurs continuously in every segment of society. The causes of social change, as well as the effects, are especially important for those involved in planning the delivery of health care services. Community nurses must recognize the forces involved in social change, a point emphasized in this chapter. In addition, the author describes the major elements of a local community, examining their role in health care planning. This "ecological approach" aims to keep plans from being divorced from the realities of community life and to ensure that their end result is not worse than the conditions planners seek to change.

PLANNING AND SOCIAL CHANGE

It has been said that the only thing constant in life is change. Yet there is great variability in man's modes of adapting to change, some men seek and savor it, others resist it; some cope readily with its consequences, others are overwhelmed by it. Societies differ markedly in how they view change and the latitudes in which they permit change to occur. In Western society change is highly valued because it is equated with progress. Indeed it is felt to be man's prerogative to change his environment, the social organization of his society and his methods of adaptation. The appetite for social change increases as social institutions no longer satisfy human needs. Western man goes to great lengths to plan his individual life, especially in anticipating its uncertainties, yet there is an aversion to planning for the consequences of our collective intervention in promoting change at the societal level.

Dubos[1] has pointed out that most of human history has been the result of accidents and blind choices. When the consequences of our interventions confront us, usually in the form of immediate crises, our solutions have generally involved piecemeal efforts in the name of social engineering. The need to develop our ability to predict, plan and thus prevent the same crises from recurring should have the highest national priority. This need was acknowledged in 1966 when a Presidential Panel of social scientists was charged with developing a set of social indicators, akin to those we have for forecasting the economy, that would serve as a barometer to aid in setting social goals and instituting programs to solve particular problems identified by the indicators.[2] The preliminary work of the Panel has not been continued.

From *American Journal of Public Health*, Vol. 63, No. 7, pp. 602–605, 1973. Reprinted by permission of the publisher and the author.

LACK OF COMPREHENSIVE PLANNING

The lack of social planning at the national level and the differing rates of change in social institutions, has created serious gaps between the purpose of some institutions and the degree to which they are effective in satisfying human needs. The structure and functions of our health institution have been, in particular, victims of social change. A growing recognition to plan led to the passage of the Comprehensive Health Planning Act (PL 89-749) in 1966.[3] With only the changeability of national political policies to guide its structure, health planning was instituted at the community level.[4] As Rogers[5] has stated "this well-intended action of Congress nor any amount of money and effort allocated to this purpose cannot be expected to produce anything but frustration and further confusion in the absence of a holistic concept of human organization." Some health planners have advocated "the whole man" approach, but nonetheless environmental health planning has been carried out independently from comprehensive health planning.[3,4] Thus, neither planning effort is ecological or comprehensive.

THE PLANNING PROCESS AT THE COMMUNITY LEVEL

An ecological approach offers a workable structure in which the planning process can be carried out at the community level. But the ecological approach necessitates teamwork across disciplines and the on-going contributions of the team toward a common goal. No single discipline has all the answers in health planning. If the planning process does not involve teamwork among planners, including the community, the plan will evolve segmentally and its implementation may, indeed, create greater problems than those which existed initially. The ecologic approach to health planning also incorporates the causes and effects of social change in the planning process. No comprehensive health plan that is implemented and forgotten, or too rigid to accommodate to the dynamics of social change, will survive long. Teamwork and the processes of social change are key elements of an ecologic approach. While the ecological approach has been verbally espoused, it has seldom been put into practice. There are some basic steps that provide practical aides to planning ecologically at the community level.

Identification of Existing Community Patterns and Potentials

A basic tenet of the ecological approach is that there is a constant striving for equilibrium between institutional goals and the needs of the people they serve as well as between institutions themselves. This state of equilibrium is never fully achieved because human behavior continually gives rise to, and is affected by, social change. How well institutions weather the effects of social change and continue to satisfy human needs determines their vitality and longevity. In the planning process it is necessary to identify those social institutions in the community that have been most adaptable and those that have been least adaptable to social change. This provides planners with some insight into community resources and attitudes toward change. It is also advantageous for planners to gain some historical perspective of institutional change in the community to fully understand present community behavior and assist in realistically planning how far the community can be expected to go. Of particular importance, however, is that this step of identifying community potentials should be oriented toward identifying *patterns*, rather than assess each community institution as an isolated entity. While community institutions do not always function in concert, the causes and effects of their actions are rarely independent of one another.

Perspective of the Community as a Total System

Pathways to health goals are not narrowly defined. They are closely related to the non-health goals of the community. Health care cannot be planned without considering how economic, political, social, religious, geographic and other factors influence its need, modes of delivery and utilization. The visibility of health problems varies from community to community and their visibility is deeply entangled with other features of community life. "Real" problems to community residents may not be the most urgent problems to outside observers. Yet the effectiveness of the planner's approach in helping the community identify more covert health needs is largely dependent upon their ability to assess the interplay of the numerous community sub-systems as they relate to the total functioning of the community. Planning is too often viewed as planning for institutions, organizations, agencies and the convenience of the people who work for them, rather than for the needs of the consumer. As Ewing[6] has pointed out, the human side of planning is grossly neglected. Planners need to divest themselves of "agency-centered" approaches if they are to effectively plan for total communities.

The Planner as Participant Observer

In order to carry out Steps 1 and 2 planners need to be participant observers. Pressing health problems always exist in the eyes of health planners. However, these pressing problems may have, in fact, a long history in the community and not be viewed as pressing issues to them. The community may present a "no problems here" response to the need for planning. The community may have workable means of coping with their problems, labeled as such by outsiders, and see no need for planning. Planning can only proceed effectively if the community establishes that its needs are not being satisfied. Planners in effect must be health educators, but they must be able to realistically present the advantages and disadvantages of planning to the community. The community should not be led to believe that planning will completely solve their problems, for as planning changes both institutions and people new needs will be created. These new needs, and consequent demands for their fulfillment, reverberate throughout all facets of the community system. New problems may arise in other social institutions as a result of having planned for health. By working with the community the health planner prepares the community for planning strategies of solution to new problems.

The planner cannot escape being a part of the community system he is planning for. Indeed he must be a participant observer in order to gain understanding of its uniqueness. While it is crucial that the planner maintain some semblance of detachment from the political intricacies of community planning, it is also essential that he plan with, not for, the community.[7]

Collection, Assimilation and Assessment of Data

Facts are obviously needed for planning, but concern with the collection of facts and more facts would seem directly proportional to the degree of uneasiness of the planner and/or the uncertainty of the community situation. Planning can easily begin and end with endless data only for the planner to find that over-powering factual evidence did not convince or sway community opinion. Viewed in another way, collecting facts is often a stop-gap measure for the planner until he feels comfortable enough with the community to begin planning. Gathering facts is also a way for the planner to convey to the community that something concrete is being done. Colt[8] aptly points out the necessity to consider some basic questions about data before they are collected, such as what kind are needed?, what kind are available?, for what purpose will the data be used?, and how reliable are they? Due to the phenomenon of social change the planner must be satisfied with yesterday's facts.

The health planner's knowledge of the community however, should not be limited to quantitative data. Indeed the multidimensioned characteristics of health encompass the entire life style of the community and its inhabitants. Kerr and Trantow[9] depict the various dimensions and relevant factors involved in defining and assessing the quality of life. Suggested methods of assessment range from the sum of the well-being status of individuals using the survey technique of Blum and his associates,[10] to indices of health and well-being,[11] to observational data which ascertains the potential of community institutions, their present effectiveness and their receptiveness to innovation and change. Indeed, the health planner's data should include a wide range of information from numerous levels in order to gain an holistic assessment of the capabilities of the community at any given point in time. As the community changes and hence its response to change, the health planner's data or knowledge of the system must also be modified. If the ecological model is followed there can be no planning for health or health services apart from the total community system which includes all of its social institutions and pattern of social organization. This is the purpose of the interdisciplinary planning team which provides the expertise for inquiry. How this team is organized, its mode of operation and degree of involvement with the community at all stages of the planning process will determine the quality of planning. It might be argued that such an interdisciplinary planning effort will not work. If professionals, however, cannot work jointly in a common effort how can professionals expect but a similar response on the part of communities? Indeed, fragmentation and specialization are at the core of the dysfunction of our health institution's current maladies and it is only realistic to project that the crises will worsen unless some coordinated effort is soon forthcoming.

Some planners have advocated the use of social indices in planning,[11,12] others have been concerned with the kinds of data to be gathered,[8,10] and still others have suggested that data be commensurate with priority areas, e.g., health service planning, health utilization, quality of health services. Some have advocated the use of urban and regional information systems for "orderly and coordination planning in improving the quality of urban life."[13] While each of these suggestions to aid in social accounting have some merit, it should be emphasized that guidelines should not be dependent solely on techniques nor should they be substitutes for goal setting. This type of social assessment needed must be geared to the uniqueness of the community and the purposes of planning. As the Presidential Panel referred to previously suggested, no set of social indicators are a substitute for rational policy and decision-making.[2]

Goal-Setting

The entire community system and planning process is dependent upon time. The community, the planner and the planning process are simultaneously undergoing change, therefore, continual evaluation is necessary from the onset. Since planning is never complete because the process produces changes which require additional planning, long-term goals are seldom reached, especially in their original form. Some short-term goals are necessary, if both the planner and the community are to experience some success for their efforts. In a "doing" society such as ours we want tangible action. If short-term results are not forthcoming, professionals often abandon their approach in favor of simple solutions or short-cuts. This action, however, jeopardizes the entire planning process, for short-term goals must be anchored to long-term ones. Some short-term goals are advantageous for another reason. Planning is both a political and subversive process. If short-term planning efforts are not successful, the alternative may be a revision of the entire system.[14] The success of short-term goals is a test of this alternative.

Implementation

Planning by "outside observers" who leave the community free of the responsibility for participating in implementing the plan will doubtlessly fail. The planner's participation in implementation will be interpreted by the community as interest in seeing the plan work. But perhaps more important the availability of the planner to aid in revising strategies of problem solution that arise during implementation will enhance the success of the plan. If the planner leaves the sole responsibility for implementation to the community, and if the community becomes overwhelmed in dealing with the problems of implementation, the plan may be abandoned. Indeed, the planner's accumulated experience with seeing

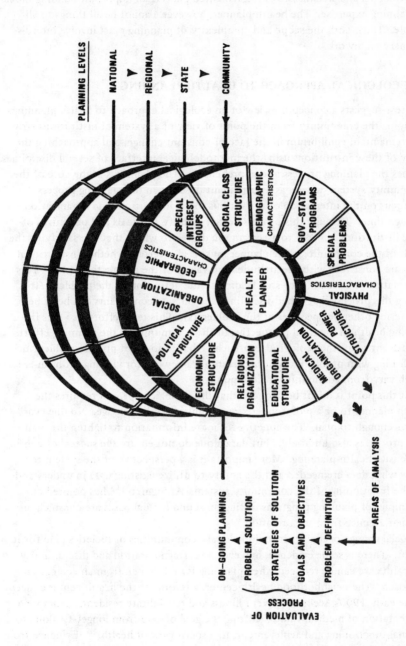

Figure 1. An Ecologic Approach to Comprehensive Health Planning.

the strengths and weaknesses of implemented plans is an important building block in planning expertise. The health planner, however, cannot be all things to all people. Thus, both the scope and complexity of planning must involve interdisciplinary teamwork.

AN ECOLOGICAL APPROACH TO HEALTH PLANNING

Figure 1 suggests a conceptual view of an ecological approach to health planning. Studying the community from the point of view of a system of institutions striving to maintain equilibrium in the face of constant change, and approaching the study of these institutions using the methodological interface of several disciplines, defines the planning process as comprehensive. The planner is at the core of the community system, where, as a participant observer in the planning process, he can focus on the interaction of the various social institutions and organizations through time. Through this process he can identify the goals and objectives of these institutions in order to ascertain the degree to which they are satisfying the needs of the community. The planner must also ascertain whether institutional goals are consistent with the attitudes and values of the people they serve. This information is a preliminary step leading to the definition of the problem. It is during this process that other disciplines and outside consultants can be of help in offering other perspectives of the problem(s). This team effort also aids in keeping health in the total perspective of the community in the planning effort. The advantage of the ecological approach is that it does not provide a blueprint for dealing with problems, rather it offers a framework for viewing problem areas which vary from community to community.

At this point it might be deduced that the ecologic approach requires the health planner to be a philosopher-king or multidisciplinary sage. No one ever knows enough to plan. The appetite for more information to tighten the planning process is also unsatiable, but data alone do not ensure the success of comprehensive health planning. More important is a perspective of the system to know what data are needed and the ability to utilize existing data in understanding the functioning of the community system. As Sigmond[15] has pointed out "examples of planning programs resting on sound factual bases are conspicuous by their absence from the literature."

Social change occurs whether individuals, communities or societies plan for it or not. There is some evidence, however, that fragmentation and discontinuity of health care can be reduced when planning is undertaken from an ecological approach. The neighborhood health center, a reform of the health center concept of the early 1900s, seeks to prevent illness and rehabilitate residents, promote a reorientation of medical values, shifting the goal of care from longevity alone to optimal functioning and achievement, to a social view of health.[16] Evidence from the Tufts-Columbia Point Health Center and other group health practice plans[17] indicates that patterns of utilization of health-care facilities are susceptible to

modification once adequate, convenient and personalized service is provided.
A health center appears to be a meaningful vehicle for consumer participation.

THE NEIGHBORHOOD AS AN ECOLOGICAL UNIT
IN HEALTH PLANNING

While the neighborhood health center provides an example of the ecological
approach applied to specific health planning problems, the Highland Park-Pierce
Neighborhood House project in southeastern Topeka is illustrative of a more
inclusive attempt to involve an isolated neighborhood in the utilization of all
types of community services.[18] The idea of this neighborhood organization
maximized the opportunity for participation of the residents and encouraged the
development of a sense of ownership, social roles, self-confidence, feelings of control over and power within the community environment, self-determination and a
choice of alternatives in matters concerning daily living. The neighborhood house
was not seen as an isolated organization nor as agency-owned (OEO). Rather it
was conceptualized as a bridge between alienated poor and uninvolved non-poor.
Of importance is the concept that the neighborhood house is the property of
neighborhood people. Thus, the neighborhood house becomes a strategy for,
and agent of, social change.

The success of the Topeka experience was due to the central dynamic structure and function of the House in accommodating resident needs and changes.
The organizational style, policies and practices of the community action agency
was broad and flexible enough to permit the growth of the House toward cooperative autonomy and indigenous leadership. While community agencies and
organizations provided financial and technical assistance, such backing was at the
invitation of the residents.

The Neighborhood House also found the professional participating consultant
useful. As he became accepted as a person, established equal status with residents,
demonstrated his willingness to learn as well as teach, and demonstrated that his
knowledge had value because it was useful, he became an effective participating
consultant and a role model. The neighborhood house staff was indigenously
chosen and manifested a firm commitment to the people of the neighborhood.
The staff was able to reach both the content and process goals of the program
and to understand and utilize for social change those conflicts that resulted in
attempts to reach the goals. Zurcher and Green[18] summarize their experience as
follows: "the participating residents appeared to be altering perceptions of themselves, the neighborhood, the 'system' and the community-at-large. Members of
the system and the community-at-large correspondingly altered their views of
Highland Park-Pierce and its residents." The principles which guided planning
for social change in Topeka are not unique, although the process of their implementation may influence the emulation of the project elsewhere.

The health planner must face several dilemmas in planning for change at the community level. He must be an advocate for the beneficial effects of planning in a society that has been uninterested in social planning. He must plan in the context of a changing system while he is trying to effect change, realizing that his insights and knowledge about the system are also changing. He cannot deny his professional role and cannot become too entangled in the politics of planning, yet he must be a participant with the community in the planning process. The perpetual cycle of planning, which creates new needs and thus more planning, places him in the difficult position of knowing when to leave the community system. Yet considering health from an ecological perspective is a recognition of the necessity for consciously planning and manipulating ways to modify the biosocial environment in a manner that forces are created that will fundamentally change the problems of the public health.[19]

REFERENCES

1. Dubos, R. *So Human an Animal.* New York: Charles Scribner and Sons, 1968.
2. *Towards a Social Report,* U.S. Department of Health, Education and Welfare, Washington, D.C., 1969.
3. Cameron, C. M. Complex Health Care Demands Planning. *J. Environ. Hlth.,* 32:34—40 (July—August), 1969.
4. Metts, A. Relationship Between Comprehensive and Environmental Health Planning. *Pub. Hlth. Rep.,* 84:647—654 (July), 1969.
5. Rogers, E. S. Public Health Asks of Sociology. *Science,* 159:506—508 (Feb. 2), 1968.
6. Ewing, D. W. *The Human Side of Planning.* New York: Macmillan Co., 1969.
7. Mott, B. J. F. The Myth of Planning Without Politics. *AJPH* 59:803—808, 1969.
8. Colt, A. M. Elements of Comprehensive Health Planning. *AJPH* 60:1194—1204, 1970.
9. Kerr, M., and Trantow, D. J. Defining, Measuring, and Assessing the Quality of Health Services. *Pub. Hlth. Rep.,* 84:415—424, 1969.
10. Blum, H. L. *Notes on Comprehensive Planning for Health.* Comprehensive Health Planning Unit, School of Public Health, University of California, Berkeley, California, 1968.
11. Gross, B. M., and Springer, M. New Goals for Social Information. *Ann. Amer. Acad. Soc. & Pol. Sci.,* 373:208—218, 1967.
12. McHale, J. Science, Technology and Change. *Ann. Amer. Acad. Soc. & Pol. Sci.,* 373: 120—140, 1967.
13. *Urban and Rural America — Policies for Future Growth.* Advisory Commission on Intergovernmental Relations. Publication A-32, Washington, D.C., April, 1968, pp. 1—29.
14. Feingold, E. The Changing Political Character of Health Planning. *AJPH* 59:803—808, 1969.
15. Sigmond, R. M. Health Planning: In Dimensions and Determinants of Health Policy. W. L. Kissick (Ed.), *Milbank Memorial Fund Quart.,* 46:91—117 (Jan.), 1968, (part 2).
16. Stoeckle, J. D., and Candib, L. M. The Neighborhood Health Center — Reform Ideas of Yesterday and Today. *New Eng. J. Med.,* 280:1385—1391 (June 19), 1969.
17. Bellin, S. S., and Geiger, H. J. Actual Public Acceptance of the Neighborhood Health Center by the Urban Poor. *J.A.M.A.,* 214:2147—2153 (Dec. 21), 1970.
18. Zurcher, L. A., and Green, A. E. *From Dependency to Dignity: Individual and Social Consequences of a Neighborhood House.* New York: Behavioral Publications, Inc., 1969.
19. Bruhn, J. G. Human Ecology in Medicine. *Environ. Res.,* 3:37—53, 1970.

Index

Accountability, 260
  in open health care system, 18
Activity(ies)
  assignment of, 29
  defined, 110
Acute care, 100
  nurse role in, 106
    expansion of, preparation for, 106—107
    with physician, 106
    present practice in, 106
Adolescent(s)
  sexual activity of, nurse's attitude toward,
      357—358
  venereal disease in, 356—362
Aged persons
  care of, past practice of, 398. *See also*
      Gerontological nursing
  family and, nurse's role in, 396
    case study for, 397—398
  institutionalization of, impact on, 400—401
Agency(ies)
  decrease in, 7
  size of, influence on community nursing
      practice, 6—7
  weaknesses in, 271
Ambulatory facilities, 9
American Nurses' Association, 4
Amputations, accidental, emergency care for,
    86
Appointment system, for primary care team,
    135
Assessment criteria, 253, 258—259
  findings in, 256—257
  method for, 253—257
  recording of family visits in, analysis of, 258
  sample for, 254
  specific patient assessment criteria,
      254—256

Behavior
  core of, 242
  cultural aspect of, 159—160, 293
    in poor, 176
    in Spanish-Americans, 160—175
    in group settings, 314—316
Birth certificates, delivery of, 6

Cancer, response to, 307
Cardiac problems, emergency treatment for,
    83—84
Care
  continuity of. *See* Continuity of care
  distributive, 1, 2, 35
  episodic, 1—2, 35
  evaluation of, 268
    of outcomes, 268
    of process of, technical issues in, 268—
        270
    of structure, 268
Case finding, in prevention of chronic disease,
    39
Child abuse
  home visits for, 385—386
  programs for, 384
    child management, parents' class, 387
    group process, 384—385
  support of mother in, 386—387
Child care. *See also* Infant care
  by mother, nurse intervention in, 373
  use of problem-oriented medical records in,
      245—252
Chinese, in America
  culture of, 189—190
  folk medicine of, 190—191
    food related to disease in, 193—194
    understanding of, 197
    use of medication, 193
    vs. Western medicine, 191—193
    Yin and Yang, 191
  food habits of, 194, 195
  health problems of, 190
  hospital admission of, 196
  main groups of, 190—191
  maternity care for, 195—196
  population of, 190
Chronic illness, 22
  adaptation to, styles of, 308
  community nurse role in, 44
    comprehensive care, 40—41
    continuity of care, 41
    homebound patient, 41—44
      economic needs of, 43—44
      environmental modification for, 43

459

460 Index

Chronic illness, community nurse role in, homebound patient—*Continued*
  health team for, 42
  meeting emotional needs in, 42—43
  physical nursing care of, 42
  in prevention of, levels, 38—40
Communication, 100
  culture and, 273—274
  on death, 306—313
  doctor-nurse, 123
  elements of, 301—302
  empathy, 275—283
  in home visits, 285—291
  interview, 299—305
  process of, 273
  skills, 273
  therapeutic intervention, barriers to, 292—298
Community
  assessment of, 415
    characteristics of
      communication, 421
      dynamics, 421—424
      physical, 416—417
      self-image, 417—419
      structure, 419—421
    health planning and, 413—414, 425—431
    for mental health purposes, 415—416
  doctor-nurse game and, 123—124
  use of retired persons in, 27
Community-action project, 88
  function of, 89
  setting of, 89
Community health nurse(s)
  employment of
    areas of, 5, 30
    increase in, 5
    settings for, 35
  generalist. *See also* Primary Care Nurse
    educational qualifications of, 32
    responsibilities of, 31
  goal of, 35
  interactional style of, 289—290
  profile of, 286
  role of. *See* Role of nurse
  specialist
    educational qualifications of, 32—33
    responsibilities of, 7, 29—30, 31—32
Community health nursing
  career development in, 33
  change in, need for, 348—349
  concepts of, 4, 37, 79
  defined, 4-5
  features of, 1-2
  future of, 7
  general scope of, 29—30
  implications for, 94—95

Community health nursing agencies. *See* Agency(ies)
Community health survey, 151
Community mental health programs. *See* Mental health services, community services
Community planning
  core committee in, 446—449
  for health care
    nurse's involvement in
      function in, 437
      method for, 437
      reasons for, 436—438
      satisfaction from, 438
    questionnaire for, 433—434
    results of, 434—436
Comprehensive care, providing of, 40—41
Comprehensive medical action, basic parts of, 246
Consumer representation, 9
Continuity of care, 41, 150
  community nurse role in, 396
  in mental health services, 50
Contract(ing), in community nursing 221—222
  beneficial effects of, 228
  defined, 222
  modification of, 227
  philosophy of, 223
  process of, 223—224
    development of plan, 225
    division of responsibility, 225—226
    establishment of goals, 224—225
    evaluation, 226
    exploration of resources, 225
    identifying of needs, 224
    renegotiation, 226—227
    setting time limit, 226
  use of, 221
Core committee, for public health unit, 449
  background of, 446—447
  decision-making process in, 449
  results of, 448—449
  setting up of, 447—448
Counseling, providing of, 100
Crisis
  defined, 230
  events related to, 295
Crisis intervention
  case study for, 296—298
  dependence in, 234, 235
  duration of, 295
  effectiveness of, 235
  in family crisis, 374
    principles in, 375
  phases of, 295—296
  steps in, 230—231

anticipation, 234
assessment, 231–232
planning, 232
techniques of, 233–234, 295
theory of, 295
Cultural acceptance, by American Indian,
182–188
Culture. *See also* Sociocultural factors
communication and, 273–274
defined, 157, 176
related to health care, 157–158

Death
communicating about, 306
barriers to, 307–308
family adjustment to. *See* Grief
feelings toward, 306
impending
adaptation to, 308
stages in, 411
communicating about
inability in, 310–311
levels of tension and, 312
methods for, 311
physician responsibility in, 312
proper timing for, 311–312
system and, 313
denial of, 307
phases of, 405
psychological aspect of, 308–309
stages of, 309–310
in young people, 310
Death rate, of poor, 175
Deliberative process. *See* Nursing process
Department of Health, Education and
Welfare (HEW), 4, 101
Dependent functions, 127
Diagnosis, 29
Diet, 100. *See also* Nutrition
reducing, related to culture, 205–206
unchanged, patterns of, 10–11
Disease. *See* Illness
Doctor. *See* Physician
Doctor-nurse game, 114, 116
communicating and, 123–124
object of, 117
origination of, 119–122
outcomes from, 118–119
preservation of, forces in, 122–123
rules of, 116–118
Drug abuse
extent of, 72
reasons for, 72
school nurse and, 70–71, 73–77
symptoms of, 76–77
Drug therapy, occupational health nurse and,
laws on, 87

Economic Opportunity Act, 9
Education of nurses
doctor-nurse game and, 121–122
related to expansion of role, 101–102, 113
problem-oriented medical record and, 242–
243
Empathy
achievement of, 283
communication of, 277–279
categories of, Nurse-Patient Empathic
Functioning Scale, 279–282
defined, 275–276
vs. sympathy, 276–277
Ethnic groups, subcultures of, 157
Expanded nurse role, 97, 102, 114

Failure-to-thrive syndrome
case study for, 376–386
community action in, 375
prevention of
child care, 373
communication, 374
crisis intervention, 374–375
family planning, 373–374
levels of, 368–369
nursing process, 369–373, 375
progenitors of, 367
interactional, 367–368
situational, 367
symptoms of, 366–367
Family
defined, 396
illness in
adaptation to, 338–339
effect of
on marriage roles, 339–344
on parent-child relationships, 344–345
on patient roles, 337–339
female role in, change in, 333–337
levels of function in, 326
adolescent, 329–330
adulthood, 330–331
chaotic, 326, 328
intermediate, 328–329
maturity, 331
problems of, emergency care for, 84–85
visits by, recording of, analysis of, 258
Family health care centers, patterns of, 9
Family nurse practitioner, 143
family study by, 143–149
Family nursing, 325
for abusive parents, 384–387
defined, 325
during death and dying, 405–411
for elderly persons, 395–403
elements of, 323–324
for failure-to-thrive syndrome, 364–382

Family nursing—*Continued*
family role in, changes in, 333–346
infant care, 348–355
for mental health problems, 389–394
model for, 327
for venereal disease in adolescents, 356–362
Female
life expectancy of, 334
professionalism of, 334–335
role in motherhood, 364–365
modern day, 334
wife-mother
as family nurse, 335–337
as patient, 342
"Free-clinic" movement, 9

Gerontological nursing
assessment of
activities of daily living, 401
emotional status, 401–402
family, 399–400
institutionalization, family reaction to, 402
impact of, 400–401
mental status, 401
nursing role, 402–403
physical, 401
defined, 395
development of, 398–399
Grief related to death, stages of, 406
anticipation, tasks in, 406–408
emancipation, tasks in, 408–409
formation of new relationships, 410–411
readjustment to social environment, tasks in, 409–410
Group action, for problem solving, 320, 321
activities in, 314
behavior in, 314
members of
concerns of, 314–316
participation by, 318–319
assumption of roles by, 319–320
self-appraisal by, 320
planning for
guidelines for, steps in, 317–318
orientation for, 317
physical arrangements, 316–317

Health. *See also* Wellness
attitudes toward, culture and, 176–177
concept of, change in, 4
defined, 21
problems of, 4
solving of. *See* Nursing process
maintenance, subsystems, 18
promotion of, 9–10
status of, in poor, 175

Health assistant(s), functions of, 132–133
Health care
barriers to, removal of, 175–181
community planning for, 432–438
concept of, 97, 112
crisis in, factors in, 12–13
facilities for, 19
influences on, Chinese-Americans and, 189–197
services
attitudes toward, understanding of, 177–178
delivery of, 29, 30
expansion of role in, impact of, 103
extending of, 99
system
changes in, 3
closed, limitations of, 13–15
goals of, 12
open
advantages of, 15, 17
model of, 16–19
need for, 13
role expansion and, 111–112
Health discipline structure, 8
Health educator, 7
Health grid, 23
Health-illness systems, related to
culture, of Spanish-Americans, 164–169
Health Inventory Technician(s), 133
Health Inventory Unit, 133
Health maintenance organization, Harvard
Community Health Plan
atmosphere in, 67
factors in, 67–68
nurse-physician team in, 66
nursing role in, 66–67
nursing triage in, 65
guidelines for, 65–66
patient-nurse encounters in, 65
problems in, 68, 69
setting of, 63–64
"telephone triage nurse" in, 64–65
Health personnel, shortage of, 12
Health planning, 1
confusion in, 428
controversies in, reasons for, 429–430
cultural approach to, 445
adapting of health care goals, 441–442
case study for, 442–444
defined, 427
ecological approach to, 455, 456–457
neighborhood organization and, 457–458
fundamental characteristics of, 428–429
methods of
creating of, 430–431
from other media, 425–427

anticipation, 234
assessment, 231–232
planning, 232
techniques of, 233–234, 295
theory of, 295
Cultural acceptance, by American Indian,
    182–188
Culture. *See also* Sociocultural factors
communication and, 273–274
defined, 157, 176
related to health care, 157–158

Death
communicating about, 306
    barriers to, 307–308
family adjustment to. *See* Grief
feelings toward, 306
impending
    adaptation to, 308
        stages in, 411
    communicating about
        inability in, 310–311
        levels of tension and, 312
        methods for, 311
        physician responsibility in, 312
        proper timing for, 311–312
        system and, 313
    denial of, 307
    phases of, 405
    psychological aspect of, 308–309
        stages of, 309–310
        in young people, 310
Death rate, of poor, 175
Deliberative process. *See* Nursing process
Department of Health, Education and
    Welfare (HEW), 4, 101
Dependent functions, 127
Diagnosis, 29
Diet, 100. *See also* Nutrition
reducing, related to culture, 205–206
unchanged, patterns of, 10–11
Disease. *See* Illness
Doctor. *See* Physician
Doctor-nurse game, 114, 116
communicating and, 123–124
object of, 117
origination of, 119–122
outcomes from, 118–119
preservation of, forces in, 122–123
rules of, 116–118
Drug abuse
extent of, 72
reasons for, 72
school nurse and, 70–71, 73–77
symptoms of, 76–77
Drug therapy, occupational health nurse and,
    laws on, 87

Economic Opportunity Act, 9
Education of nurses
doctor-nurse game and, 121–122
related to expansion of role, 101–102, 113
problem-oriented medical record and, 242–
    243
Empathy
achievement of, 283
communication of, 277–279
    categories of, Nurse-Patient Empathic
        Functioning Scale, 279–282
    defined, 275–276
    vs. sympathy, 276–277
Ethnic groups, subcultures of, 157
Expanded nurse role, 97, 102, 114

Failure-to-thrive syndrome
case study for, 376–386
community action in, 375
prevention of
    child care, 373
    communication, 374
    crisis intervention, 374–375
    family planning, 373–374
    levels of, 368–369
    nursing process, 369–373, 375
progenitors of, 367
    interactional, 367–368
    situational, 367
symptoms of, 366–367
Family
defined, 396
illness in
    adaptation to, 338–339
    effect of
        on marriage roles, 339–344
        on parent-child relationships, 344–345
        on patient roles, 337–339
    female role in, change in, 333–337
levels of function in, 326
    adolescent, 329–330
    adulthood, 330–331
    chaotic, 326, 328
    intermediate, 328–329
    maturity, 331
problems of, emergency care for, 84–85
visits by, recording of, analysis of, 258
Family health care centers, patterns of, 9
Family nurse practitioner, 143
family study by, 143–149
Family nursing, 325
for abusive parents, 384–387
defined, 325
during death and dying, 405–411
for elderly persons, 395–403
elements of, 323–324
for failure-to-thrive syndrome, 364–382

Family nursing—*Continued*
  family role in, changes in, 333—346
  infant care, 348—355
  for mental health problems, 389—394
  model for, 327
  for venereal disease in adolescents, 356—362
Female
  life expectancy of, 334
  professionalism of, 334—335
  role in motherhood, 364—365
    modern day, 334
  wife-mother
    as family nurse, 335—337
    as patient, 342
"Free-clinic" movement, 9

Gerontological nursing
  assessment of
    activities of daily living, 401
    emotional status, 401—402
    family, 399—400
    institutionalization, family reaction to, 402
      impact of, 400—401
    mental status, 401
    nursing role, 402—403
    physical, 401
  defined, 395
  development of, 398—399
Grief related to death, stages of, 406
  anticipation, tasks in, 406—408
  emancipation, tasks in, 408—409
  formation of new relationships, 410—411
  readjustment to social environment, tasks in, 409—410
Group action, for problem solving, 320, 321
  activities in, 314
  behavior in, 314
  members of
    concerns of, 314—316
    participation by, 318—319
    assumption of roles by, 319—320
    self-appraisal by, 320
  planning for
    guidelines for, steps in, 317—318
    orientation for, 317
    physical arrangements, 316—317

Health. *See also* Wellness
  attitudes toward, culture and, 176—177
  concept of, change in, 4
  defined, 21
  problems of, 4
    solving of. *See* Nursing process
  maintenance, subsystems, 18
  promotion of, 9—10
  status of, in poor, 175

Health assistant(s), functions of, 132—133
Health care
  barriers to, removal of, 175—181
  community planning for, 432—438
  concept of, 97, 112
  crisis in, factors in, 12—13
  facilities for, 19
  influences on, Chinese-Americans and, 189—197
  services
    attitudes toward, understanding of, 177—178
    delivery of, 29, 30
      expansion of role in, impact of, 103
    extending of, 99
  system
    changes in, 3
    closed, limitations of, 13—15
    goals of, 12
    open
      advantages of, 15, 17
      model of, 16—19
      need for, 13
    role expansion and, 111—112
Health discipline structure, 8
Health educator, 7
Health grid, 23
Health-illness systems, related to culture, of Spanish-Americans, 164—169
Health Inventory Technician(s), 133
Health Inventory Unit, 133
Health maintenance organization, Harvard Community Health Plan
  atmosphere in, 67
    factors in, 67—68
  nurse-physician team in, 66
  nursing role in, 66—67
  nursing triage in, 65
    guidelines for, 65—66
  patient-nurse encounters in, 65
  problems in, 68, 69
  setting of, 63—64
  "telephone triage nurse" in, 64—65
Health personnel, shortage of, 12
Health planning, 1
  confusion in, 428
  controversies in, reasons for, 429—430
  cultural approach to, 445
    adapting of health care goals, 441—442
      case study for, 442—444
  defined, 427
  ecological approach to, 455, 456—457
    neighborhood organization and, 457—458
  fundamental characteristics of, 428—429
  methods of
    creating of, 430—431
    from other media, 425—427

nurse involvement in, 439–440
programs for, 439, 442
studies on, 440–441
shortcomings in, 427
Health team, composition of, 29
Home visit(s)
for abusive parents, 383–386
communication in
client and, situations in, 285–286
findings in, categories of
nurses' interacted styles, 289–290
obscuring of legitimate concerns, 288
ritualistic performance, 290–291
unshared long-range goals, 287–288
nurses' profile in, 286
Hospital, admission to, of Chinese-Americans, 196
Hospital-based services, 7

Illness. *See also* Chronic illness; Mental illness
classification of, in Spanish-American culture, 166–167
impact of
adaptation to, family and, 338–339
on female roles, 333–346
on marriage roles, 339–344
on parent-child relationships, 344–345
on patient roles, 337–339
Independent action, inhibition of, 122
Independent functions, 126
Independent nurse practitioner
community response to, 154–155
locale for, 151
need for, 150
philosophy of, 155–156
progress in, 155
start of practice of
answering service for, 152
financial outlay, 153
partnership in, 151–152
policies in, 152–153
public announcement of, 153–154
Indian, American. *See also* Navaho Indian
cultural acceptance of, methods for, 182–184
establishing rapport, 185–186
evaluating teaching methods, 187–188
explaining values, 186–187
maternal nursing and, lactation and, 202
white community attitude toward, 183
Infant(s), maternal deprivation, consequences of, 365–366
failure-to-thrive syndrome, 366–367
Infant care, community nurse role in, 355
facilities for, 351–352

meeting needs of
family unit and, 349–350
newborn, 349
in premature infant, 350–351
nursing process, 352–355
Injury(ies)
crushing, emergency care for, 86–87
lacerations, emergency care for, 82–83
occupational
examples of, 80–81
initial treatment for, 79–80
in manufacturing industry, 80–85
in nonmanufacturing industry, 85–87
Inservice education, by community nurse, approach to, 90–91
Interdependent functions, 127
Interview
components of, 299–301
defined, 299
elements of communication in, 301–302
techniques of
application of, factors in, 304–305
nonverbal, 304
verbal, 303–304

Leadership, need for, doctor-nurse game and, 123
Licensing laws, state, related to expansion of role, 102
Life functions, 100
Locomotion, 100
Long-term care, 100
nurse's function in, 107–108
expansion of, preparedness for, 108–109
with physician, 108
present practice of, 118
services of, 107

Malpractice insurance, 152
Manpower, shortage of, 113
Marriage role, impact of illness on, 339–344
Maternity nursing
for Chinese-Americans, 195–196
Navaho culture and, 198–204
Medicaid, 6, 60
Medical records librarian, 262
Medical student training, doctor-nurse game and, 119–121
Medicare, 6
Medication, administration of, 100
Mental health services
community assessment for, 415–416
community nurse role in, 394
in aftercare, 47–51
areas of, 46
communication with hospital, 51–52

Mental health services, community nurse role
        in—*Continued*
    as consultant, 49—50, 52—54, 89—90,
        91—94
    goals, establishment of, 52
    group process, 53
    inservice education, 90—91
    mental health facility, 46
    plan of action in, 48—49
    community services, 46
        consultation and helping plan, 391—392
        development of, 294—295
        family involvement in, 392
        follow-up clinic, 393
        group activities, 393
        group counseling, 392—393
        hospital, admission for, 389, 390
        individual counseling interviews, 392
        operational flow, 390
        personal problem center, 390—391
        termination planning, 393
Mental illness, 22
    impact of, on marriage roles, 340, 342—343
Motherhood, pressures for, society and, 364—
        365

Navaho Indian
    attitudes of, related to hospitalization, 199,
        200, 203
    maternity nursing and
        approach to, 199
        recommendations in, 199—200, 201
        beliefs in, 198—200, 203
        childbirth, cultural attitudes toward, 200,
            201
        handling of newborn, 203-204
        medical practices of, 202
Neighborhood centers, 9
Nonhealth-oriented setting, community
        nurse role in, 88—95
Nonaccepting, reaching of, 9
Nurse. *See* Doctor-nurse game;
        Physician, interprofessional
        relations; Role of nurse; *and
        specific specialty relationship with
        physician*
Nurse clinician specialists, 137—138
    in primary care, 138
Nurse practitioner programs, 137
Nursing
    defined, 395
    elements of, extension of role in, 103—109
    functions of, 261—262
    implications of, Spanish-Americans and,
        169—173
Nursing audit, 268
    basis for, 260—261

committee for
    action of, 262—263
    composition of, 262
    findings of, 263—265
        assessment of, 265
    defined, 261—262
    findings of, 271
    method for, 266
    operational issues in, 270—271
    results of, 266
    technical issues in, 268—270
Nursing care
    assessment of. *See* Assessment criteria
    quality of
        agency concern in, 267
        evaluation of, approaches to, 268
        weaknesses in, 271
Nursing practice
    categories of, 99—100
    elements of, 100
Nursing process
    assessment criteria in, 253—259
    background of, analytic components of,
        217—218
    contracting in, 221—229
    crisis intervention, 230—235
    emphasis of, 213
    for infant care, 355
        checklist for, 352—353
        evaluation of, 354
        implementation of, 354
        nursing formulation, 353—354
    method of, 215
    analytical components of
        convergence of interest, 217, 218—219
        establishment of an execution set, 217
        establishment of an initiating set, 217,
            219—220
        fulfillment of charter, 218
        legitimation and sponsorship, 217
        background of, 216
        outline for, 218—220
        relevant person in, 215
            identifying of, 216
    for prevention of families who fail to thrive
        data collection for, 370—371
        goals
            levels of, 368—369
            setting of, 372
        inferential nursing diagnosis, 371—372
        initiating events for, 369
        intervention, 372—373
    problem-oriented medical record in, 236—
        252
    steps in, 213
    through group action, 314—321
    use of, 213

Nutrition. *See also* Diet
  teaching of, 176
Nutritionist, 7

Obesity, cultural stigma of, 205—206
  combating of, 208—210
  degree of, 206—207
  reasons for, 206, 207—208
  reducing diet, related to culture, 205—206
  results of, 208
Occupational health nurse
  responsibility of
    determining cause and effect, 80
    first aid training by, 81
    in manufacturing industry, 81—85
    in nonmanufacturing industry, 85—87
    transportation of patient, 80
    treatment by, 79—80
Occupational health setting, manpower in,
    waste of, 6
Office of Economic Opportunity, 184

Parent(s)
  abusive. *See* Child abuse
  -child relationship, effect of illness on,
    344—345
Patient
  assessment of. *See* Assessment criteria
  consideration of, in open health care
    system, 17—18, 19
  family study of, by family nurse practi-
    tioner, 143—149
  illness and, role changing during, 337—339
  Primary Care Team and
    entry into, 133, 134
    relationship with, 133—135
  relationship with nurse, 178
Patient advocacy
  administration role in, 59—60
  community nurse role in, 64
    in achieving patient independence, 57—
      58
    necessity of, 61—62
    reporting inhumanities, 56—57
    shift in priorities, 58—59
    in social-political relationships, 61
  goals of, 56
  patient in, as center of care, 60
  philosophy of, 55—56
Physical therapist, 7
Physician, 7
  attitudes of, medical school training and,
    119—121
  interprofessional relationships. *See also*
    Doctor-nurse game
  expansion of role and, 102—103
  in primary medical care practice, 131, 136

shortage of, relief of, 135—137
  training of. *See* Medical student training
Physician's assistant, 8, 66
Planning. *See also* Community planning;
    Health planning
  comprehensive, lack of, 451
  defined, 425
  method of, steps in, 425—426
  planners in, as participant observers, 452—
    453
  process, at community level, 451
    data for, 453—454
    goal setting, 454
    identifying of existing patterns and
      potentials, 451—452
    implementation, 454, 456
    perspective of, 452
  social change and, 450
Poor
  building trust of, 179—180
    by discussion, 180—181
  death rate of, 175
  health status of, 175
Poverty, culture of, 176
  powerlessness in, 177—179
  related to health care, 175
Primary care, 100
  dimensions of, 104
  ideal of, defined, 140—141
  need for, 125
  nurse responsibility in preparedness for,
    105—106
    with physician, 105
  present practice in, 104—105
  practicing physician in, 136
  satellite clinics for, 245
Primary Care Assistant(s) (PCA), function of,
    131, 132
Primary Care Nurse (PCN), 126, 139
  decision making by, 131
  education of, 138—139
  function of, 126
    dependent, 127
    independent, 126—127
  need for, 137—138
  Primary Care Team and, model for, 130, 131
  qualifications of, for selection, 127—128
  role of, in health action, 134
  training of, 126, 128—130
Primary Care Team, 139—140
  appointment system in, 135
  effect of, on physician manpower shortage,
    135—137
  establishment of, 125—126
  function of, model for, 130, 131
  nurse-patient ratio in, 137
  organization of, 132

Primary Care Team—*Continued*
  patient and
    entry in, 133, 134
    relationships in, 133—135
Problem-oriented medical record (POMR),
        135, 236, 243—244
  advantages of, 135, 240, 241—242, 250—
        251
  aspects of, 236
  chart audit, 249—250
  in community child health care, 247
    establishment of, 246
    nursing assignment and progress notes,
        247—248
    problem list, 246, 248—249
  components of, 246
    data base, 237—239
    problem assessment and plans, 240
    problem list, 239
  flow chart for, 241
  future of, 251
  impact on nursing education, 242—243
  nursing implications of, 243
  philosophy of education and, 236—237
Problem-solving process. *See* Nursing process
Program planning. *See* Health planning
Psychiatric treatment, traditional, criticism of,
        293—294
Public health
  community and, 4
  community nursing and, 1
  concept of, 29, 97
  manpower for, lack of, 5
  nursing services for, personnel in, 30
Public health nursing. *See* Community
        Health Nursing
Public health team
  expansion of, 7—8
  health discipline structure of, 8

Rapport, establishment of, 185—186
Record-keeping. *See also* Nursing audit;
        Problem-oriented medical record
  Problem-Oriented Record System, 135
  as a source of information, 263, 269
Rehabilitative care, in prevention of chronic
        illness, 39—40
Restoration, 18
Role of nurse, 35—36, 100—101
  achieved, 111
  assigned, 111
  defined, 110
  expansion of, 110
    barriers to, 110, 112—113
    conclusions and recommendations in,
        101—109
    independent nurse practitioner and, 155—156

strategies for, 114—115
  fulfillment of, barriers to, 113—114
  influences on, 113
  theories on, 110—111

School nurse, work with drug abusers, 70—71
  approach to, 72
  in counseling, 74—75
  in obtaining parents' cooperation, 75—76
  in prevention, 73—74
  in recognition of symptoms, 76—77
  in treatment, 75
School nursing, manpower in, waste of, 5
Self-realization, related to wellness, 26—27
Sex education, in combating venereal disease,
        358—360
Sexual activity, of adolescents, nurse's atti-
        tude toward, 357—358
Sexual roles, related to doctor-nurse game,
        123
Shock, emergency treatment for, 79—80
Social services, role expansion and, 110, 111
Sociocultural factors, related to therapeutic
        intervention, 293—295
Spanish-Americans
  cultural context of
    aspects of, 160—161
      economic, 163—164
      political, 163
      religious, 162
      social and kinship, 161—162
  health-illness systems, 164—169
  health services for, planning of, 172—173
  nurse and, relationships with, 169—173
Staff nurse, function of, 446—447
Stress, cultural influences on, 157
Sympathy vs. empathy, 276—277

Teaching, of health care, evaluation of, 187—
        188
Team, primary care, 126, 130
"Telephone triage nurse"
  qualifications for, 64—65
  value of, 64
Therapeutic intervention
  barriers to, factors in, 293—295
  crisis intervention, 295—298
  success of, factors in, 294
  techniques of, 292
Therapy, 29
Trust, building of, 179—180
  goals in, 180—181

Values, cultural, understanding of, 186—187
Venereal disease, in adolescents, 356
  counseling for, nurse's role in, 361
  suggestions for, 361—362

epidemic proportions of, 356–357
sex education on, 358
  new approaches to, 360–361
treatment of, services for, short-comings of,
    359–360

Weed system. *See* Problem-oriented medical
    record (POMR)
Well-child center, waste of manpower in,
    5–6
Wellness, 29

axis of interest toward, 21
  need for, 22
behavior, 18
factors in, 26–27
high-level
  factors in, 27–28
  health grid of, 23–24
levels of, 21, 22
  quantifying of, 26
spirit of man in, 24–26
Wellness-oriented health worker, 18